174

Cases in

Medicine

Atlas and Commentary

174
Cases in
Medicine
Atlas and Commentary

Raghavendra Bhat MD FRCP (Glasgow)

Professor and Chairman, Internal Medicine
Ras Al Khaimah Medical and Health Sciences University
Ras Al Khaimah
UAE
e-mail: nita2005bhat@yahoo.co.in

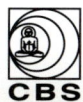

CBS

CBS Publishers & Distributors Pvt Ltd

New Delhi • Bengaluru • Chennai • Kochi • Kolkata • Mumbai
Hyderabad • Jharkhand • Nagpur • Patna • Pune • Uttarakhand

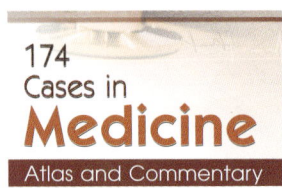

ISBN: 978-93-89565-92-8

Copyright © Author and Publisher

First Edition: 2021

Published by Satish Kumar Jain and produced by Varun Jain for

CBS Publishers & Distributors Pvt Ltd
4819/XI Prahlad Street, 24 Ansari Road, Daryaganj, New Delhi 110 002, India
Ph: 011-23289259, 23266861, 23266867   Fax: 011-23243014   Website: www.cbspd.com
e-mail: delhi@cbspd.com; cbspubs@airtelmail.in
Corporate Office: 204 FIE, Industrial Area, Patparganj, Delhi 110 092
Ph: 011-49344934   Fax: 011-49344935   e-mail: publishing@cbspd.com; publicity@cbspd.com

Branches

- **Bengaluru:** Seema House 2975, 17th Cross, K.R. Road,
  Banasankari 2nd Stage, Bengaluru 560 070, Karnataka, India
  Ph: +91-80-26771678/79   Fax: +91-80-26771680   e-mail: bangalore@cbspd.com
- **Chennai:** 7, Subbaraya Street, Shenoy Nagar, Chennai 600 030, Tamil Nadu, India
  Ph: +91-44-26680620, 26681266   Fax: +91-44-42032115   e-mail: chennai@cbspd.com
- **Kochi:** 42/1325, 1326, Power House Road, Opp KSEB, Ernakulam Kochi 682 018, Kerala, India
  Ph: +91-484-4059061-67   Fax: +91-484-4059065   e-mail: kochi@cbspd.com
- **Kolkata:** 6/B, Ground Floor, Rameswar Shaw Road, Kolkata 700 014, West Bengal, India
  Ph: +91-33-22891126, 22891127, 22891128   e-mail: kolkata@cbspd.com
- **Mumbai:** 83-C, Dr E Moses Road, Worli, Mumbai 400018, Maharashtra, India
  Ph: +91-22-24902340/41   Fax: +91-22-24902342   e-mail: mumbai@cbspd.com

Representatives

• **Hyderabad**	0-9885175004	• **Jharkhand**	0-9811541605	• **Nagpur**	0-9421945513	• **Patna**	0-9334159340
• **Pune**	0-9623451994	• **Uttarakhand**	0-9716462459				

Printed at Nutech Print Services, Faridabad, India

_to_

_the countless patients who gave me priceless
knowledge which went a long way in shaping my career.
Some of them were encountered at Government Wenlock Hospital,
Mangalore, during my long association with the institution during my
tenure at Kasturba Medical College, Mangalore.
Others were encountered in the course of my busy clinical practice.
These images promote first hand learning facilitated by the
accompanying discussion in the Question–Answer format.
I am ever grateful to these people who selflessly helped the
cause of learning, the least I can do is to dedicate this work to them!_

Preface

L earning internal medicine has many angles—direct learning from books, referring to journals, seeing patients, attending rounds, discussing with teachers, interns, postgraduate students and fellow students and other resources. It is rightly said that "A picture is worth a thousand words". Not only the concept is clarified but the retention is also made easy. Chinese and Malaysian students in my alma mater (KMC Manipal, Mangalore) owned cameras (which was rarity) and took pictures of patients and made notes. This was my first exposure for this method of learning. I liked it very much but could not do it as I did not own a camera and left it at that. Much later I bought a camera and started to collect patient images for learning and teaching. I improvised that by using questions and answers to discuss these images. I have also included pictures contributed by some of my postgraduate students during and after the completion of their training. I am grateful to them. This book has some of the images collected from all these sources.

This book is a great source of essential and accurate information needed for updating particularly to achieve excellence—facilitate learning for entrance examinations and facilitate leaning for undergraduate and postgraduate students and anyone who wants to learn more.

I thoroughly enjoyed each moment of collection of the images and preparing this book. I hope the reader enjoys it too and uses it for advancement of learning and knowledge.

Raghavendra Bhat

Contents

Contents

Cases in Medicine

xii

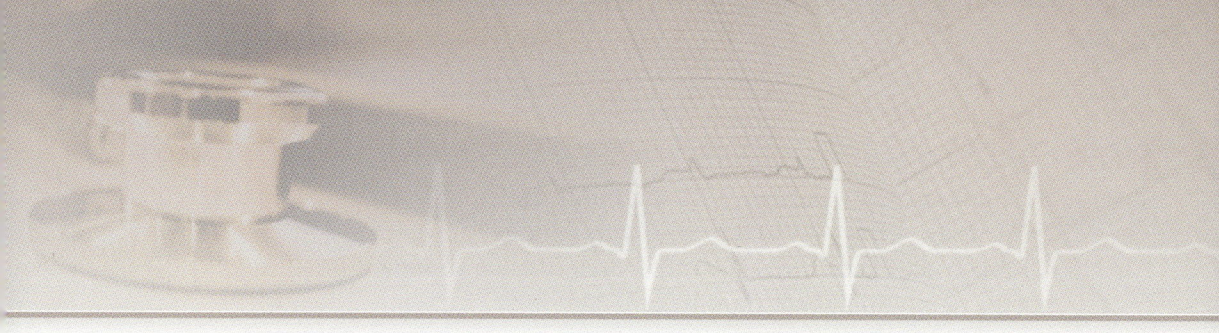

1. Xanthelasma Palpebrarum

Word meaning—yellow foil

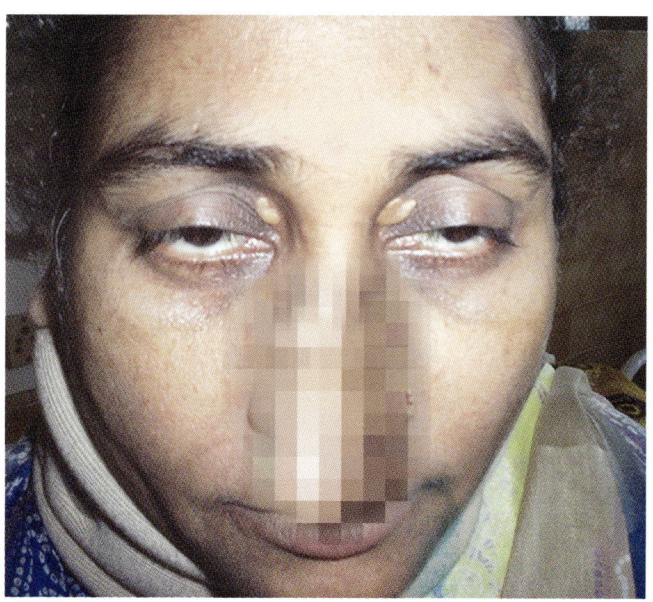

Quiz 1

What are xanthelasmas?

Multiple, yellowish orange slightly elevated plaques seen in nasal portions of upper eyelids (inner canthi) associated in about 50% with a lipid abnormality.

Quiz 2

What are the clinical manifestations of elevated blood lipid levels?

Clinical manifestations of elevated blood lipid levels:

1. *Eruptive xanthomas:* Red yellow papules on buttocks—triglycerides >1000 mg/dL
2. *Tendinous xanthomas:* Achilles, patella, triceps tendons +/– cutaneous xanthomas. Associated with familial essential cholesterolemia. Look for corneal arcus
3. *Lipemia retinalis:* Cream colored blood vessels in the fundus associated with elevated triglyceride (TG) levels >2000 mg/100 ml.

Quiz 3

Discuss the approach to a patient with dyslipidemia.
Look for dyslipidemia: Elelvated LDL (usually in younger adults).
Also look for coronary artery disease, atherosclerosis, and diabetes mellitus.
Examine other family members (familial).

Quiz 4

What are the conditions associated with hyperlipidemias?
a. *Elevated TC (total cholesterol), reduced HDL*
   • Obesity
   • Beta blockers
b. *Elevated TC, TG*
   • Diabetes
   • CKD
   • OC
c. *Elevated TC*
   • Hypothyroid
   • Nephrotic syndrome
   • Obstructive liver disease
   • Cushing's syndrome
   • CST therapy
d. *Elevated TG, HDL*
   Alcohol

Quiz 5

What are the conditions where TG (triglyceride) is reduced?
Hyperthyroidism, cirrhosis, malignancy.

Quiz 6

What are the examples of organ involvement in hyperlipidemias?
a. *Skin and subcutaneous tissue*
   Xanthomata—Increased cholesterol
              Cutaneous: Homozygous-familial
              Tendinous: Tendo Achillis, elbow
   Xanthomata—Increased triglycerides
              Eruptive: Pruritic Buttocks, elbow
              Striate: Orange yellow papules on palmar crease—type III
              hyperlipidemia
              Tuberous: Pinkish red, large nodules bony
              Prominences: Type III hyperlipidemia
b. *Eyes*
   Eyelid: Xanthelasma palpebrarum
   Corneal arcus (increased cholesterol); corneal opacity (reduced HDL)
   Fundus: Lipemia retinalis

c. *Heart*
   Accelerated atherosclerosis: Angina pectoris, acute MI—increased cholesterol/increased TGs (type III hyperlipidemia).
d. *Liver*
   Hepatomegaly: Increased cholesterol, LCAT deficiency—target cells in PS
e. *Enlargement of liver and spleen (hepatosplenomegaly)*: Increased TGs
f. *Pancreas*
   Acute pancreatitis: TG >1000 mg/100 ml
g. *Others*
   Arthritis: Increased cholesterol—homozygous FH.

Quiz 7

What are the various treatments available?
Methods of treatment available
a. *Trichloroacetic acid peel:* No scar
b. *Laser*
c. *Cryotherapy*
d. *Drugs*
   - *Statins:* HMG CoA reductase inhibitors—reduce cholesterol—Atorva, Simva, Prava, Pitava and Rosuva. Statins or reduce LDL, increase HDL.
     Reduce: TG
     Side Effects: Muscle pain, rhabdomyolysis, liver failure
   - *Ezetimibe:* Cholesterol transporter blocker—inhibits intestinal and biliary absorption of cholesterol by blocking the passage across the intestinal wall. Reduces LDL
   - Cholestyramine, colesevelam, colestipol bile acid binding resins—decreased enterohepatic circulation of bile acid—anion
     Exchange resin—binds to bile acids in SI
     Prevents hepatic conversion of cholesterol into bile acids
   - *Fibrates:* Finofibrate
     PPAR alpha agonists—peroxisome proliferative activated receptor
     alpha agonists—reduce LDL, increases HDL
   - *Nicotinic acid:* Reduces total mortality—reduces cholesterol, VLDL, LDL
     FFA; increases HDL
   - *Orlistat:* Reduces TG only; acts by GIT lipase inhibition.
   - *PCSK0 inhibitors*: Proprotein convertase subtilisin/kexin type 9 (PCSK9) is a proteolytic enzyme that indirectly regulates serum LDL cholesterol (LDL-C) by causing the destruction of LDL receptors.
   - *Inclisiran*: A small-interfering RNA (siRNA) therapy that uses the body's RNA interference process to selectively block the production of the PCSK9 protein in the liver.

Quiz 8

Give some examples of external markers of metabolic disorders
Some examples of external markers of metabolic disorders
1. *Kayser-Fleischer ring* seen as corneal rings of grey color (in dark color eyes) and brown color (in light color eyes)—seen in Wilson's disease due to excessive copper (resulting from ceruloplasmin deficiency) leading to ectopic deposition in organs including the eyes (liver, myocardium, kidneys, basal ganglia are other sites).

Cases in Medicine

3

2. *Angioid streaks:* Irregular grey lines radiating from the optic disc seen in Paget's disease of the bone, pseudoxanthoma elasticum (may be associated with blue sclera) Ehlers-Danlos disease, sickle cell anemia.

3. *Cherry red spots:* Sphingolipidoses (Niemann-Pick disease, Tay-Sachs disease) due to abnormal deposition of sohingolipid in the ganglion cells within the macula.

4. *Blue/black sclera:* Alkaptonuria

5. *Gouti tophi:* Deposited adjacent to the affected joint.

2. Periorbital Hyperpigmentation

OBSERVATION

Generalised hyperpigmentation with remarkable periorbital pigmentation also involving the bridge of the nose.

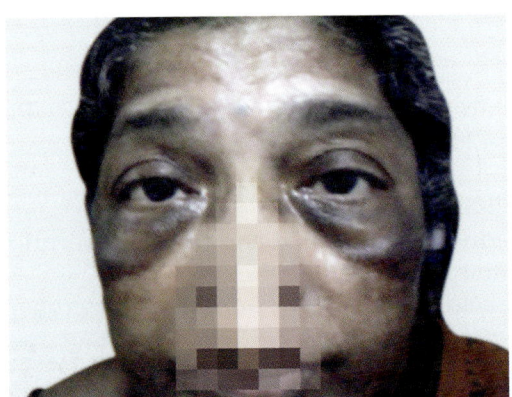 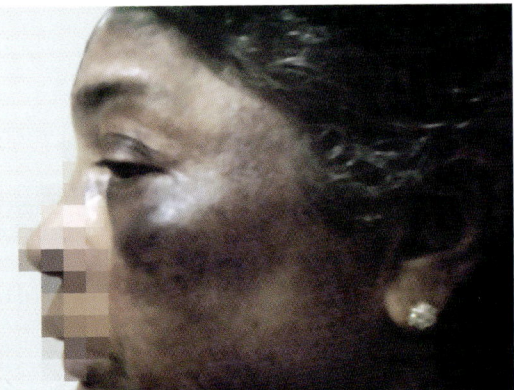

Quiz 1

What are the locations of various causes of hyperpigmentation?

a. *Generalised:* Endocrine Addison's, Cushing's, primary biliary Cushing's, Nelson's syndrome-Follows bilateral adrenalectomy, thyrotoxicosis, carcinoid, acromegaly, acanthosis nigricans
   Metabolic: Hemochromatosis sometimes follow a repeated blood transfusions
   Malnutrition: Pellagra
   Chronic infections: TB, kala azar, pinta
   Malabsorption syndrome
   Malignancy: Non-metastatic manifestation, Sezary syndrome, Hodgkins, malignant melanoma
   Congenital: Neurofibromatosis, Chediak-Higashi, Hermansky-Pudlák, Waardenburg syndrome
   Cirrhosis: Primary biliary—xanthomas + pruritus + melasma
   Racial
   HIV associated
   CTD: Dermatomyositis, scleroderma
   Drugs: Minocycline, clofazamine, amiodarone, busulfan
   Toxin: Arsenic, phenol

b. *Face:* Melasma ("mask of pregnancy")

c. *Abdomen:* Linea nigra—pregnancy
d. *Lips and buccal mucosa:* Peutz-Jeghers syndrome
   Drugs: Cloroquine, HCQS, quinidine, zidovudine, tetracycline, chlorpromazine; Smokers' melanosis
e. *Knuckles:* Vitamin B_{12} deficiency
f. *At the site of contact:* Chemicals—ointments containing mercury
   Chemicals taken systemically: Salicylates, cisplatin, bleomycin
   Ochrnosis—due to homogentisic acid accumulation in alkaptonuria. Can also be acquired exposure to phenols, HCQSs + Urine turns black on standing
g. *Palm and palmar creases:* Addison's disease
h. *Recent scars:* Addison's disease.

Quiz 2

What is melasma?
Chloasma (melanoderma/melasma—brown patches of irregular shape and size seen on the face/body also called "mask of pregnancy")—due to increase in estrogen and progesterone.

Quiz 3

What are the various mechanisms of hyperpigmentation in melasma and other causes?
1. *Drugs:* Ocs (containing estrogen/progesterone) though melasma—pigmentation of sun exposed skin most commonly seen in pregnancy, anticonvulsants, psoralens, perfumes
2. Pituitary (MSH induced)
3. Cushing's syndrome (ACTH induced), ectopic ACTH secretion in oat cell ca bronchus.
4. *Addison's disease (where ACTH levels are high):* MSH is a by-product of ACTH synthesis from POMC (pro-opiomelanocortin);
5. Hypothyroidism with increase in MSH can also cause it.

Quiz 4

Give list of syndromes causing oral pigmentation.
1. *Peutz-Jeghers syndrome:* Oral pigmentation + Hamartomatous GI polyps + AD + CHR19 STK11 (LKB1) Gene + Intussusception
2. *Cronkhite-Canada syndrome:* GI polyps + Alopecia + Spotty pigmentation + Neurologic manifestations.

Quiz 5

What is acanthosis nigricans (AN).
Hyperpigmentation + velvety thickening of skin involving flexures—axilla, groin, neck
Types: Malignant
       Non-malignant
a. *Malignant:* Severe cutaneous features—ca of GIT, ovaries, pancreas, lung, liver, uterus, urinary bladder, gall bladder. May be associated with cutaneous papillomatosis, pruritus (40%)

b. *Non-malignant*
  - *Insulin resistant type:* Associated with obesity
  - *Familial type*
  - *Congenital syndromes:* Lawrence-Seip syndrome
  - *Drug induced*

3. Hyperpigmentation of the Palmar Creases

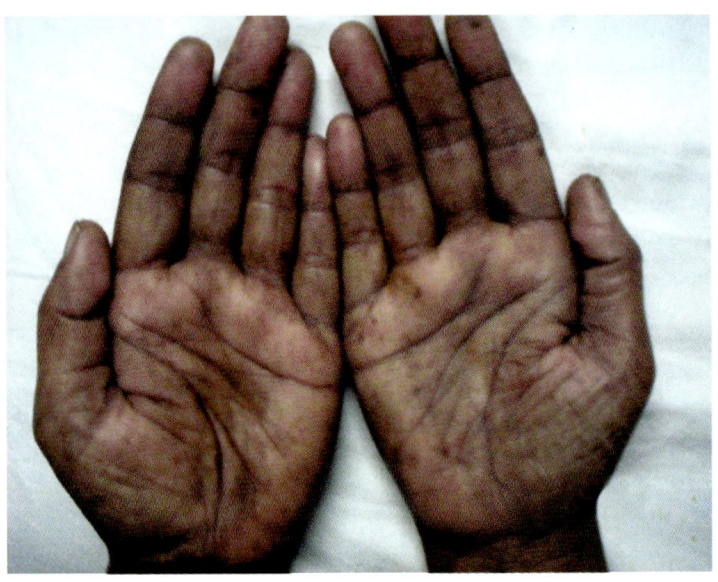

Addison's disease: Look for pigmentation of skin, mucosa (oral cavity), nipple and areola (recent) scars. Blood pressure (SBP <90), anemia, general weakness.

Look for tuberculosis, malignancy (may be due to metastasis into the adrenals), autoimmune cause

Addison's diseases: MSH induced

Cushing's disease: ACTH induced

MSH is a by-product of ACTH synthesis from POMC (pro opiomelanocortin)

Malnutrition: Vitamin B_{12} deficiency—knuckle pigmentation

Coeliac disease

Porphyria

Mercury poisoning: Ointments containing mercury

Nelson's syndrome

4. Clubbing of Fingers

Hippocratic Fingers

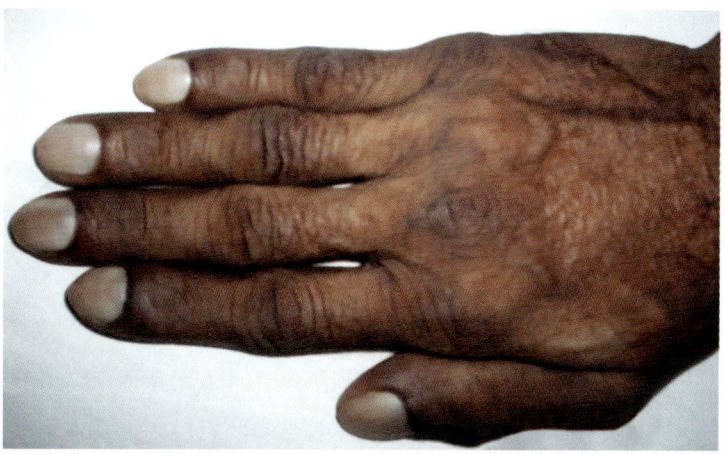

Quiz 1

What are the stages of clubbing?

Stage 1: Convexity and glossiness increases with loss of angle at the nail bed.

Stage 2: Hypertrophy of the tissues with increased fluctuation at the nail bed.

Stage 3: Bulbous swelling at ends of fingers—parrot beak, drumstick clubbing.

Stage 4: Pulmonary osteoarthropathy—bony changes involving wrist and ankle associated with distal bone pain and joint pain. Clubbing was first noticed by Hippocrates as the sign of disease.

Quiz 2

Which bedside test is suggestive of clubbing?

Schamroth test—usually a small lozenge-shaped window is visible when the distal phalanges are apposed.

Obliteration of this window suggests presence of clubbing.

Quiz 3

What are the mechanisms of clubbing?

1. Vasodilatation
2. Metabolic—platelet derived growth factor and hepatocyte growth factor.

Quiz 4

What are the causes of clubbing?

Causes of clubbing:

1. *Lung (about 80%)*: Ca bronchus, lung abscess, empyema, bronchiectasis, complications/sequelae of TB, COPD, ILD.

2. *Heart and vascular (about 10–15%):* CCHD, infective endocarditis, LA myxoma, infected abdominal aortic graft.
3. *GIT:* Primary biliary cirrhosis, Crohn's, malabsorption
4. *Idiopathic:* Cause not known in up to 60%
5. *HPOA:* Hypertrophic pulmonary osteoarthropathy—a special form of clubbing characterised by clubbing associated with periosteal and synovial thickening-associated with lung cancer.

Quiz 5

What are the causes of HPOA?
Syn: Marie-Bamberger syndrome
1. Idiopathic—Tauraine-Solente-Gole syndrome
2. Familial pachydermoperiostosis
3. *Acquired:* Carcinoma bronchus, lung abscess, pleural mesothelioma

Quiz 6

What is Primary HPOA?
Primary HPOA: Tauraine-Solente-Gole syndrome seen without lung disease. Due to decreased PG E2 breakdown.

Quiz 7

What are the causes of unilateral clubbing?
Unilateral clubbing: Axillary artery aneurysm, subclavian vein aneurysm, aortic aneurysm, PDA with R to L shunt with right sided aortic arch.

Quiz 8

What are the causes of unidigital clubbing?
Unidigital clubbing: Median nerve injury.

Quiz 9

What causes differential clubbing?
Differential clubbing: PDA with PH clubbing in LL > UL.

Quiz 10

What causes rapid clubbing?
Rapid clubbing: Lung abscess, ca bronchus.

Quiz 11

What is pseudoclubbing?
Pseudoclubbing
1. Apparent clubbing in people of African desent.
2. *Thyroid acropachy:* Painful, no nailfold edema, X-ray shows subperiosteal new bone formation of soap bubble type (as against linear deposition in usual HPOA)
3. *Pachydermoperiostosis:* Coarse, thick, deeply furrowed skin on forehead, scalp, face + increased sweating on palm and sole + AD inheritance + bony changes
4. Scleroderma

5. Acromegalic bone enlargement
6. *Acro-osteolysis:* Pseudoclubbing seen in people working with vinyl chloride. Distal digits acquire a flattened and bulbous shape due to collapse of the soft tissues as a result of destruction of distal phalanges. The nail bed angle is normal.
7. *Nail breaking:* Nail curved + hyponychial angle preserved + loss of pulp tissue.

Quiz 12

What are very rare causes of clubbing?
Cardiac: Atrial myxoma
Pulmonary: AV malformation, mets
Mediastinal lymphoma, thymoma; achalasia cardia
Extrathoracic: Thyroid ca, purgative abuse, pachydermoperiostosis.

5. Cyanosis

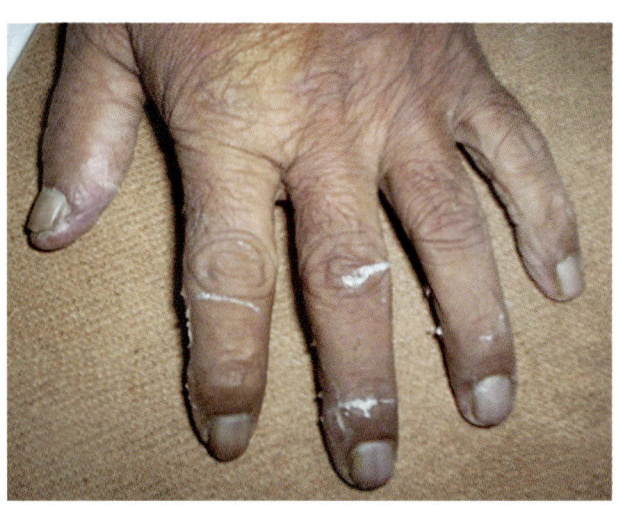

Quiz 1

What is cyanosis?
Bluish/purplish hue of skin and nailbed and mucus membranes due to incease in reduced hemoglobin more that 5 gm/dl in the capillary blood.

Quiz 2

What is the pathophysiology of cyanosis?
Deoxyhemoglobin (which looks bright red when viewed directly) looks bluish when viewed in the capillaries through a translucent layer of epithelium.

Types
a. Central
b. Peripheral

Quiz 3

What are the mechanisms of cyanosis?

Mechanisms:

a. Central cyanosis
   1. *Hypoxic hypoxia:* Obstructive airways disease—COPD, severe asthma
   2. *Shunt hypoxia:* Cyanotic congenital heart disease, AVM, hepatopulmonary syndrome (in cirrhosis of the liver)
b. Peripheral cyanosis

   Overutilization hypoxia/stagnant hypoxia—vasoconstriction, Raynaud's disease, low cardiac output.

Quiz 4

What are Pseudocyanosis/Mimics of cyanosis?

1. Replacement cyanosis—met- /sulfhemoglobinemia. Not true cyanosis.
2. *Pigmentary cyanosis:* Due to abnormal pigment (like methemoglobin, sulfhemoglobin)—not due to reduced oxygen
3. Enterogenous cyanosis

   Apparent cyanosis due to absorption of toxic materials like nitrates from the intestines resulting in met- or sulfhemoglobin—chocolate color.
4. Carbon monoxide poisoning—carboxy hemoglobin—cherry red color
5. Argyria

   Skin deposits of metallic silver—silver containing topical antiseptics slate grey color. Does not blanch on pressure (true cyanosis might).

Quiz 5

What is red cyanosis?

Seen in patients with polycythemia vera.

Quiz 6

Why does cyanosis come easily in patients with polycythemia?

A minimum of 5 gm/dl of reduced hemoglobin is required for the cyanosis to develop. Hence, it is very rare and unlikely in anemia and very easy to develop in patients with polycythemia.

Quiz 7

What is "tardive cyanosis?" (cyanosis tardiva)

In potentially cyanotic conditions with shunts, no cyanosis occurs when the cyanosis is L to R. When there is a reversal of the shunt however, that is later in the disease, the cyanosis may start appearing initially on exertion hence the term tardive cyanosis.

Quiz 8

Why does cyanosis occur easily in polycythemia and hardly ever in severe anemia?

Cyanosis occurs easily in polycythemia and almost never in severe. Anemia as at least 5 grams of reduced hemoglobin are required and it is simply not available in severe anemia.

Quiz 9

What are the three stages of Raynaud's phenomenon?
1. Pallid phase of blanching—arteriolar spasm
2. Cyanotic phase of arteriolar spasm + dilated venule and capillary bed filled with poorly oxygenated blood
3. Hyperemic phase—dilated arteriole and AV shunts.

Quiz 10

What is acrocyanosis?
Chronic, painless cyanosis of usually several fingertips seen in possible connective tissue disorders.

Quiz 11

What is differential cyanosis?
Cyanosiss LL > UL seen in PDA with shunt reversal (R to L shunt), PDA with aberrant right subclavian artery.

6. Clubbing with Cyanosis—TOF

OBSERVATION

Cyanosis of all four limbs associated with clubbing

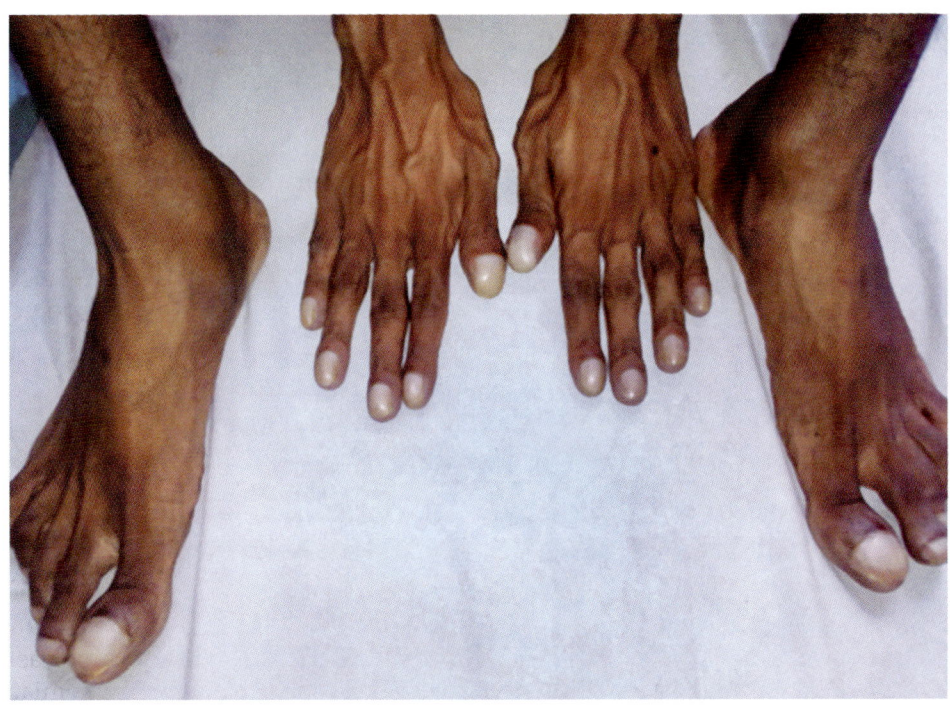

Quiz 1

What conditions are associated with coexisting clubbing and cyanosis?

a. *Cardiac:* CCHD

b. *Vascular:* AVM (congenital and acquired) (localized, as a part of systemic disease)

c. *Pulmonary:* ILD

d. *Special situations*

a. *Cardiac*
   1. Fallot's tetralogy
   2. Shunt reversal (R to L)—Eisenmenger syndrome in ASD/VSD/PDA

b. *Vascular*
   1. AVM—congenital localized limbs, lung
   2. Acquired—as a requirement for hemodialysis, bullet injury
   3. As a part of systemic disease—hepatorenal syndrome

c. *Pulmonary*
   ILD

d. *Special situations*
   Bronchiectasis—usually associated with clubbing only. Cyanosis indicated collaterals between pulmonary and bronchial arteries—very rare situation.

7. Bald Tongue

OBSERVATION

Sides of the tongue show indentation with the teeth marks + surface of the tongue has lost papillae → bald tongue

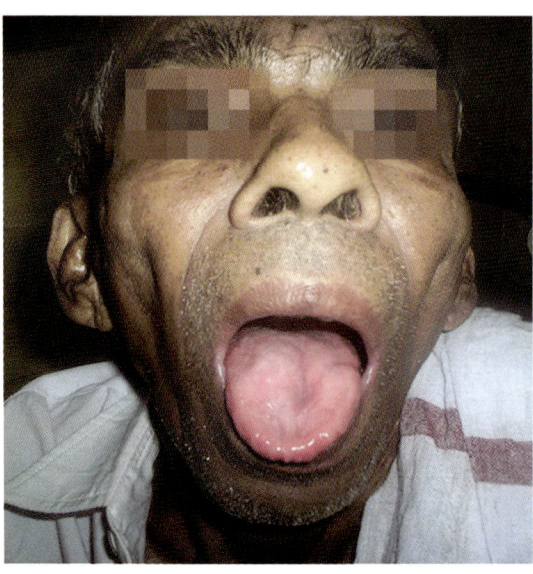

Cases in Medicine

Quiz 1

What is bald tongue? How does the tongue become bald?
Normally papillae regenerate and the surface of the tongue remains rough: In iron deficient states the regeneration of the papillae is inadequate giving rise to a smooth surface due to lack of papillae → bald tongue. Similar changes are also seen in the remaining GI tract resulting in secondary malabsorption worsening the state of iron deficiency.

Quiz 2

What are the markers of iron deficiency?
Koilonychia
Bald tongue
Pallor (non-specific): Anemia—microcytic hypochromic type with anisocytosis and poikilocytosis
PICA (specific).
Esophageal webs may be associated with dysphagia—Paterson-Kelly syndrome or Plummer-Vinson syndrome which is premalignant.

Quiz 3

What is the commonest mechanism of iron deficiency anemia?
Chronic blood loss—the cause for which may vary from place to place.

Quiz 4

What is the peripheral smear finding of iron deficiency anemia?
Microcitic (MVV <80), hypochromic (MCHC <32) RBCs with anisocytosis and poikilocytosis.

Quiz 5

What are the D/Ds for microcytic hypochromic anemia?
1. Iron deficiency = Reduced serum iron + increased iron binding capacity + reduced ferritin + no stainable bone marrow iron.
2. Anemia of chronic disease = Reduced serum iron + reduced iron binding capacity + increased ferritin + increased bone marrow stainable iron.
3. Thalassemia = Increased serum iron = Normal iron binding capacity + increased ferritin + increased bone marrow stainable iron + target cells (Mexican hat cells) in PS.
4. Sideroblastic anemia = Ringed sideroblasts in the bone marrow (containing accumulated iron as unique mitochondrial ferritin) + Failure to utilize iron.
5. Lead poisoning = Anemia + basophilic stippling + colicky abdominal pain + wrist drop + encephalopathy + optic neuritis.

8. Erythema of Upper Part of the Body—Chest and Face

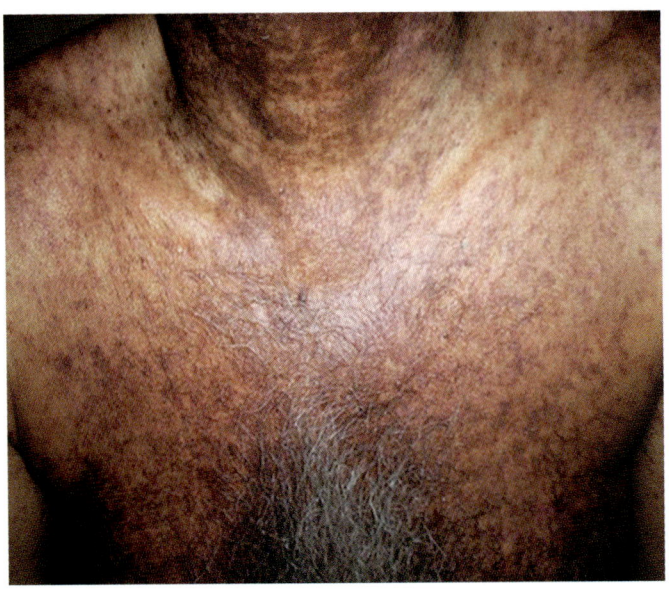

Quiz 1

What history would you take in patient with flushing of face and upper body?
History of alcohol, exposure to heat, emotional upset (emotional blushing), fever, exercise menopause (climacteric flushing, chills, insomnia, palpitations)—HRT with estrogen helps. Adrenergic and opioid pathways might have a role—Alpha 2 adrenergic blockers and naloxone may have an additive effect; UV light exposure, steroid therapy.

Quiz 2

In what situation a diabetic may get upper body flushing and erythema?
Autonomic neuropathy diabetes mellitus + Antabuse like reaction with chlorpropamide (AD inheritance).

Quiz 3

What are the features of carcinoid syndrome? How can the flushing be blocked?
Look for carcinoid syndrome: Head and neck flushing, tachycardia, diarrhoea, wheezing, hypotension, abdominal cramps. Urine 5-HIAA is high. Flushing can be blocked with octreotide (somatostatin analogue (SC/IV).

Quiz 4

What is the value of urine examination?
Value of urine examination is alcohol and 5-HIAA (for carcinoid).

Quiz 5

Which foodstuffs can induce these features?
Food stuffs: Spicy foods, chinese restaurant syndrome due to monosodium glutamate; tyramine, histamine, aldehyde, nitrites, potassium metabisulphite (associated with wheezing).
Hot beverages—by a countercurrent heat exchange mechanism involving anterior hypothalamus.

Quiz 6

Which type of food poisoning can induce these features?
Ciguatera food poisoning due to ciguatoxin (not destroyed by heat), flushing, vomiting, diarrhea, abdominal pain, dysaesthesia of tongue, teeth and gingivae, ataxia. The syndrome is self limiting and may last for as long as years!

Quiz 7

Which are the endocrine causes of these features?
Endocrine: Pheochromocytoma (hypertension, sweating, chest discomfort).

Quiz 8

What is systemic mastocytosis?
Mastocytosis (abdominal pain, diarrhea, hypotension,urticaria pigmentosa) Darier sign—urticaria on stroking.

Quiz 9

What are the features of anaphylaxis?
Anaphylaxis (vasodilatation resulting in erythema and "feeling hot" hypotension, urticaria, angioedema).

Quiz 10

Which malignancy can induce these features?
Medullary carcinoma of thyroid (protracted flushing, persistent discoloration, telangiectasia of face and arms, thyroid nodule, elevated calcitonin levels).

Quiz 11

Which hematologic condition can give rise to these features?
Polycythemia rubra vera: Red face and upper body flushing—ruddy complexion.

Quiz 12

Which drugs have to be suspected?
Chlorpropamide, tetracycline, doxycycline, hydrochlorothiazide.
Photosensitive eruptions—usually in exposed areas.

Cases in Medicine

9. Hand Deformity

OBSERVATION

1. Symmetrical, involving fingers and wrist—MCP and IP joints involved.
2. Thumb deformity present.
3. Wrist involved (ulnar deviation). Usually follows chronic inflammation—rheumatoid arthritis.
4. Also notice shiny stretched skin, prominent veins, hyperpigmentation involving dorsum of the hand and knuckles.
5. Observe flexion deformities at the DIP joint.

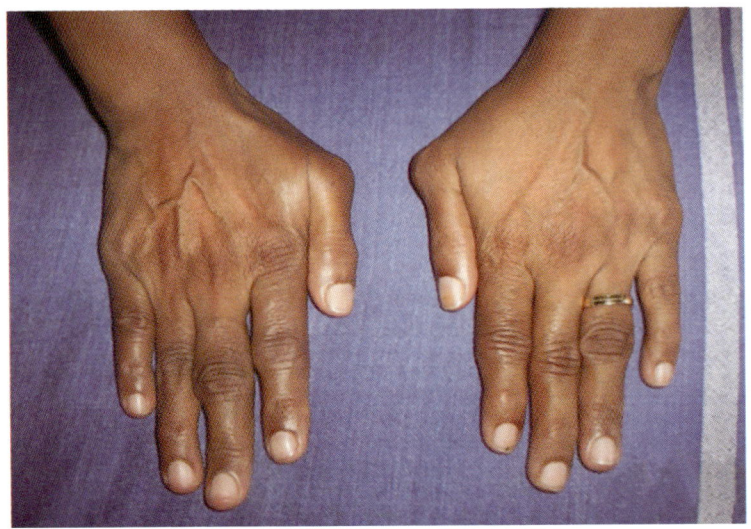

Quiz 1

What is the inference of all these findings?
Deforming rheumatoid arthritis.

Quiz 2

What else do you observe at the distal IP joint?
Nodules—Heberden's nodules suggesting osteoarthritis.

Quiz 3

What are Heberden's nodes?
Persistent non-tender subcutaneous nodules seen in the distal IP joints—related to osteoarthritis.

Quiz 4

What are Bouchard's nodules?
Persistent non-tender subcutaneous nodules at the proximal IP joints—also related to osteoarthritis.

Quiz 5

Describe subcutaneous nodules seen in patients with rheumatoid arthritis?

They are tender persistent subcutaneous nodules at flexor and extensor tendons of hand, sacrum, Achilles tendon, olecrenon. Other sites for the rheumatoid nodules include sclera, lungs, and myocardium.

They may be associated with deforming arthritis, and extra-articular manifestations

Quiz 6

How do these differ from subcutaneous nodules of rheumatic fever?

Subcutaneous nodules of rheumatic fever are non-tender, transient, seen on extensor surfaces of arm, forearm, hand, tips of vertebrae, and angles of scapula. They may be associated with other features of rheumatic fever, murmurs.

Quiz 7

What are the extra-articular manifestations of RA?

1. Subcutaneous nodules
2. Serositis: Pleural effusion (low glucose), pericardial effusion
3. Hand: Subcutaneous nodules, longitudinal nail ridges, clubbing (associated lung fibrosis), splinter hemorrhages (vasculitis), palmar erythema.
   Vasculitis: Cyanosis, Raynaud's phenomenon, cryoglobulinemia, Livido reticularis, splinter hemorrhages
   Leg ulcers, pyoderma gangrenosum, ankle edema
4. Eye: Episcleritis, scleral nodule, keratoconjunctivitis sicca (Sjögren's syndrome), retinal vascular involvement
5. Lymphadenopathy: LN proximal to involved joint—histologically resembles giant follicular lymphoma, lymphoma
6. Immunosuppression: Infected leg ulcers, pneumonia
7. Nerves
   Peripheral nerves (PN): Carpal tunnel syndrome, mononeuritis multiplex (vasculitis)
   CNS: Ischemic stroke (medium size vessel vasculitis)
   Muscle: Myositis, polymyositis, vasculitis
8. CVS
   Pericardial effusion, myocarditis, endocarditis, MR, coronary arteritis
9. RS
   Pleural effusion, pulmonary fibrosis, PH, adenocarcinoma, rheumatoid nodules in lung, pneumonitis (with methotrexate trt)
10. Syndromes
    a. Sjögren's syndrome: RA + xerostomia + xerophthalmia
    b. Still's disease: Juvenile RA + fever with rash
    c. Felty's syndrome: Severe RA arthritis + splenomegaly + thrombocytopenia + leukopenia
11. Systemic
    Fever, fatigue, lymphadenopathy, anorexia, weight loss, drug side effects (CST, methotrexate)

Quiz 8

How do you decide that the disease is active?
Joints: Pain, morning stiffness
ACCP (anti-cyclic citrullinated polypeptide) antibodies—diagnostic
Positive rheumatoid factor
Elevated ESR
Elevated CRP
Blood: Eosinophilia + lymphocytosis

Quiz 9

What are the complications of RA?
1. *Joints*: Deformity, subluxation, dislocation, septic arthritis
   Atlanto-axial dislocation
2. Amyloidosis AA—malabsorption, renal failure
3. Anaemia of chronic disease
4. Leg ulcers
5. Scleromalacia perforans
6. Sepsis—septic arthritis, pneumonia
7. Vasculitis
8. Malignancies—adenocarcinoma (lung), lymphoma

Quiz 10

List the drugs used in the management of RA and the important complications of some of them?
1. *Antimalarials*: Chloroquin, HCQs, side effects (SE) rash, retinopathy
2. *Sulfasalazine*: SE rash, oligospermia, nausea, dizziness, headache
3. *Methotrexate* (*purine antagonist*): SE lung-pneumonia, fibrosis; liver—fibrosis, failure; neutropenia
4. *Penicillamine*: SE obliterative bronchiolitis, glomerulonephritis, anemia, thrombocytopenia, myesthenia gravis, myositis
5. *Leflunomide*: Pyrimidine antagonist—SE hypertension, diarrhea, liver damage
6. *Infliximab*: TNF alpha antagonist
7. *Etanercept*: TNF alpha receptor antagonist
   SE opportunistic infections—TB, fungal, bacterial septicemia
   Autoimmunity—SLE, MS
8. Azathioprine
9. Mycophenolate mofetil
10. Cyclophosphamide
11. Cyclosporine A
12. Chlorambucil
13. *Gold:* Sodium aurothiomalate
14. IM/oral SE rash, nephrosis, renal failure, diarrhea

10. Herpes Zoster

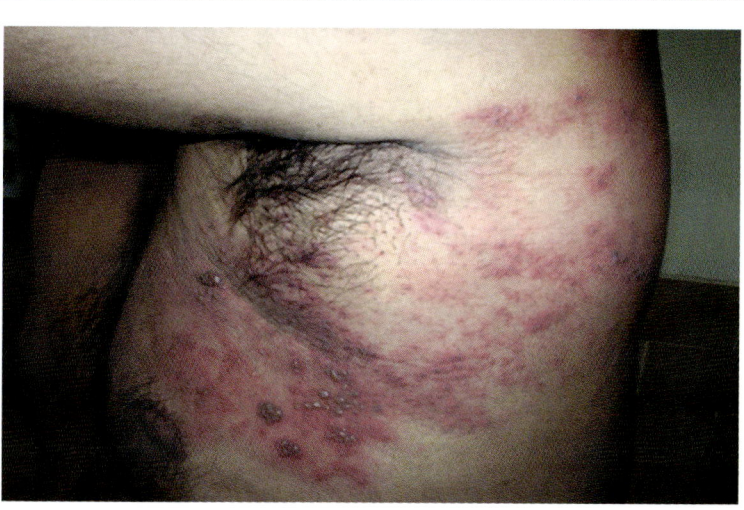

Quiz 1

What are the observations?

1. Vesicles and erythema
2. Unilateral, dermatomal distribution on the left side

Quiz 2

What is the most likely diagnosis?

Herpes zoster

Quiz 3

What is the cause?

Activation of the latent varicella zoster virus in the dorsal root ganglion. This results in pain in the area of nerve root distribution.

Burning pain may precede the vesicles.

The vesicles strictly follow dermatomal distribution and do not cross the midline. They are found more on the trunk than the limbs (more dermatomes than the limbs).

Usually affects sensory roots—dysaesthesia, pain may be caused.

Motor roots can be affected, e.g. facial palsy, limb weakness, urinary retention.

Quiz 4

What is Ramsay Hunt syndrome?

Synonyms: Zoster oticus, geniculate zoster

Painful varicella zoster infection presenting with vesicular eruption on pinna with facial palsy + vesicles sometimes seen on hard palate + loss of taste in anterior 2/3rd of tongue + pain in the ear.

Cases in Medicine

Name some syndromes associated with herpes zoster.

1. Ramsay Hunt syndrome.
2. Orbital apex syndrome involving apex of the orbit and cavernous sinus by the herpes virus through trigeminal nerve ganglia.
3. Guillain-Barre syndrome following herpes zoster—rare.
4. *Oglive syndrome:* Acute colonic pseudo-obstruction usually due to a medical condition which is extra-abdominal—herpes zoster.
5. Herpes zoster ophthalmicus—a vesicle on the nose is a strong predictor of herpes zoster ophthalmicus.
6. Herpes zoster ophthalmicus with orbital pseudotumour.
7. Post-herpetic depigmentation.
8. Herpes zoster oticus—involving the ear.

11. Post-herpetic Depigmentation

OBSERVATION

Depigmentation—stricty unilateral, dermatomal distribution.

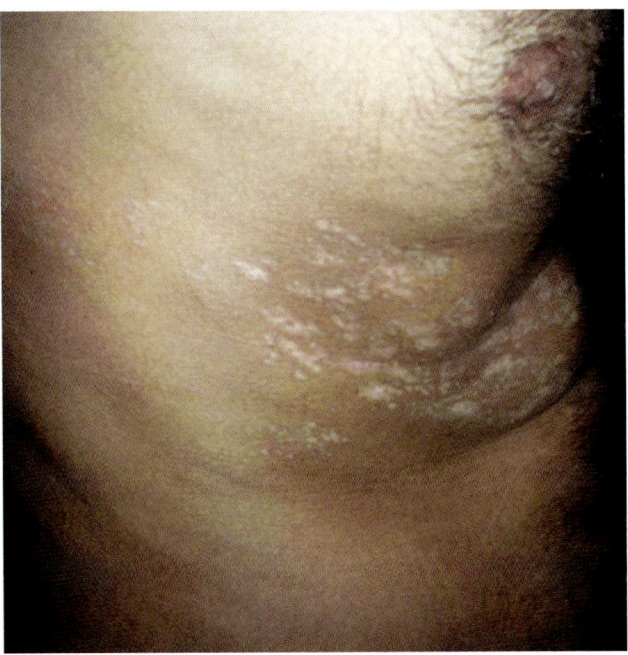

What is the likely diagnosis?

Post-inflammatory depigmentation following herpes zoster.

Quiz 2

What are the complications of herpes zoster?

Complication	Sites of zoster virus multiplication
1. Post-herpetic neuralgia (PHN)	Sensory ganglion
2. Bacterial superinfection	Sensory ganglia
3. Blindness following Herpes zoster ophthalmicus	Cranial nerve II, III, VI
4. Facial palsy	Cranial nerve VII
5. Aseptic meningitis	Cranial nerve V
6. Motor neuropathy	Any sensory ganglia
7. Transverse myelitis	Vertebral ganglia
8. Vasculopathy (encephalitis)	Cranial nerve V
9. Ramsay Hunt syndrome	Cranial nerve VII (geniculate ganglion) with spread to Cranial nerve VIII

Quiz 3

What are the indications for the use of antiviral drugs?

a. Age >50
b. Pain moderate/severe
c. Rash severe
d. Involvement of face/eye
e. Other complications of herpes zoster
f. Immunocompromised state

Quiz 4

Whish are the antiviral drugs used?

a. *Immunocompetent*
   1. Acyclovir
   2. Famciclovir
   3. Valacyclovir
   4. Brivudin

b. *Immunocompromised*
   1. Acyclovir
   2. Foscarnet

12. Palmar Creases

OBSERVATION

Asymmetric palmar creases: Single palmar crease unilateral (seen only on the right hand). Usually called simian crease.

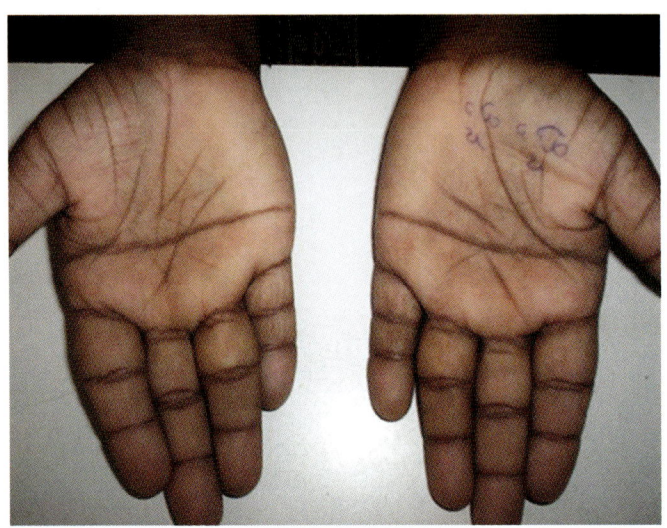

Quiz 1

What is a simian crease?

Simian crease—single transverse palmar crease formed by the fusion of proximal and distal palmar creases. Resembles transverse flexion crease seen in the monkeys (simian). Seen commonly in Down syndrome (50%)–not pathognomonic; and 5% normal people.

Quiz 2

What is sydney crease?

Sydney crease: A variation in proximal palmar crease—an elongated proximal palmar tranverse crease reaching the ulnar side of the palm—seen in Down syndrome, rubella embryopathy.

Quiz 3

Where do you find yellow palmar creases?

Yellowish palmar creases seen in type 3 beta hyperlipoproteinemia.

Quiz 4

Where do you find diagonal ear lobe crease?

Diagonal ear lobe crease: Possible association with coronary artery disease.

Frank's sign is a diagonal crease in the ear lobe extending from the tragus across the lobule to the rear edge of the auricle and is believed to be indicative of cardiovascular disease and/or diabetes.

13. Zidovudine Nails

OBSERVATION

Black coloured nails.

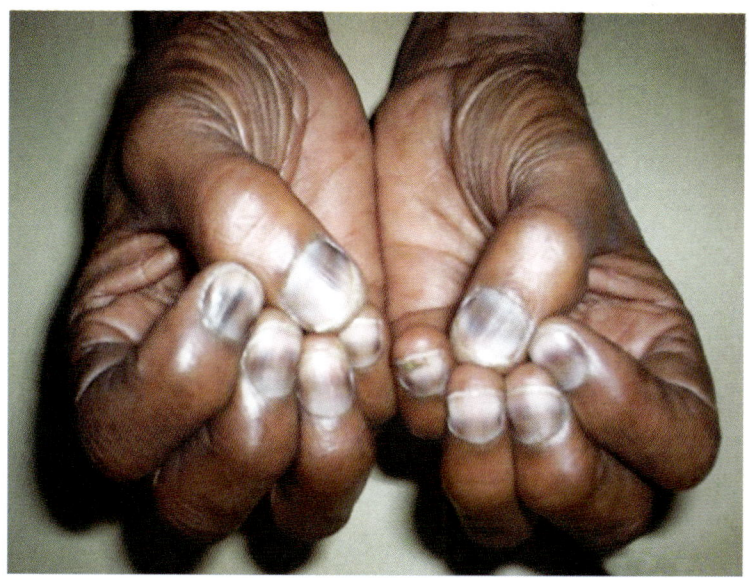

Quiz 1

What is the cause of this discoloration?

Hyperpigmentation of the nails and skin—patient on zidovudine therapy (anti-retroviral therapy).

Other side effects seen with zidovudine therapy—anemia.

Quiz 2

What are the various causes of nail discoloration?

Various causes of nail discloration

a. *Black nails*
Zidovudine, subungual bleeds
b. *Black longitudinal streaks*
Peutz-Jeghers syndrome
c. *Yellow nails*
Nail patella syndrome—lymphedema + pleural effusion
d. *Yellow droplet lesion*
Psoriasis
e. *Splinter hemorrhages*
Infective endocarditis, vasculitis, scurvey

f. *Blue lunulae*

Argyria, Wilson's disease, antimalarial therapy

g. *Red lunulae*

Carson monoxide poisoning

h. *White nails*

Hypoalbuminemia—cirrhosis

i. *Half and half nails*

Terry nail—red brown distal end—cirrhosis, diabetes, CCF

Lindsay nails—distal brown (melanin)—renal failure.

14. Pseudohypertrophy of the Calf

OBSERVATION

Both calf muscles appear big

Pseudohypertrophy of the calf

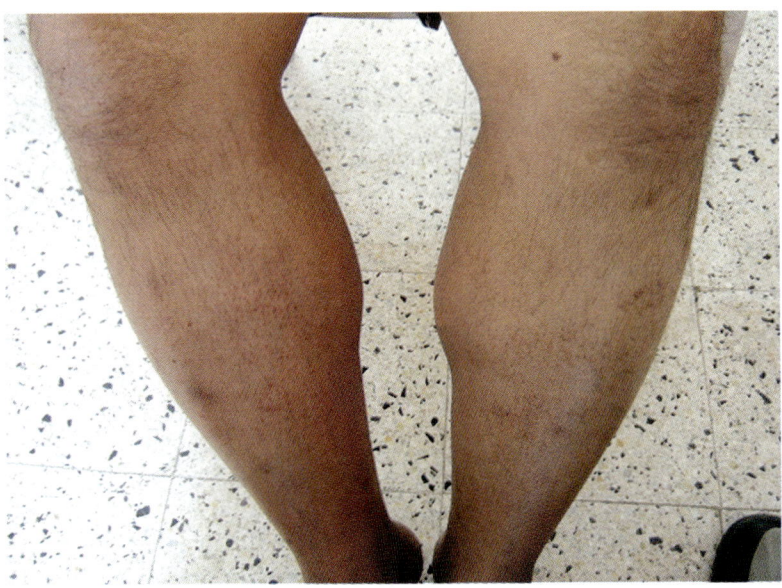

Quiz 1

What is pseudohypertrophy?

Pseudohypertrophy is the term used when the increase in the size of the organ or the part of the body is NOT due to increase in the number/size of specific functional elements but due to presence of some other tissue—fat/fibrous tissue.

Pseudohypertrophy may be compensatory—due to increase in the leg girth with compensatory enlargement of weak muscles (where hypertrophy is due to muscle tissue) or to replacement fibrosis where the increased girth is also significantly contributed to by the fat tissue.

Quiz 2

What are the causes of pseudohypertrophy?
Causes of pseudohypertrophy include:
1. Duchenne's muscular dystrophy
2. Myhre syndrome—short stature, brachydactyly, deafness, mental retardation, facial dysmorphism, striking muscular build.
3. Kocher-Debré-Semelaigne syndrome—hypothyroidism related pseudohypertrophy of calf muscles in pediatric age group.
4. Amyloid related to systemic amyloidosis.

Quiz 3

What is the new contemplated use of calf muscles?
As LV assist device—research in progress.

15. Wound Myiasis

OBSERVATION

Larvae of housefly coming out of the ulcer.

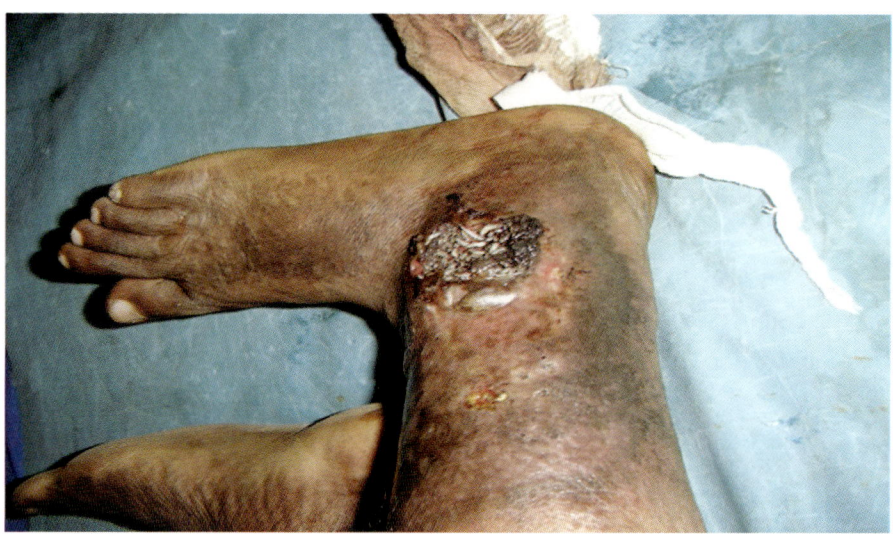

Quiz 1

What is myiasis?
Infection due to invasion of tissues or cavities of the body by larvae of dipterous insects, e.g. housefly larvae.

Quiz 2

Larvae of house fly seen teeming in the wound. This is an example of wound myiasis.

Quiz 3

What is the importance?

The larvae are directed at dead and necrotic tissue, which is the principle of using larva in the maggot therapy.

Quiz 4

What are the other forms of myiasis?

Other forms of myiasis include—ocular, oral, nasopharyngeal, auricular, urogenital, cutaneous, furuncular, rectal, gastric, etc.

Quiz 5

What is pseudomyiasis/accidental myiasis?

Pseudomyiasis results from
1. Accidental swallowing of larvae through food (cheese flies in cheese).
2. Accidental deposit of eggs on oral/genitourinary openings.

16. Heberden's Nodes

OBSERVATION

Nodules at the distal interphalangeal joints—**Heberden's nodes.**

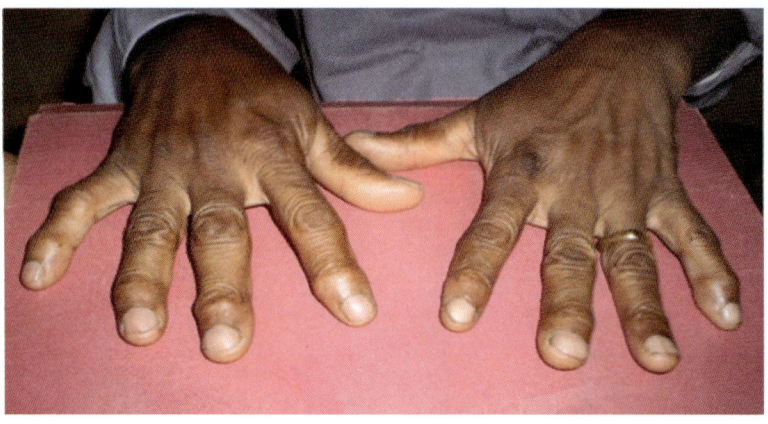

Quiz 1

What are Heberden's nodes?

Heberden's nodes are persistent , non-tender nodules seen at the distal IP joints in osteoarthritis.

Quiz 2

What are Bouchard's nodes?

Bouchard's nodes are persistent, non-tender, subcutaneous nodules seen in relation to the proximal IP joint in osteoarthritis.

Quiz 3

What are the other nodes associated with arthritis?

Other nodes associated with **arthritis—Haygarth's nodes, Osler's nodes,** gouty tophi.
Subcutaneous nodules associated with rheumatic fever and rheumatoid arthritis.

Quiz 4

What are Haygarth's nodes?

Haygrath's nodes: Exostoses from the articular surface or periosteum of bone near the joints or fingers seen in RA.

Quiz 5

What are Osler's nodes?

Osler's nodes: Circumscribed, painful swellings seen in the skin/subcutaneous tissue of hands and feet in subacute bacterial endocarditis.

Quiz 6

What are gouti tophi?

Gouti tophi are deposits of uric acid/urates near joints, external ear cartilage, kidneys in gout.

Quiz 7

What are neurofibromata?

Neurofibromata—type I NF von Recklinghausen's disease of nerves. Autosomal dominant (AD) inheritance. Gene locus-17q11—NF 1 gene.
II NF associated with bilateral acoustic neuomas, meningiomas.
AD inheritance. Gene locus 22q11-NF 2 gene.

Quiz 8

What are Xanthomas/Xanthelasma?

Xanthomas are depositions of yellowish cholesterol—rich material that can appear anywhere in the body containing accumulated lipids in large foam cells of skin. They could be palmar, tendon, or tuberoeruptive types.
Xanthelasmas are a sharply demarcated yellowish collections of cholesterol underneath the skin deposited as elevated plaques usually on or around the inner canthus of upper eyelids.

Quiz 9

What are ivory osteomas?

Ivory osteomas in Gardner's syndrome. Osteomas are benign, slow growing masses of mature, lamellar bone arising from skull or mandible.
Gardner's syndrome: Colonic polyposis with tendency for malignancy, ivory osteomas skull. AD mutation at APC (adenomatous polyposis coli) gene at chromosome 5q. Can be familial.

Quiz 10

What type of subcutaneous nodules may be seen in mycobacterial infection?

Cutanoues tuberculosis due to atypical mycobacteria presenting as subcutaneous nodules.

Cases in Medicine

What is erythema nodosum?

Erythema nodosum: Painful nodular lesions on the extensor surfaces of lower extrimities coming in crops can be accompanied by arthralgia, fever. Self limiting can recur.

Associated with drug reactions (sulfa, penicillin), leprosy, TB, sarcoidosis, acute rheumatic fever.

17. Dilated Veins around the Umbilicus

OBSERVATION

Dilated, varicose veins radiating from the umbilicus are seen. This appearance is due to engorged paraumbilical veins radiating from the umbilicus to join the systemic veins.

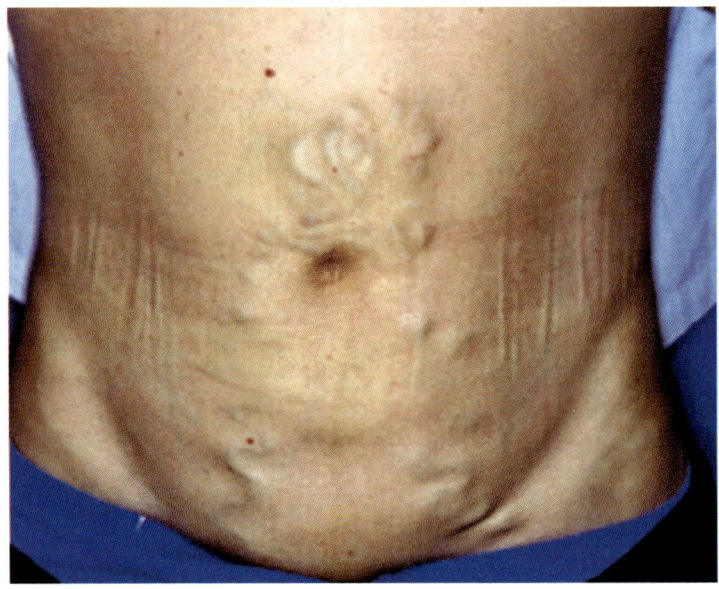

Quiz 1

What is "Caput Medusae"?

When seen all round the umbilicus (which is rare), it is called caput medusae—due to apparent similarity to (mythological) Medusa's hair which was once turned into snakes by (mythological) Athena.

Quiz 2

Where do you find dilated veins around the umbilicus?

The dilated veins can be seen in Cruvilhier-Baumgarten syndrome—cirrhosis of the liver with patent umbilical and paraumbilical veins and varicose periumbilical veins.

Auscultation over the dilated tortuous veins may reveal a venous hum.

Cases in Medicine

Quiz 3

What are the other features of Cruvilhier-Baumgarten syndrome?
1. Portal systemic encephalopathy
2. A continuous bruit—"Bruit de diable" Devil's noise/Nuns murmur
   Location: Xiphoid process, umbilicus
   Radiation—precordium, back
3. Systolic accentuation—sitting up, inspiration
4. Murmur disappears on firm pressure.

Quiz 4

What are the various differential diagnosis for a hum on the liver?
Differential diagnosis: Hum on the liver
1. Bruit de diable
2. Very vascular tumour of the liver
3. Compression of the portal vein by the enlarged LN.

Quiz 5

Why do you get dilated veins around the umbilicus in cirrhosis of the liver?
Due to loss of the hepatic architecture, blood flow inside the liver gets obstructed resulting in a low velocity high resistance flow. Paraumbilical veins cannot empty into the liver and, therefore, anastomosis with systemic veins which now carry abnormally more blood resulting in dilated, tortuous veins around the umbilicus. The direction of flow is normal—away from the umbilicus.

Quiz 6

What happens in extra-hepatic obstruction of veins?
Paraumbilical veins open, carry the blood from abdominal wall to the liver—the direction of blood flow is towards the umbilicus that is to say towards the umbilicus (reverse of normal).

Quiz 7

What are the sites of important portocaval anastomosis?
1. On the anterior abdominal wall
   Umbilical veins with abdominal wall veins
   Can produce caput medusae and Cruvilhier-Baumgarten syndrome
2. In the retroperitoneum
   Veins of retzius connecting intestinal veins with retroperitoneal branches of IVC
3. Coronary azygos system—gastric veins with esophageal veins (which empty into the azygos venous system)
   Dilatation can result in esophageal varices
4. At the junction of rectum and anal canal
   Inferior mesenteric vein communicates with hemorrhoidal veins (which empty into hypogastric veins)
   Dilatation can result in internal/external hemorrhoids.

18. Buffalo Hump

OBSERVATION

A rounded bulge of fat seen behind the neck on the upper portion of the back—dorsocervical.

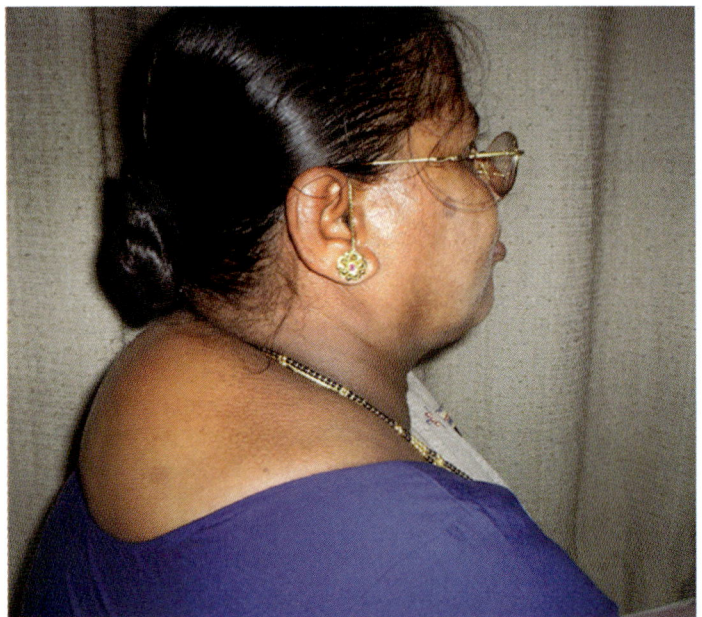

Quiz 1

What is buffalo hump?

Abnormal fat deposition that occurs between the shoulders in the upper portion of the back below the neck in Cushing's syndrome and other causes of hypercorticalism.

Quiz 2

What is the mechanism of production of Buffalo hump?

Due to the redistribution of body fat—lipodystrophy—causing a visible and palpable fatty elevation in the upper portion of the back below the neck. It is persistent and non-tender. Other places where such deposits occur include midsection, upper back, face (moon face).

Quiz 3

Which conditions can cause it?

It can be seen in:

a. Cushing's syndrome
b. Cushing's disease

c. Obesity

d. Diabetes mellitus

e. Drugs also can cause it—corticosteroids, some ARVs.

Quiz 4

What can sometimes mimic the buffalo hump?

Kyphoscoliosis can mimic the buffalo hump—particularly in patients with weak bones—osteoporosis.

19. Generalized Maculopapular Rash with Photosensitivity

OBSERVATION

Generalized rashes with erythema. Patient gave a history of photosensitivity.

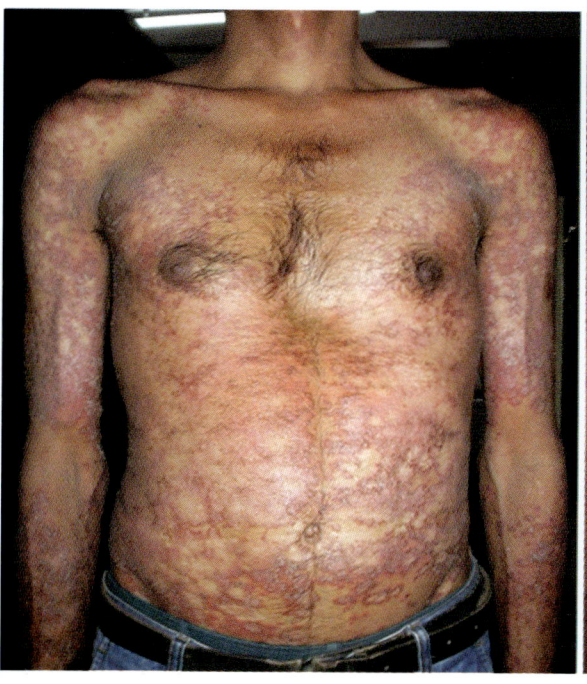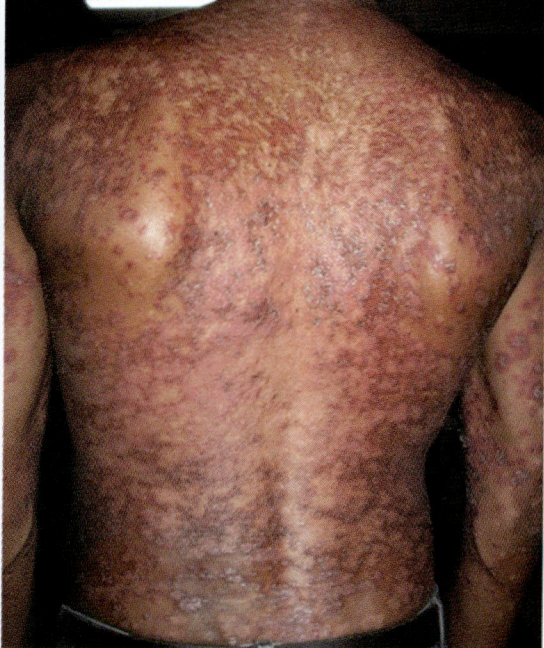

Quiz 1

What are the causes of such situations?

Consider

a. Drug reactions (ART—niverapine, ATT—pyrazinamide, actinomycin-D, dapsone), doxycycline

b. SLE

c. Psoriasis

d. Photosensitivity.

20. Arcus Senilis

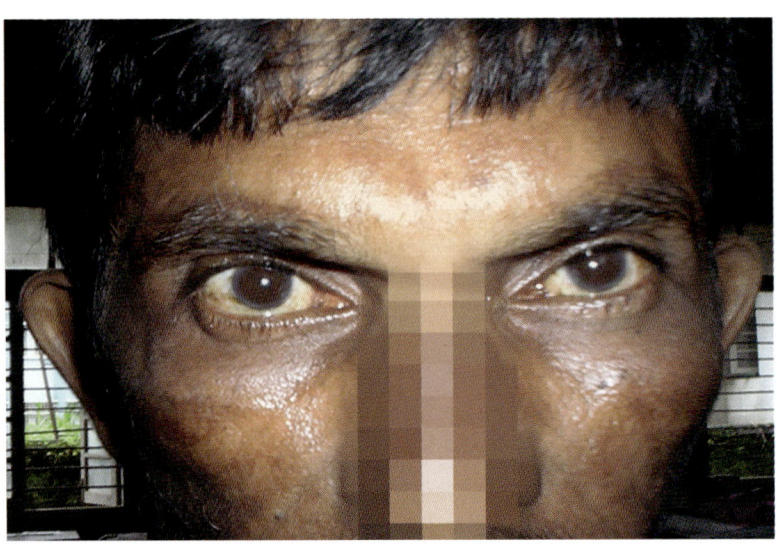

Quiz 1

What is arcus senilis?
Corneal arcus—greyish yellow crescentic (circular) band of about 1.5 mm width within the outer margin of the cornea.

Quiz 2

What is the mechanism of development of arcus senilis?
Deposition of lipids at corneoscleral junction.

Quiz 3

What are the differences between the arcus senilis and Kayser-Fleischer ring?
KW ring is is a brown ring due to abnormal copper metabolism due to ceruloplasmin deficiency resulting in ectopic deposition of excessive copper in the viscera—liver, eye, basal ganglia, myocardium and kidneys.
Differences:
1. No gap between the KF ring and the periphery of cornea.
2. Situated in the deeper layer of the cornea.

Quiz 4

What are the conditions where the KF rings can be found?
a. Wilson's disease: Ceruloplasmin deficiency, altered copper metabolism, deposition at the level of Descemets' membrane at the corneoscleral junction—pathognomonic.
b. Intraocular foreign body.

Quiz 5

What is the significance of arcus in the young patients?

Premature corneal arcus in the young patients below the age of 40 years particularly when associated with xanthelesma is likely to be associated with familial hypercholesterolemia. Premature arcus is also associated with coronary artery disease.

Quiz 6

Where does the KF ring start?

10 o'clock to 2 o'clock position.

Quiz 7

What is the importance of unilateral corneal arcus?

Association with carotid artery stenosis on the opposite side (the side where there is no arcus) if ocular hypotony and artificial eyes are excluded.

Quiz 8

Can the KF ring disappear?

Yes

a. After chelation therapy.

b. After a successful liver transplant.

Examples of other Ocular Markers of Systemic/Internal Disease

1. Marfan's syndrome—superior dislocation of the lens.
2. Homocystinuria—inferior dislocation of the lens. Can be associated with coronary, cerebral, renal artery thrombosis.
3. Pinguecula—raised yellowish white areas around the limbus.
   Seen in Gaucher's disease.
4. Retinal phacomas and glial masses (on retinoscopy) in tuberous sclerosis (AD). Triad— adenoma sebaceum, MR, epilepsy.
5. Angioid streaks—irregular grey lines radiating from the optic disc. Seen in pseudoxanthoma elasticum, Paget's disease, sickle cell disease, Ehlers-Danlos syndrome.
6. Cherry red spots in sphingolipidosis—Niemann-Pick, Tay-Sachs disease—abnormal sphingolipid accumulation in the ganglion cells in the macula.
7. Blue sclera—osteogenesis imperfecta, pseudoxanthoma elasticum, alkaptonuria.
8. Hyperteliorism—can be associated with Leopard syndrome, Noonan's syndrome, PS with ASD, Hurler's syndrome (gargoylism), supravalvular AS.

Cases in Medicine

21. Complications of Tobacco use

OBSERVATION

Incompletely opened mouth, stained teeth, growth in the posterior part of the mouth, staining of tongue.

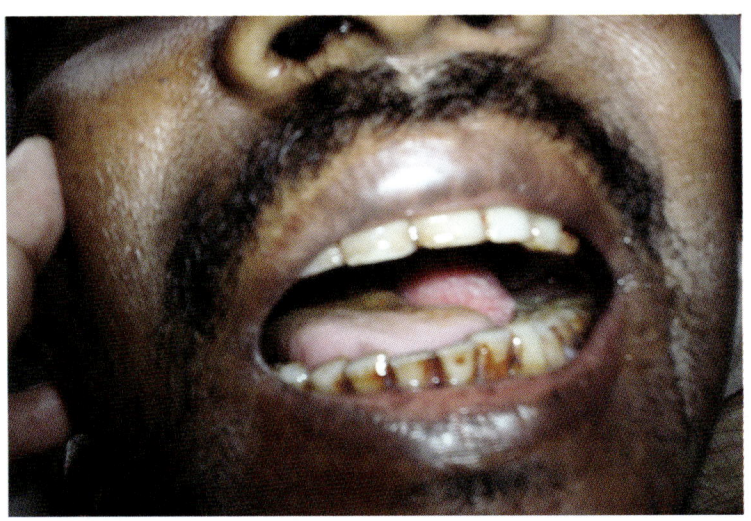

Quiz 1

What is the inference?

Staining of teeth: Central teeth stained by smoking; lateral and other teeth stained by chewing tobacco.

Staining of tongue:

Growth in the oral cavity—possibly malignant

Inability to open the mouth completely suggests—submucus fibrosis.

Quiz 2

What are the types of tobacco use and misuse?

Types of tobacco use include

a. Smoked tobacco

b. Smokeless tobacco
   1. Snuff
   2. Chewing tobacco (cheni, gutka—held in the mouth between teeth and cheek)
   3. Toothpaste

22. Elephantiasis

OBSERVATION

Gigantic right lower limb below the knee with increase in the girth and thickness of skin and subcutaneous tissues, formation of nodules, loss of anatomic landmarks, depigmentation, hyperpigmentation.

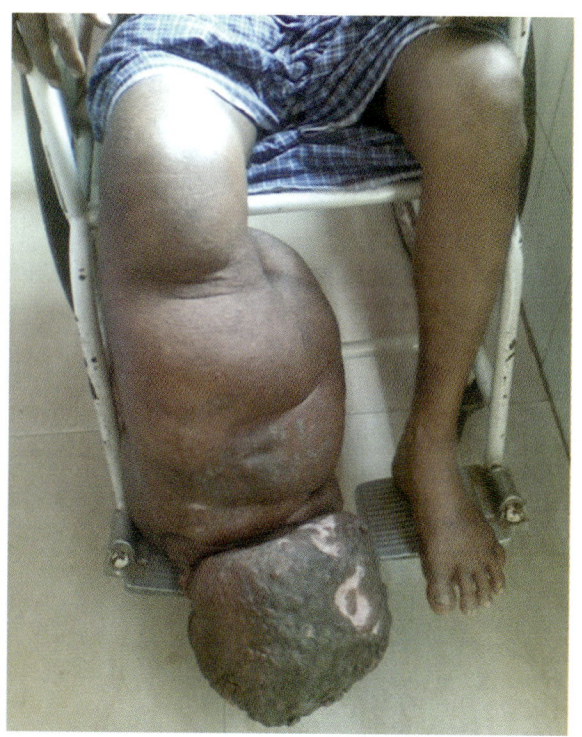

Quiz 1

What is elephantiasis?
Hypertrophy, enlargement, fibrosis of the skin and subcutaneous tissues of lower limbs/scrotum/vulva.

Quiz 2

Which sites can elephantiasis develop?
Lower limb, upper limb, breast, vulva, scrotum, penis.

Quiz 3

What are the changes seen in elephantiasis?
Increase in limb girth, increase in thickness of skin and soft tissues, hypertrophy of soft tissues, nodularity, ulceration, depigmentation, hyperpigmentation.

Quiz 4

What are the causes of elephantiasis?

a. Elephantiasis is usually due to filarial worms *Wuchereria bancrofti*, *Brugia malayi*.
b. Other factors blamed include Wolbachia bacteria in the worm, host immune response, opportunistic infections.
c. Chronic oedema is due to the obstruction of the lymphatic system and involvement of lymph nodes by the parasite.

Quiz 5

What is the mechanism of elephantiasis?

Lymphatic obstruction—filarial. Non-filarial etiolofies include lymph node removal, irradiation, agenisis of lymphatics (Milroy's disease), foreign body occluding the lymphatics (silica dust).

Quiz 6

What is Podoconiosis?

Podoconiosis is non-filarial elephantiasis.
Non-filarial elephantiasis seen in Kenya, Rwanda, Tanzania, Burundi, Sudan, Egypt.

Quiz 7

What is the mechanism of podoconiosis?

Due to persistent contact with irritant soils—red clay rich in alkali metals—sodium and potassium and associated with volcanic activity.

Quiz 8

What are the complications of lymphedema and podoconiosis?

Complications:

a. Tendency for ulceration
b. Secondary infection
c. Mechanical restriction of movements

Cases in Medicine

23. Malar Rash

In Latin mala means jaw or cheek bone.

OBSERVATION

Butterfly rash on the face involves the bridge of the nose, shape resembles that of a butterfly.

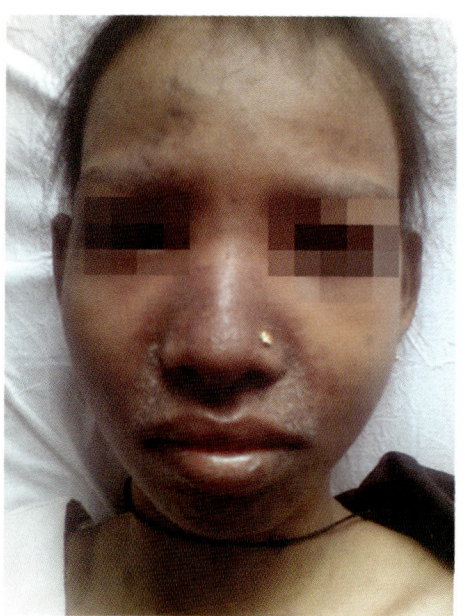

Quiz 1

What are the causes of malar rashes?

Causes of malar rash include SLE—photosensitive rash involving the bridge of the nose, sparing the nasolabial folds; is macular, non-pruritic.

This is an example of an atypical rash. Only 30% of patients with SLE have typical rashes.

Differential Diagnosis

a. Pellagra—due to chronic niacin deficiency (due to reduced intake of niacin/lysine or increased intake of leucine; or due to altered metabolism in carcinoid syndrome).

b. Dermatomyositis—connective tissue disorder with inflammation of muscle and skin. More classically erythematous rashes are found on the upper eyelid (heliotrope rash) and back/upper chest—Shawl sign—with photosensitivity. Similar erythematous lesions may be found on the malar region as well.

c. Bloom syndrome—congenital telangiectatic erythema (mainly butterfly distribution), photosensitivity, proportionate dwarfism, dolichocephaly, tendency for malignancy. Androgen receptor (AR) mutation in BLM (bloom syndrome) gene on chromosome 15q. Chromosomes are excessively unstable and there is predisposition to malignancy.

Cases in Medicine

37

d. Lyme disease due to tick *Borrelia burgdorferi*.

e. Erysipelas due to streptococci can cause painful malar rash.

f. Seborrheic dermatitis—scaly lesions on skin and malar rash.

g. Extreme sun exposure in sensitive people.

24. Photosensitive Rashes on the Front of the Same Patient

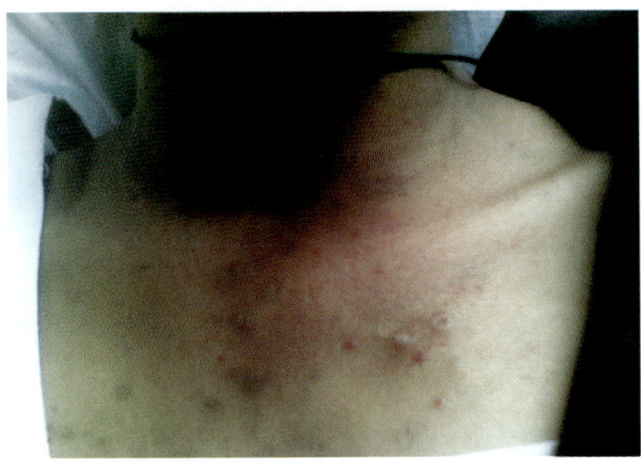

25. Pectus Excavatum

OBSERVATION

A hollow (congenital deformity) seen on the lower part of the chest with abnormal development of ribs and sternum resulting in posterior displacement of the xiphoid cartilage.

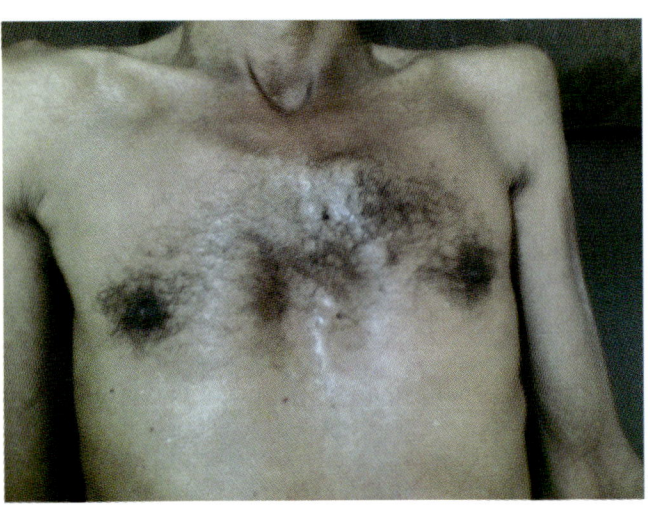

Quiz 1

What is it known as?
Pectus excavatum.

Quiz 2

What are the effects of pectus excavatum?
Can press on and displace the heart.
It can result in:
a. Cardiac—increased RV pressure, palpitations
b. Respiratory—breathlessness, reduced respiratory function
c. Chest pain
d. Back pain
e. Psychological effects—anxiety, avoid people.

Quiz 3

What are the syndromes associated with pectus excavatum?
Associates syndromes: Marfan's syndrome, straight back syndrome, spinal muscular atrophy coeliac disease.

26. Polythelia—Accessory Nipples

OBSERVATION

At least six nipples seen on the right side and three on the left side—accessory nipples/ polythelia.

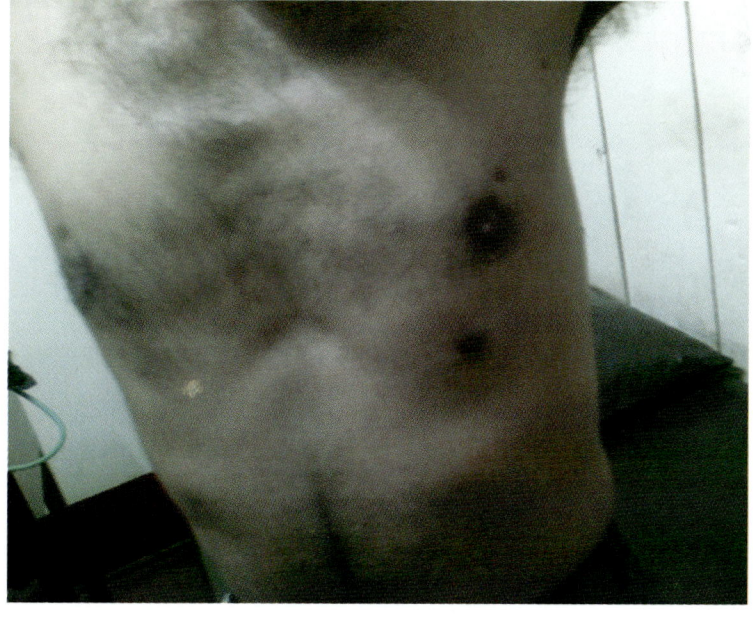

Quiz 1

What is the embryology of the development of nipples and polythelia?

Milk lines developing from epidermis give rise to breasts and nipples.

 Milk lines start in the armpit and curve forwards through the location of regular nipples and descend obliquely to the groin.

Quiz 2

Historically what was the importance of polythelia?

A third nipple was considered to confirmation that the lady is a witch!

Quiz 3

How many nipples do you see in this patient?

At least nine! (six on right side and three on left side).

Quiz 4

Which gene and syndrome are associated with this anomaly?

An important gene associated with supernumerary nipples is DHODH—Dihydroorotate dehydrogenase (quinone).

 Known to be associated with Hailey-Hailey disease.

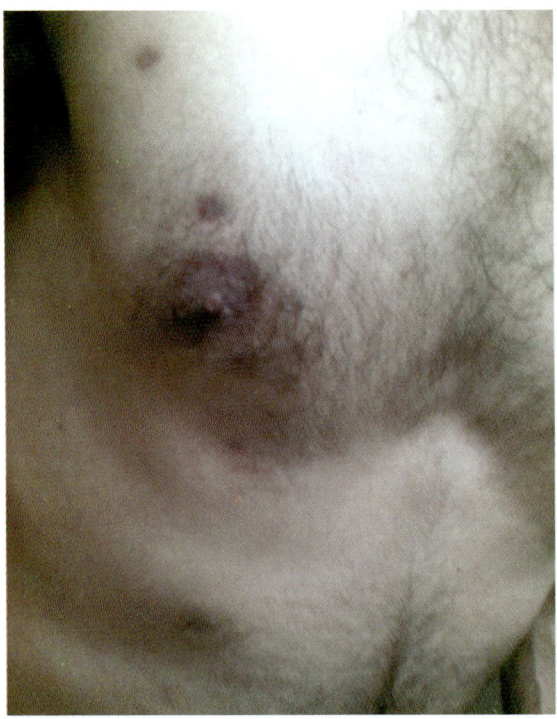

How many nipples can you see in this patient?

At least six on the right side!

And at least three on the left side!

27. Unilateral Ptosis

OBSERVATION

Unilateral ptosis on the right side with extensive blackish discoloration of the upper eyelid and below the lower eyelid (black eye) suggesting subcutaneous bleed—possibly traumatic.

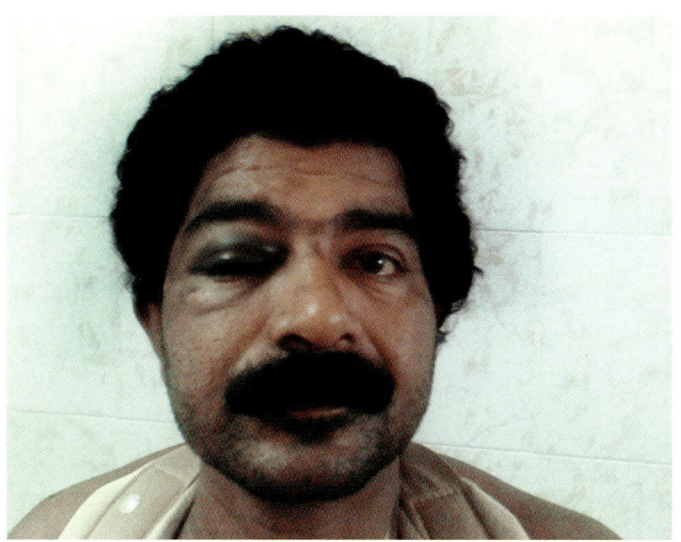

Quiz 1

What are the other causes of unilateral ptosis?

Other causes of unilateral ptosis:

a. Diabetes mellitus

b. Brain tumor

c. Horner's syndrome in pancoast tumor

d. Berry aneurysm

e. Local lid causes—like neurofibromas, hematoma (mechanical ptosis)

f. Congenital ptosis—may be unilateral (usually bilateral). Associated anomalies include—congenital facial diplegia, external ophthalmoplegia, lingual palsy, club foot.

Quiz 2

What is Marcus Gunn phenomenon and what is its significance?

Marcus Gunn jaw winking phenomenon due to misdirection of III nerve fibres, is characterised by synkinesia with abnormal ocular movements—upward jerking associated with chewing/sucking in the nursing children. This phenomenon is an example of pathological congenital synkinesis.

This condition can be associated with—amblyopia, anisometropia, strabismus.

Inheritance pattern AD with incomplete penetrance.

Quiz 3

What is inverse Marcus Gunn phenomenon?

This is a condition where the eyelids close upon opening the mouth (reverse of the Marcus Gunn Phenomenon).

Quiz 4

How do you identify myasthenia gravis as the cause of ptosis?

By using edrophonium injection IV—remarkable improvement will be seen in 30 seconds and worsening shortly thereafter.

Quiz 5

What are the features of ptosis due to Horner's syndrome?

The other findings could include—wasting of sternomastoid—clavicular head (XI nerve involved); Wasting of trapezius (XI, XII nerves)—lesion could be on the base of the skull.

Hoarseness of voice with gradual involvememnt of XI, XII nerves could be due to a neurofibroma of the XII nerve.

Partial unilateral ptosis without frontalis overreaction and with small pupils and dysphagia could be at the brain stem.

Quiz 6

When do you suspect functional ptosis/pseudoptosis?

One sided drooping of the eyelid (on the side of ptosis) and an overreaction of the frontalis muscle on the other side.

Quiz 7

Which mid brain lesions can cause ptosis?

Vascular, encephalitic, MS.

Ptosis with headache may be due to an aneurysm in the circle of Willis—most often a PCA aneurysm.

Ptosis without headache may be due to syphilis (tabes dorsalis) and diabetes.

Quiz 8

What are the features of tabes dorsalis?

Joints—painless range of increased abnormal movements—neuropathic joint, AR pupil, ptosis (usually bilateral).

Quiz 9

What are the differential diagnosis of abnormally increased joint movement range?

a. Ligament laxity syndromes, e.g. pseudoxanthoma elasticum;

b. Hypotonia—LMN paralysis, cerebellar lesions, posterior column lesions (like tabes dorsalis).

28. White Flaky Lesions in the Throat

OBSERVATION

Extensive, white flaky lesions on the throat and the tongue.

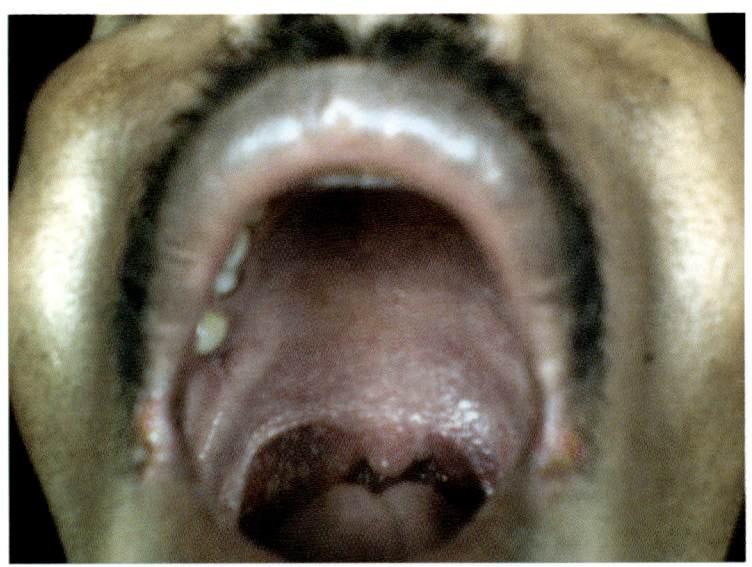

Quiz 1

What diagnosis do these observations suggest?
Suggestive of candidiasis (oral thrush)

Quiz 2

What are the causes of oral candidiasis/thrush?
Causes:
a. Diabetes mellitus
b. AIDS
c. Corticosteroid therapy
d. Chemotherapy for malignances
e. Prolonged antibiotic therapy

Quiz 3

What are the characteristic features of these lesions?
They appear white and scaly and are painful.
   Can be removed. Removing however, can expose bleeding spots.

What are the types of oral candidiasis?

a. Primary oral candidiasis
  - Acute pseudomembranous
  - Chronic pseudomembranous, erythematous
  - Candida associated lesions
b. Secondary oral candidiasis
  - Oral manifestation of systemic mucocutaneous candidiasis, e.g. thymic aplasia, candidiasis endocrinopathy syndrome
  - Hyperplastic, plaque like nodular
  - Denture related, angular stomatitis.

29. Chylous Ascites

OBSERVATION

Milky white fluid (obtained during abdominal paracentesis).

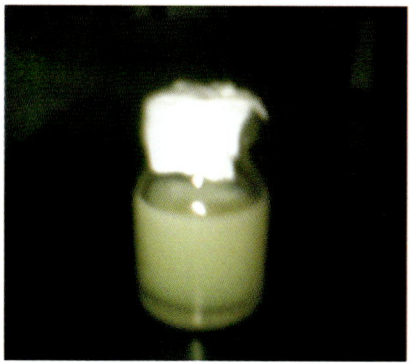

Quiz 1

This milky white fluid was obtained during abdominal paracentesis. What is it?
Chylous ascites.

Quiz 2

What is chyle?
Chyle is alkaline white, odourless liquid rich in protein (>50 gm/litre), triglycerides (4–40 gm/litre).

   Chyle leaks are rare.

Quiz 3

What are the various manifestations of chyle leak?
Chyle leak can manifest variably as
a. Chylothorax/chylous effusion—thoracic cavity

Cases in Medicine

b. Chylous ascites—peritoneal cavity

c. Chylous pericardial effusion—pericardial cavity

d. Externlal chyle draining fistula.

Quiz 4

What are the causes of chyle leaks?

The causes of chyle leaks include:

a. Lymphoma

b. Trauma—penetrating injury

c. Blockage of lymphatics due to adult filarial worms

d. Lymphangiectasia

Quiz 5

What are the various modalities of treatment available?

Rx for chyle leaks

a. Omit fat (FFA) from diet

b. Octreotide

c. Pleurodesis—for chylothorax.

30. Bilateral Short 2nd and 3rd Metatarsals

OBSERVATION

2nd and 3rd metatarsals are short.

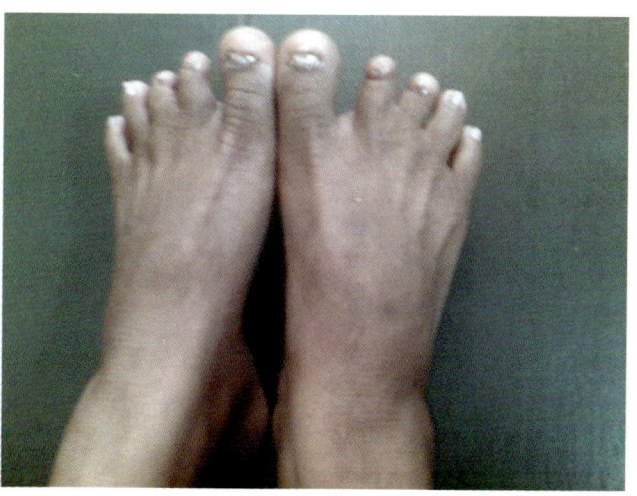

Quiz 1

What is this condition known as?

This condition is known as brachymetatarsia-1 or more abnormally short metatarsals.

What are the conditions/syndromes associated with short metatarsals?

a. Morton's syndrome—1 metatarsal abnormally short-results in discomfort and callusing of metatarsal head.
b. Turner's syndrome—4th metatarsal short
c. Pseudohypoparathyroidism—3rd and 4th metatarsals short
d. Pseudopseudohypoparathyroidism—3rd and 4th metatarsals short
   "Knuckle knuckle dimple dimple syndrome."

31. Koilonychia (Spooning) of Nails

OBSERVATION

Spoon-shaped nails—koilonychia best seen in the nail of the great toe.

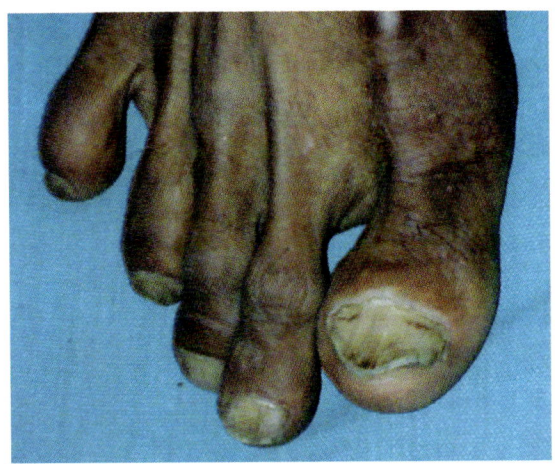

Quiz 1

What is the significance of koilonychia?

It indicates iron deficiency and is suggestive of iron deficiency anaemia if associated with anaemia.

Quiz 2

What are the various features of iron deficiency?

a. *Nails:* Platynychia (flattening), koilonychia (spooning)
b. *Tongue:* Bald tongue (atrophy of filiform papillae)—reversible with treatment; sore tongue, angular stomatitis
c. *Pharynx, esophagus:* Dysphagia, esophageal webs (Plummer Vinson syndrome/Paterson Kelly syndrome)—premalignant (carcinoma of the postcricoids area can result)
d. *Stomach:* Achlorhydria, gastritis

e. *Pica (abnormal craving for non-food items)*: Pagophagia (eating ice) seen in 50% of patients with iron deficiency—reversible.

f. Amenorrhea in severe iron deficiency

h. *Beeturia*: Pink to red colored urine after ingestion of beets.

Quiz 3

What are the lab featuers of iron deficiency?

a. PS—microcytic hypochromic anemia with anisocytosis, poikilocytosis; thrombocytosis (reversible);

b. BM—iron stores severely reduced or absent; erythroid hyperplasia

c. Serum ferritin—reduced;
   Serum iron binding capacity—increased;
   Serum transferrin saturation—low;
   Soluble transferring receptor—high.

Quiz 4

What are the newly proposed markers of iron status?

a. sTfR—soluble transferring receptor

b. SQUID (liver iron)

c. Hepcidin

d. ZPP—erythrocyte zinc protoporphyrin

e. CHr—content of hemoglobin in reticulocytes.

32. Vitiligo

OBSERVATION

Extensive areas of depigmentation on the hands.

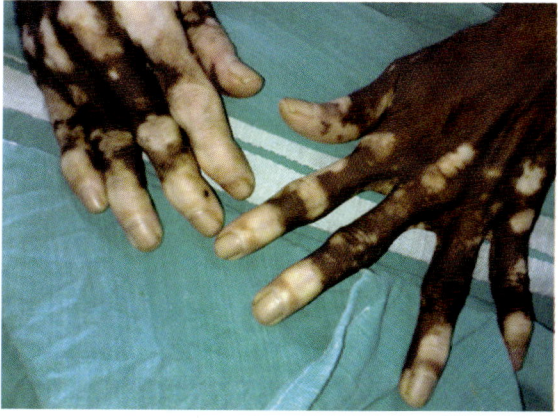

Quiz 1

What is the diagnosis?

Vitiligo 1 involving multiple fingers.

Quiz 2

What are the causes of vitiligo?

a. Autoimmune

b. Genetic

c. Viral

d. Oxidative stress

Quiz 3

What is the mechanism of vitiligo?

Damage to or death of melanocytes—the pigment forming cells-resulting in areas of depigmentation. May involve small areas initially and then gradually enlarge. Hairs may not be involved.

Quiz 4

What are the clinical features of vitiligo?

Invovement of face, hands, lower limbs (classically knees and dorsum of the feet) wrists; orifices-around mouth, eyes, nostrils, genitalia, umbilicus.

   Mood disorders like depression in stigmatized patients.

Quiz 5

What are the conditions that can be associated with vitiligo?

Usually autoimmune disorders: Pernicious anemia, achlorhydria, diabetes mellitus, Addison's disease, thyroid problems.

Quiz 6

What are the differential diagnosis of vitiligo?

a. *Pityriasis versicolor*: Initial lesions after sunlight exposure, perifollicular depigmentation. Late lesions may be more difficult to identify.

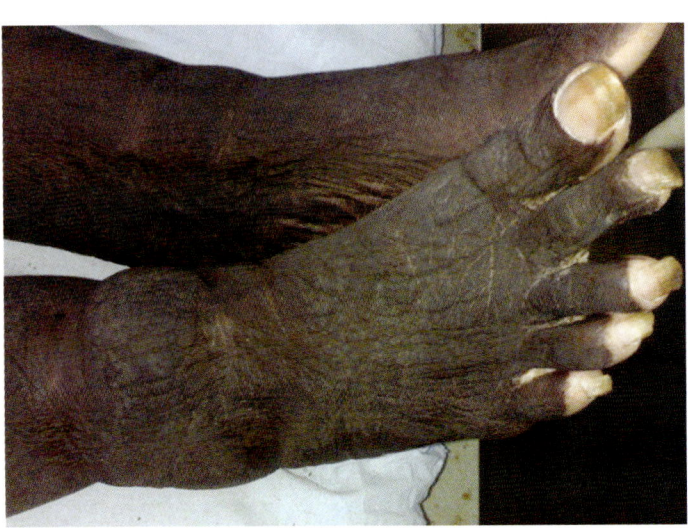

b. *Albinism*: Complete lack of melanin due to absence of enzyme tyrosinase involved in tyrosine metabolism associated with:
  - Intolerance to sunlight
  - White skin and hair
  - Pink iris
  - Impaired vision
  - Nystagmus, optic nerve hypoplasia, astigmatism
c. *Tuberculoid leprosy*: Solitary asymmetric skin lesions
d. Postinflammatory depigmentation
e. *Piebaldism:*
  - AD inheritance
  - White forlock, triangular white macule on forehead
f. Primary adrenal insufficiency

33. Barbiturate Blisters

OBSERVATION
1. Blisters on the extensor surface of forearm, arm, fingers (index middle and ring)
2. Patient had barbiturate overdose with suicidal intent.

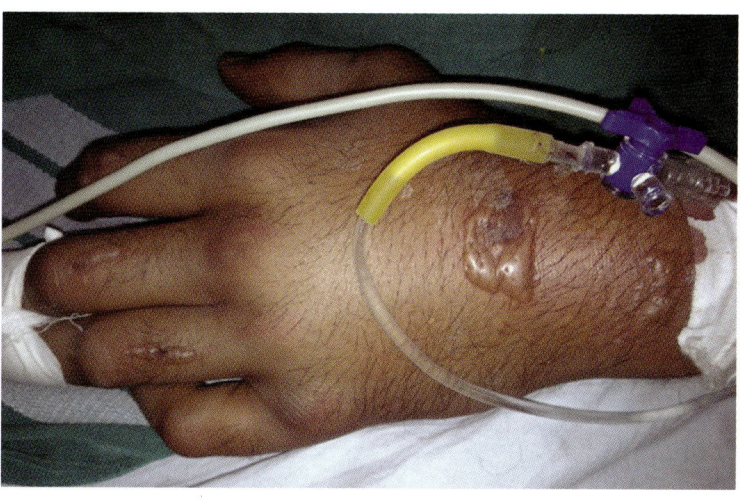

Quiz 1

What is the diagnosis?
Barb blisters/barbiturate blisters due to suicidal overdose of barbiturates.

Quiz 2

What is the mechanism of barbiturate blisters?
Increased porphyrins, pressure necrosis, hypotension, infection, use of vasoactive drugs, all have been contemplated.

Quiz 3

What is the importance of this finding in a comatose patient/a patient with H/o poisoning?
Highly suggestive of barbiturate as the etiological factor.

Quiz 4

What are the differential diagnosis for blisters in the situation of acute poisoning?
1. Barbiturates
2. TCAs—tricyclic antidepressants
3. Carbon monoxide
4. Benzodiazepines

Quiz 5

What is the importance of general examination in situation of acute poisoning?
a. *Temperature*
   Hypothermia: Phenobarbitone, phenothiazine, TCAs
   Hyperthermia: Amphetamine, ecstacy, MAO inhibitors, cocaine, atropine derivatives
   Theophylline, serotonin syndrome
b. *Pulse*
   Tachycardia/Irregular pulse—overdose with salbutamol, antimuscarinics, quinine, phenothiazines
   Chloral hydrate, cardiac glycosides
c. *Pupils*
   Dilated: Sympathomimetics, anticholinergics, TCA
   Constricted: Opiates, cholinergics
   Unequal: Head injury
d. *Other eye signs*
   Strabismus: Carbamazepine
   Papilloedema: Carbon monoxide, glutethimide, methanol
   Nystagmus: Phenytoin
e. *Muscle rigidity:* Amphetamines, ecstacy
f. *Breath odour*
   Ketones: DKA, alcoholic ketoacidosis
   "Bitter almond": Cyanide
   "Garlic like": Organophosphorus, arsenic
   "Rotten egg": Hydrogen sulfide
g. *Perioral acneform lesions:* Solvent abuse
h. *Mouth:* Dry: Anticholinergics
   Excessive salivation: Parasympathomimetics

34. Marked Conjunctival Congestion + Subconjunctival Hemorrhage—Leptospirosis

OBSERVATION

1. Marked conjunctival suffusion
2. Subconjunctival hemorrhages

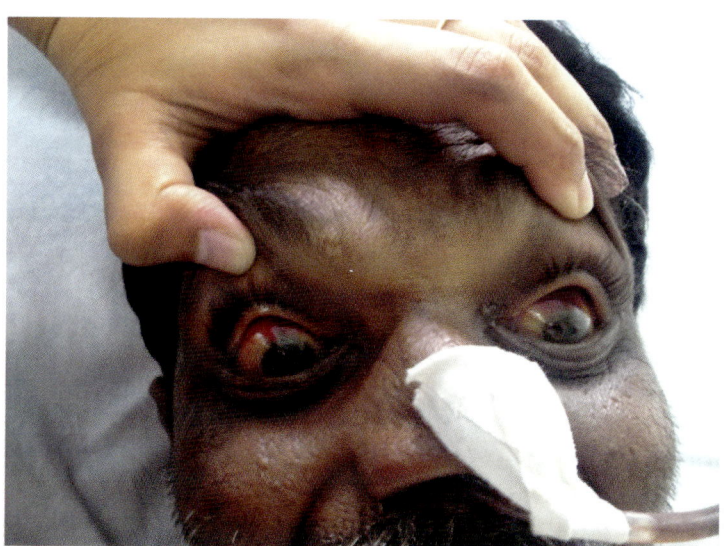

Quiz 1

What are the various possibilities?

Leptospirosis to be considered first particularly if associated with jaundice. Other conditions to be considered inclede:

1. Dengue fever sometimes can cause these features due to thrombocytopenia
2. Other causes of thrombocytopenia also must be considered, if these are ruled out-ITP,
3. Acute leukemias can rarely present with subconjunctival haemorrhage and so can bone marrow suppression.

Quiz 2

What is leptospirosis?

A zoonosis spread by contamination of water with infected rat's urine—organisms entering the body through breaches in skin, mucosa, conjunctiva.

Quiz 3

What are the synonyms of leptospirosis?

Synonyms: Weil's syndrome, canicola fever, canefield fever, 7-day fever, rat catcher's yellows, pretibial fever, black jaundice, Fort Bragg fever.

Quiz 4

Which are the occupations prone for this zoonosis?

Farmer, vetenary doctors, anomal handlers, butchers.

Quiz 5

What are the C/F?

IP-7 to 10 days

a. *Symptoms:* Fever, myalgia, fatigue, headache, jaundice, hematuria.

b. *Signs:* Fever; muscle tenderness (calf), lymphadenopathy (axillary, cervical), hepatitis (jaundice); hemorrhages—subconjunctival, hematuria; meningitis, renal failure.

Quiz 6

What are the differential diagnosis?

a. *Hemorrhagic fevers:* Dengue, Congo cremian fever.

- *Hepatitis:* Viral (enzyme creatine phospholipase is raised in leptospirosis and not in viral hepatitis), alcoholic hepatitis.
- *Severe multisystem febrile conditions:* Typhoid fever, sevre Falciparum malaria, septicaemia, rickettseosis.

Meningitis

Lobar pneumonia mimic—pulmonary haemorrhage.

Quiz 7

What is severe form of leptospirosis known as?

Severe forms of leptospirosis is called Weil's disease/Weil's syndrome—myocarditis with hypotension, acute renal failure, altered sensorium, pulmonary hemorrhage, acute hepatic failure, coagulation failure.

Quiz 8

What are the late complications and sequellae?

Vasculits (edema, liver failure, kidney failure, uveitis), interstitial nephritis (renal failure), DIC, myocarditis, pericarditis, uveitis, meningitis.

Quiz 9

What are the drugs used in the treatment?

a. *For active disease:* Penicillins (including CP, ampicillin, amoxycillin)

   Cephalosporins: Cefataxime, ceftrioxone

b. *For cure:* Doxycycline

OBSERVATION

1. Puffiness of face—swellings around the lower portion of the eye
2. Swellings of lips
   Following multiple bee stings

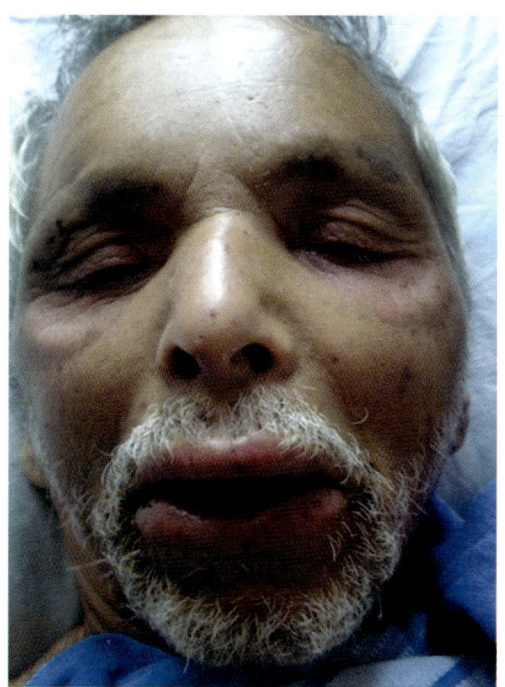

Quiz 1

What is the diagnosis?

Progressive disfiguring angioedema following multiple bee stings.

Quiz 2

What are the observations now?

1. Slight reduction in the puffiness of the face
2. Lips are involved and have started to swell

Diagnosis of progressively increasing disfiguring angioedema secondary to multiple bee stings likely.

Cases in Medicine

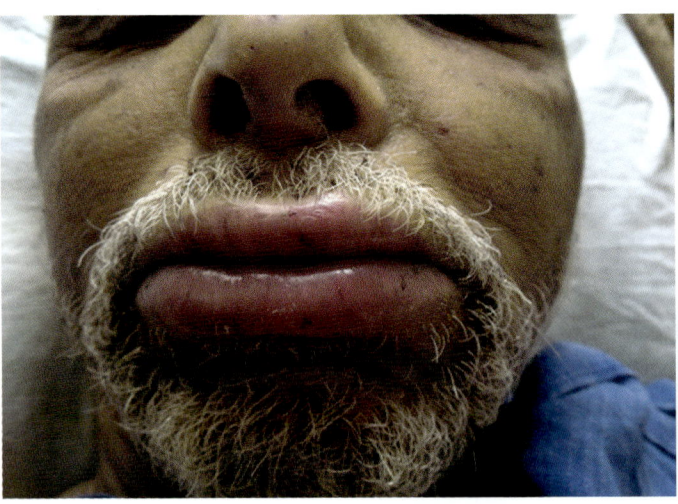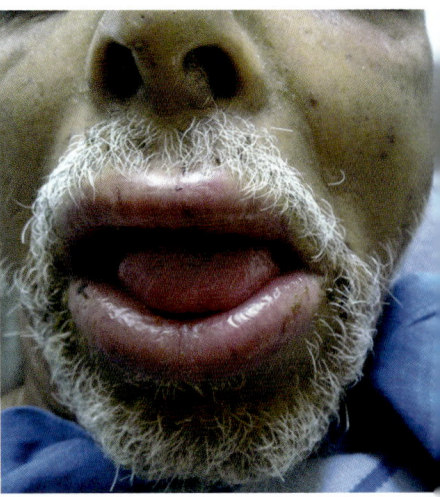

Quiz 3

What are the observations now?

1. Progressively increasing swelling of the lips.
2. Now the tongue is also involved.

There was however, no involvement of larynx (choking) and bronchi (wheezing).

Quiz 4

What are the types of hereditary disfiguring angioedema?

- Type I due to C1 esterase inhibitor deficiency (C1INH decreased levels) 85% cases.
- Type II due to inactive C1 esterase inhibitor (normal levels but decreased function of C1INH 15% cases.
- Type III due to periodic accumulation of bradykinin through alternative mechanisms—C1INH normal. May be linked to many situations—XD inheritance (females affected) pregnancy and use of hormonal contraception; mutations on factor XII gene.

Quiz 5

What are the acquired types of angioedemas?

1. *Acquired type 1*: AAE-I—linked to underlying lymphoproliferative disorder which destroy the function of C1 inhibitor. No family history
2. *Acquired type 2*: AAE-II—autoantibodies presrnt (for no apparent reason) destroy the C inhibitor.
3. *Idiopathic:* Swelling and hives persist beyond 6 weeks. Rule out thyroid dysfunction.
4. *Non-histaminergic (INAE):* Angioedema without urticaria; no relationship to infections parasites, autoimmune disorders. No response to H1 antihistaminics and CST
5. *Allergic:* Commonest form—swelling (face, lips, tongue, limbs), urticaria, hives due to external cause—bee stings (as in this patient), cold, heat, drugs, latex, etc. Throat (larynx may be involved.

   Drugs blamed include—bupropion, vaccines, SSRIs, Cox II inhibitors, antidepressants NSAIDs, statins, proton pump inhibitors.

6. *ACE inhibitor induced:* Captopril, enalapril, ramipril and others). Swelling can involve throat, lips, tongue, hands, feet, genitals, intestines. Usually no urticaria. If urticaria is present, ACE inhibitor induced angioedema is unlikely. Due to accumulation of bradykinin and hence no response to H_1 antihistamincs, H_2 antihistaminics and CST. Stopping the drug is the main treatment. Can also be seen with ARBs.

Quiz 6

What are the lab findings related to the complement system in HAE?

HAE-I: Low levels of C1 inhibitor; C4 low; C1, C3, C1q—normal

HAE-II: C1 inhibitor levels—normal/high but dysfunctional

HAE III (HAE with normal C1 inhibitor): Complement system normal

AAE-I: Low levels of C1 inhibitor and C4. C1q may be reduced

AAE-II: Similar to AAE-I

Idiopathic: Normal

INAE: Normal

Allergic: Normal

ACE Inhibitor induced: Normal

Quiz 7

What is the treatment?

1. *Hereditary type I* (HAE-I): C1 inhibitor concentrate—brand Cinryze® for prevention—IV use/ self use IM.

   Brand: Berinet for treatment—facial, laryngeal, abdominal attacks. Can be used IV/IM (self use)

   Kallikrein inhibitor: Kalbitor—SC use in patients >16 years

   Bradykinin inhibitor: Bradykinin receptor antagonist (Firazyr brand)—SC for acute attacks in patients >18 years.
2. Hereditaty type II (HAE-II) treatment similar to HAE I.
3. Hereditary angioedema with normal C1 inhibitor. Use HAE therapies
4. *Acquired type I (AAE-I):* Treat underlying lymphoproliferative disorder. Prevention of episodes by antifibrinolytics, tranexamic acid and EACA. Long term treatment—androgens.
5. Acquired HAE type II (HAE-II). Attack prevention—antifibrinolyitcs—tranexamic acid, EACA. Immunosuppressive therapy may help.
6. *Idiopathic:* Antihistamines (mainstay); DHEA; L thyroxine (for thyroid dysfunction); prednisolone
7. *Non-histaminergic (INAE):* Antifibrinolytic agents—tranexamic acid, EACA
8. *Allergic:* Avoid known allergens. Antihistamines, adrenaline injection.
9. *ACE inhibitor induced:* Stop the offending drug, CST, injection adrenaline do not help. Inhaled adrenaline may prevent complete airway closure.

Cases in Medicine

36. Clinodactyly

OBSERVATION

Curvature of the fifth finger towards the fourth finger.

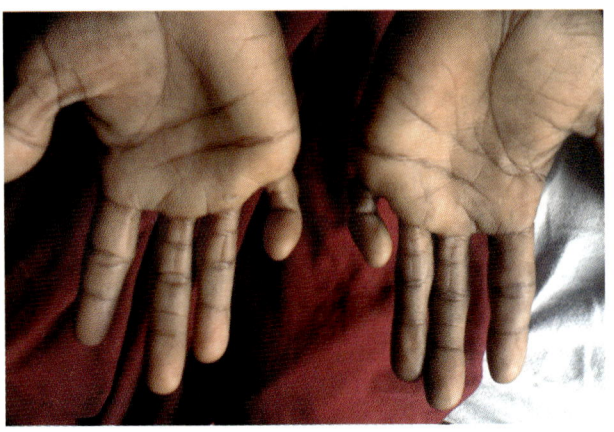

Quiz 1

What is this deformity called?
Clinodactyly or congenitally curly toes.
Can be seen in hands/toes: When syndactyly involves 3rd, 4th, 5th toes.

Quiz 2

What is the mechanism of this deformity?
Due to a radial angulation at the IP joint in the radioulnar/palmar planes of usually 5th finger.
This is because the middle phalanx of 5th finger is distinctly short and more so on the radial side (compared to the ulnar side) giving an abnormal 15 to 30° angulation for the distal phalanx.

Quiz 3

What are the conditions known to be associated with clinodactyly?
Associations include:
1. Down syndrome (80% patients)
2. Russel: Silver syndrome—Dwarfism, hypoglycemia, lack of subcutaneous fat, precocious puberty, GERD
3. *Feingold syndrome:* Microcephaly, syndactyly, short palpebral fissure, atresia of esophagus/ duodenum.
   Due to mutations in MYCN gene on the short arm of chromosome 2 (2p24.1).

Quiz 4

What is the possible inheritance pattern?

AD

Quiz 5

What is the X-ray finding?
X-ray shows brachymesophalangy of little finger.

Quiz 6

What is Char syndrome?
PDA + facial dysmorphism + curved little finger.

Quiz 7

What are short limb syndromes?
Rhizomelia: Shortening of the proximal part of the limb.
Mesomelia: Shortening of the middle part of the limb.
Acromelia: Shortening of the distal part of the limb.
Amelia: Birth defect of lacking one or more limbs.
AD inheritance
Quantitative cartilaginous defect
Advanced paternal age has a role
Pelvis: Width > Depth—"Champagne glass" appearance of the pelvic outlet
Neurologic complications
a. Due to nerve root compression
b. Due to spinal cord compression

37. Candidiasis of the Tongue

OBSERVATION

Flaky, white lesions on the tongue—oral thrush

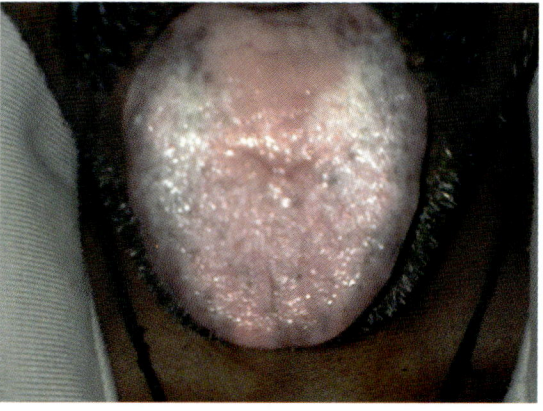

Cases in Medicine

Quiz 1

What are the various causes of discolourations of the tongue?
Differential diagnosis discoloration of the tongue
a. White tongue

b. Black hairy tongue

c. Magenta colored tongue

Quiz 2

What are the causes of white tongue?

a. *White tongue*
  1. White milky flakes. Leave bleeding surface on attempted removal.
     Seen in—AIDS, diabetes mellitus, debilitating illness, cancer, poor oral hygiene, drugs (corticosteroids, cytotoxic chemotherapy, prolonged antibiotic therapy)
     Autoimmune endocrine conditions like primary hypoparathyroidism and diabetes can be associated with it.
  2. White coated tongue may be seen in acute peritonitis
  3. Leukoplakia—white patches on tongue and oral cavity—Premalignant
  4. Hairy leukoplakia can be seen in patients with AIDS
     Geographic tongue—irregular red and white patches.

Quiz 3

What are the causes of black hairy tongue?

b. *Black hairy tongue:* Due to keratin accumulation on the elongated filiform papillae (resembling hairs) on the dorsum of the tongue.
   Black colored tongue: May be due to bismuth therapy, Addison's disease, Peutz-Jeghers syndrome

c. *Magenta colored tongue*
  1. *Roboflavin deficiency:* Magenta colored sore tongue with spreness of the angles of the mouth and the lips
  2. Scarlet/Beefy tongue in niacin def and some other B complex factor def
  3. *Scarlet fever:* Strawberry tongue—bright red tongue

Quiz 4

Where do you find a blue/bluish purple tongue?

Central cyanosis—the colour may be seen on the undersurface of tongue, lips, buccal mucosa.

Quiz 5

Where do you get a bald tongue?

Bald tongue—normal coloured tongue with loss of papillae.

Intestines also can become "bald" due to loss of villi resulting in reduced absorption.

OBSERVATION

Generalised hyperpigmentation with specifically increased pigmentation around the knuckles.

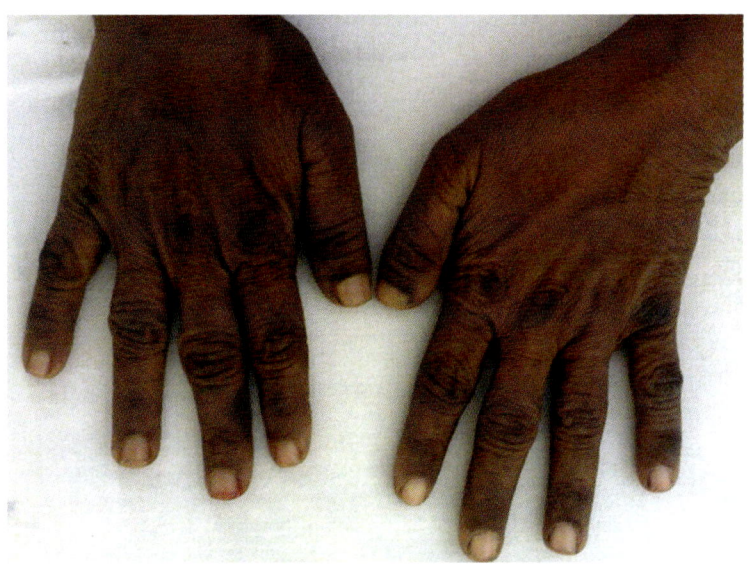

Quiz 1

What are the various mechanisms of hyperpigmentation? Give examples.

Various mechanisms of hyperpigmentation:

1. *Increased melanin:* Café au lait spots, post-inflammatory hyperpigmentation
2. *Incresed ACTH, MSH, and melanin:* Addison's disease
3. *Increaed melanocytes:* Acanthosis nigricans
4. Incresed melanin or melanocyte with sun exposure
5. *Iron deposition:* Hemochromatosis
6. *Hemosiderin deposition:* Diabetic dermopathy.

Quiz 2

What are the mechanisms of hyperpigmentation?

a. *Increased melanin:* Incresed MSH, ACTH Addison's
   Increased melanin: Café au lait spots, post-inflammatory hyperpigmentation
b. *Increased hemosiderin:* Diabetic dermopathy
c. *Increased iron deposition:* Hemochromatosis
d. *Increased melanocytes:* Acanthosis nigricans, photosensitivity

Quiz 3

What is the differential diagnosis for knuckle hyperpigmentation?
Differential diagnosis for knuckle hyperpigmentation
1. Vitamin B_{12} deficiency

Quiz 4

What are the differential diagnoses for oral, acral, nail, skin pigmentations?
a. *Peutz-Jeghers syndrome*: Polyposis coli—premalignant
b. *McCune-Albright syndrome:* Polyostotic fibrous dysplasia, Café au lait spots, precocious puberty
c. *Leopard syndrome:* Lentigenes; ECG abnormalities (BBB); ocular hypertelorism; pulmonary stenosis; abnormal genitalia; retarded growth; dearness (SN)
d. *Gardner syndrome*
e. *Cronkhite-Canada syndrome*
f. LAMB *syndrome:* Lentigenes, atrial myxomas, blue naevi. Cutaneous, cardiac, endocrine involvement. Familial myxomas seen.
g. Drug-induced hyperpigmentation
h. Friction induced
i. Heavy metal poisoning

39. Differential Diagnosis: Hyperpigmentation of Palmar Creases

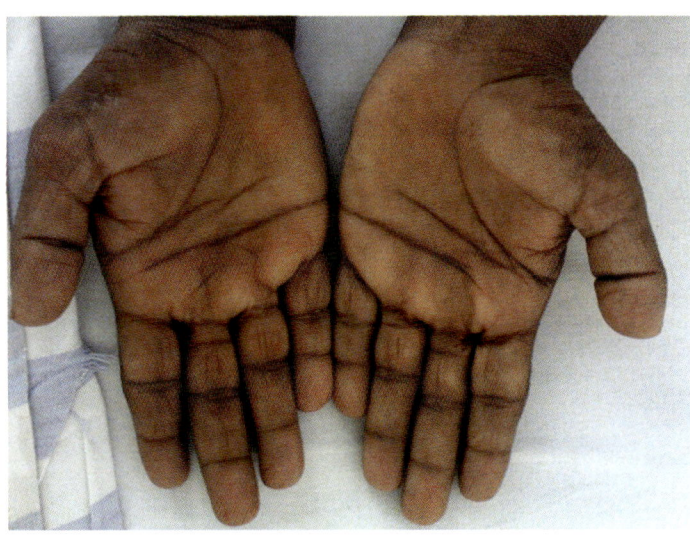

1. *Addison's disease sites:* Buccal mucosa, cheek, recent scars, nipple and areolas, genital skin. Hyperpigmentation is absent in secondary and tertiary Addison's disease.

Various presentations of Addison's disease
a. *Acute primary adrenocortical insufficiency:* Waterhouse Friedrichsen's syndrome.

b. *Chronic primary adrenocortical insufficiency:* Secondary to disseminated TB or autoimmune.

c. Secondary adrenal insufficiency due to deficiency of ACTH produced by the pituitary gland.

d. *Tertiary adrenal insufficiency:* Due to the deficiency of CRH produced by the hypothalamus.

e. *Autoimmune polyendocrine syndrome:* Addison's + type I diabetes + Hashimoto's thyroiditis with goiter + vitiligo.

f. *Schmidt syndrome:* Addison's disease with Hashimoto's thyroiditis.

Lab evidences

Hypoglycemia, hypercalcemia, hyponatremia, hyperkelemia, eosinophilia, metabolic acidosis.

40. Herpes Zoster

OBSERVATION

Multiple vesicles and erythema suggesting active infection.

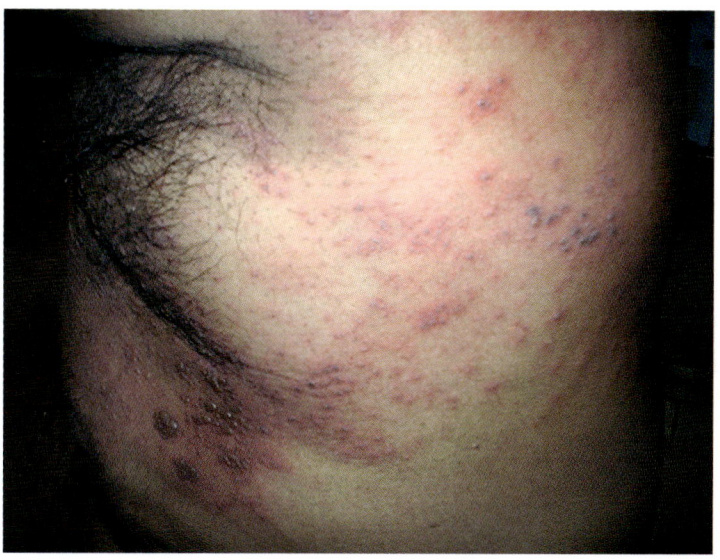

Quiz 1

What is the mechanism of herpes zoster (Hz) infection?

Reduction in the level of T cell immunity of VZV-resulting in reactivation of the virusus after chickenpox infection (which reside in the multiple sensory ganglia and establish a lifelong latency).

Quiz 2

What are the risk factors for HZ?

Risk factors, which increase with age, include:

a. Women > men

b. Whites > blacks

c. Family H/o herpes zoster (Hz)

d. Immunocompromised people with reduced T cell immunity.

Quiz 3

When do you get to see HZ in childhood?
Patients getting chickenpox *in utero* or in early infancy when the cellular immune system is not fully mature.

Quiz 4

When do you get to see severe HZ? (also increased risk of infection)
Immunocompromised patients with severe reduction in T cell immunity

a. Organ tansplants/hemopoietic stem cell transplants

b. Patients receiving immunosuppressive therapy

c. Patients with lymphoma, leukemia
   Patients having HIV infection

Quiz 5

What is post-herpetic neuralgia (PHN)?
Pain persisting after the resolution of the rash for >90 days; can persist long; can interfere with daily activities; can produce fatigue, depression, social withdrawal.

Quiz 6

In which patients do you see PHN?
10 to 50% of HZ patients particularly after the age of 50 years
Those who had severe pain at onset,
Severe rash
Large number of lesions

Quiz 7

What are the neurologic complications of HZ?

a. Bell's palsy

b. Ramsay Hunt syndrome

c. Transverse myelitis

d. Aseptic meningitis

e. Cerebral infarction (granulomatous vasculitis)

f. Cranial polyneuropathy.

Quiz 8

What are the ophthalmic complications of HZ?
HZ ophthalmicus—due to involvement of V1
Keratitis' scleritis
Uveitis

Quiz 9

What are the manifestation of HZ in immunocompromised patients?

Disseminated skin lesions

Acute/chronic outer retinal necrosis

Veruccous skin lesions

Aciclovir resistant VZV

Multiple organ involvement—lung, liver, brain, GIT—hepatis, pancreatitis

Quiz 10

What are the symptoms of HZ?

a. Prodromal—preceding the rash

   Fever + tingling/itching/pain for 2 to 3 days

b. *The rash:* Dermatomal distribution (thoracic/trigeminal/lumbar/cervical)—does not cross the midline

   Macule/papule → vesicles → pustules

   New lesions appear for 3 to 5 days

   Rash dries with crusting in 7 to 10 days

   In immunocompromised patients—rashes may disseminate and viremia and new rash appearance can last for even up to 15 days.

Quiz 11

What is zoster sine herpete?

Prodromal features not followed by rash. May lead to unnecessary anxiety and diagnostic procedures.

Quiz 12

What are the various types of pain and other sensastions associated with HZ?

Paresthesias: Burning and tingling

Dysaesthesia: Altered/painful sensitivity to touch

Allodynia: Pain associated with non-painful stimuli

Hyperaesthesia: Exaggerated/prolonged response to painful stimuli

Pruritus

Cases in Medicine

63

41. Herpes Zoster Infection

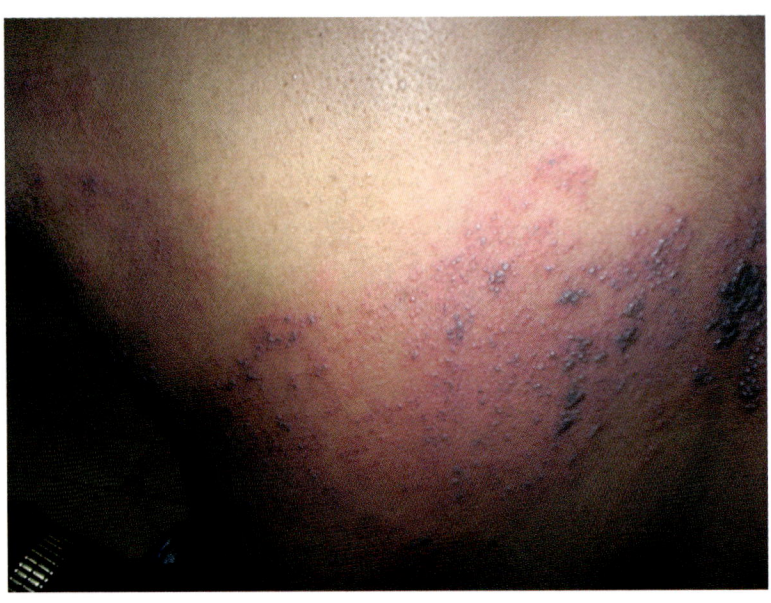

Quiz 1

What are the modalities to prove the diagnosis?

Diagnostic modalities particularly when the rashes are atypical include:

a. Direct immunofluoroscence assay—for VZV antigen—sensitivity 82%; specificity 76%.
b. PCR assay—for VZV DNA in the cells at the base of the lesions—sensitivity 95%; specificity 100%.

Quiz 2

What are the mimics of HZ infection?

a. Herpes simplex infectiuon—can recur in dermatomal distribution making an erroneous diagnosis of "recurrent herpes zoster".
b. Atypical lesions with disseminated skin lesions—specific testing for both HS and HZ may be useful.

Quiz 3

What tests are available for the diagnosis of CNS infections?

a. *CNS vasculopathy:*
   PCR of the CSF
   Titre of anti-VZV antibody in CSF > in blood

b. Visceral herpes zoster (in immunocompromised patients)—PCR assay of blood

For example, hepatitis, pancreatitis in the absence of rash

c. *Zoster sine herpete:* PCR assay for VZV in the blood/CSF.

Quiz 4

Which antiviral drugs are used for the treatment of HZ?

a. *Guanosine analogues:* Aciclovir, valacyclovir, famciclovir

Blood levels (oral bioavailability) are more in valacyclovir and famciclovir on TID dose than acyclovir for HZ; sensitivity of aciclovir % doses for HZ is less than that for HS

Indications for treatment with antiviral drugs:

- Age > 50 years
- Pain—moderate/severe
- Rash—severe
- Face/eye involvement
- Other complications of HZ
- Immunocompromised state

b. *Glucocorticoids:* Low dose prednisolone tapering doses

- May reduce time taken for complete jealing
- May reduce PHN
- Avoid in patients with DM, hypertension, peptic ulcer, osteoporosis
- Particularly useful in the management of CNS complications like—Bell's palsy, CNS vasculopathy.

c. *Pain releivers*

- NSAID
- OPIOIDs—oxycodone
- Gabapentin
- Lidocaine patches
- TCA

42. Swellings around the Neck

OBSERVATION

Two swellings—one in front of the neck and the other just above the right clavicle.

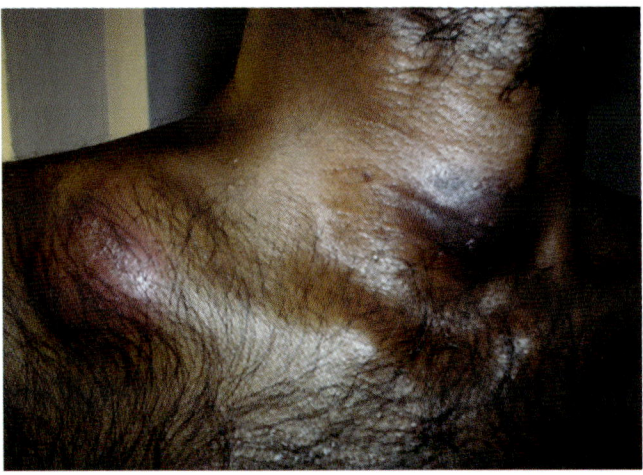

Quiz 1

What are the tissues of origin of the swellings?

Swellings are located at the known lymph node regions—lymph nodes including the delphian lymph nodes are related to the isthmus of thyroid gland; another is in the supraclavicular region.

Quiz 2

Which conditions are associated with LN enlargements in these regions?

Conditions where enlargement of these LN is seen:

a. Tuberculosis

b. HIV

How do you distinguish lymphoma—Hodgkin from non-Hodgkin?

Non-Hodgkin's lymphoma is suggested by the following findings:

1. *Facial nerve LMN involvement:* LN are situated between the 2 lobes of the parotid gland
2. CNS involvement
3. Hyperuricaemia
4. Involvement of the Waldeyer's ring—constituted by—lingual tonsil (A), lingual tonsil (P), tubal tonsil, palatine tonsil (L)
   Also notice some redness—signs of inflammation in the region of the LN.
5. Involvement of thyroid gland, parotid gland
6. Involvement of unusual lymphatic sites—Waldeyer's ring, small intestine, mesenteric and para-aortic LN, tonsils
7. Involvement of extralymphatic sites—lung, pleura, nervous system, etc.

Quiz 3

What is Marfan's law?

Healing of localized tuberculosis (e.g., cervical TB) protects against further development of pulmonary tuberculosis.

43. Massive Parotid Swelling—Pleomorphic Adenoma

OBSERVATION

Massive enlargement of the parotid gland on one side.

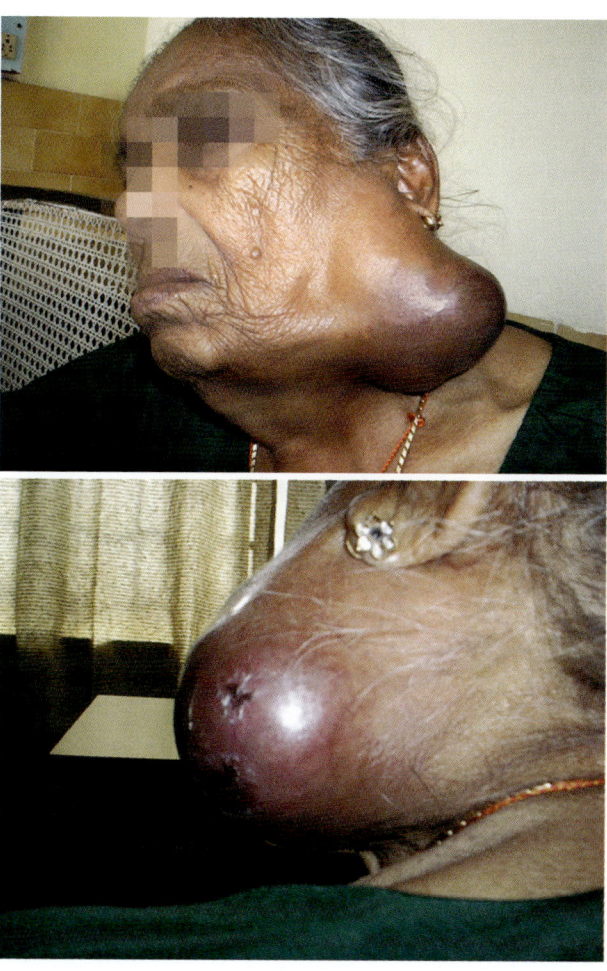

Quiz 1

How do you say it is arising from the parotid gland?

1. Location of the swelling—preauricular/retromandibular
2. Ear lobe elevated

Quiz 2

What are the causes of massive swelling arising from the parotid gland?

Causes of massive swelling arising from the parotid gland include:
• Pleomorphic adenoma.

Quiz 3

How do you suspect malignancy?

The possibility of malignancy is suspected when
1. Involvemement of the facial nerve—unilateral
2. Large fixed parotid mass
3. Skin involvement
4. LN involvement
5. Trismus

Quiz 4

What is the relation of LN to the parotid gland?

LN are situated in between the two lobes of the parotid gland.

Quiz 5

What are the sites from which the mets go to the parotid gland?

Sites from which the mets go to the partid gland:
Anterior scalp, periocular, temporal, malar regions.

44. Burr Holes

OBSERVATION

Healed scars of three burr holes, two on the left side and one on the right side.

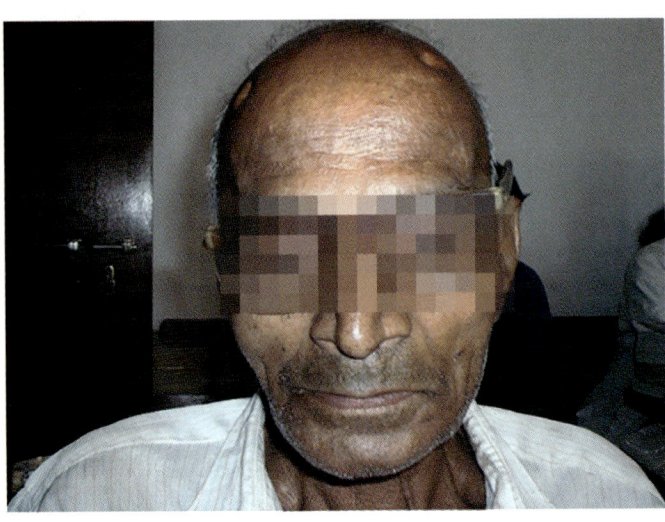

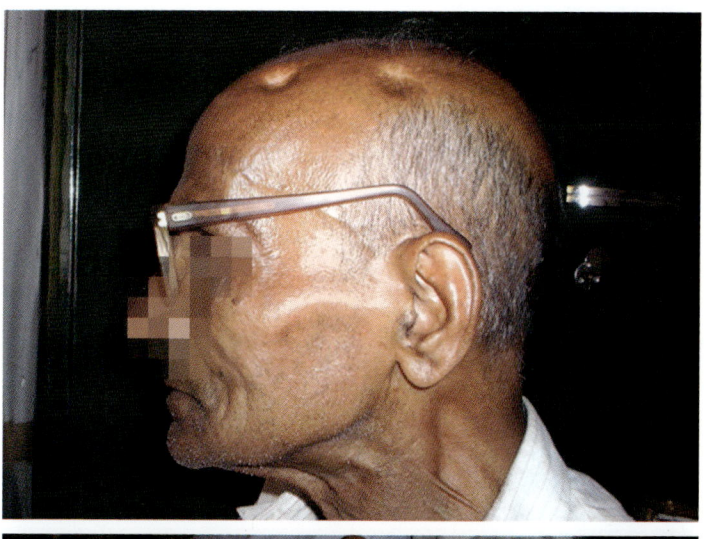

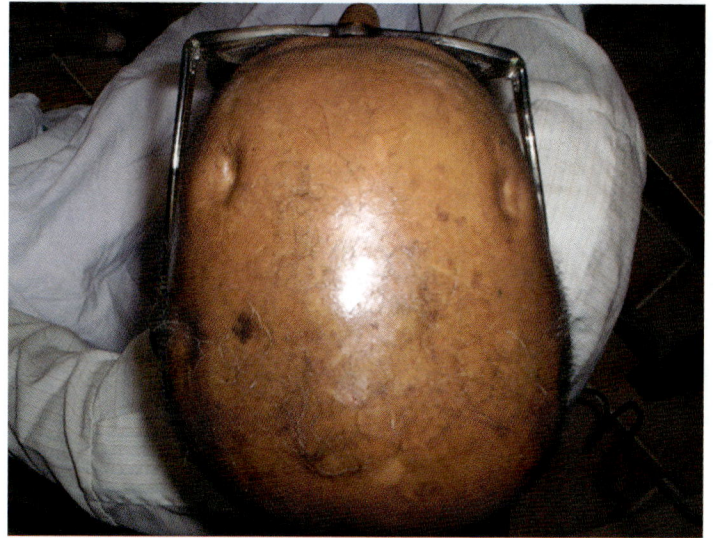

Quiz 1

What is the inference of this observation?

Before the advent of CT scan, otherwise unexplained neurologic deficit in the form of hemiplegia , particularly after trauma, when a possibility of subdural hematoma was seriously considered, burr holes were bored in the skull to let out the collected blood hence to relieve the pressure with a fond hope of reversing the neurologic deficit—a procedure known as trephining which is probably the oldest recorded surgery.

Quiz 2

What must have been the sequence of events in this patient?

This person must have had a right sided hemiplegia and therefore the burr holes were first trephined on the left side. Obviously the result must have been negative and therefore you also find burr hole on the right side which must have been done subsequently—a phenomenon of contrecoup injury can explain this (which must have been suspected). However, you find only 1 burr hole on the right side explaining the possibility of the clot being found and evacuated from there which must have made the surgeon feel that there is no need for another burr hole. Clot found, evacuated, the patient must have fully recovered, In fact, when he used to consult me he was neurologically fit and fine.

45. Single Palmar Crease on the Right Side

OBSERVATION

The palm of the right hand has only one single palmar crease instead of two creases as seen on the palm of the left hand of the same patient.

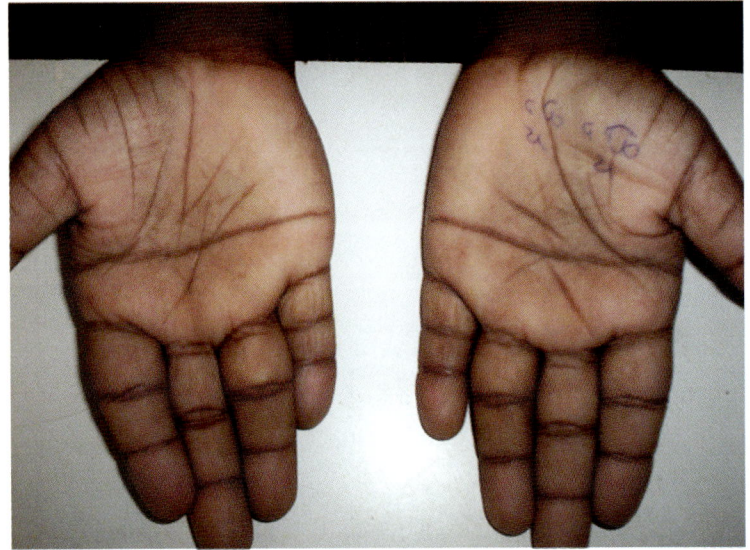

Quiz 1

What is such a palmar crease called?
Simian crease

Quiz 2

What are the conditions in which a Simian crease is found?
- Normal people (up to 1 in 30);
- Down syndrome (trisomy 21);
- Aarskog-Scott syndrome (XR);
- Fetal alcohol syndrome;
- Cri du chat syndrome (chromosome 5);

- Kleinefelter syndrome;
- Noonan's syndrome (chromosome 12);
- Patau syndrome (chromosome 13);
- Edward's syndrome (chromosome 18).

Quiz 3

What is Sydney line?

When the proximal transverse crease extends beyond the midline axis of the 5th finger towards the ulnar border of the palm.

Quiz 4

Which are the conditions where the Sydney line is seen?

- Down syndrome
- Congenital rubella
- Acute leukaemia
- Alzheimer's (some cases)
- Psychological disordes including schizophenia.

46. Flushing of Face

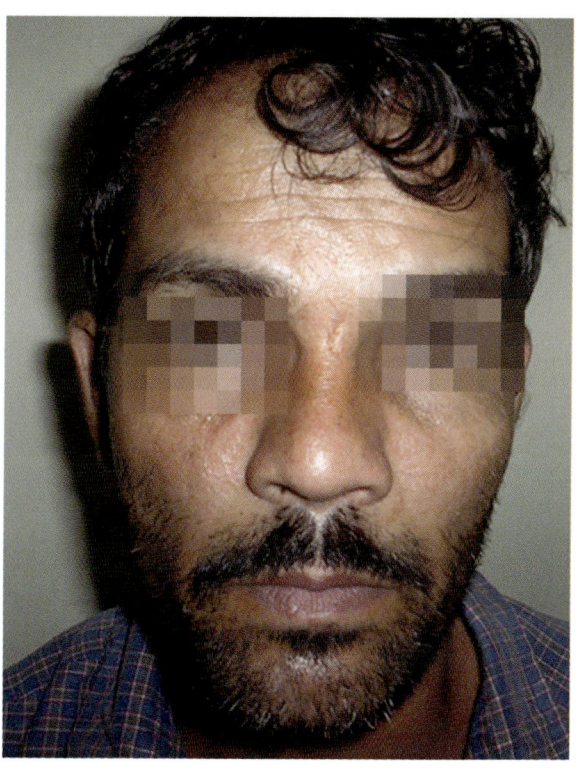

47. Flushing of Face and Upper Body

OBSERVATION

Flushing of face

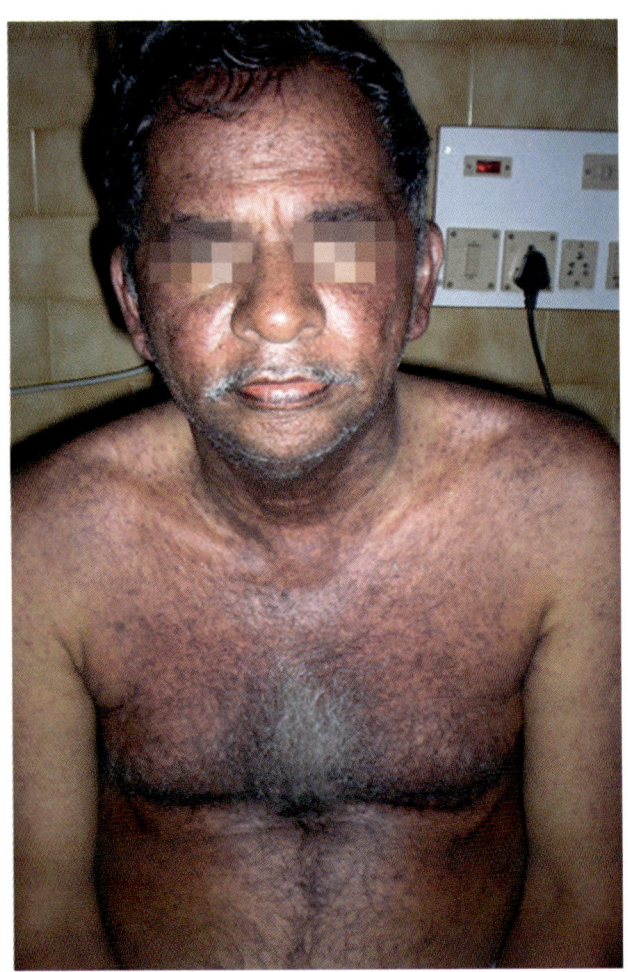

Quiz 1

What are the causes of flushing of the face?

Flushing of face is visible redness of face accompanied by warmth

The causes include:

a. Fever
b. Alcohol
c. Benign cutaneous flushing
d. Menopause

Cases in Medicine

e. Carcinoid
f. Pheochromocytoma
g. Mastocytosis
h. Anaphylaxis
i. Medullary carcinoma thyroid
j. Pancreatic cell tumor (VIPoma)
k. Renal cell carcinoma
l. Neurologic causes
m. Drugs
n. Rare causes

Quiz 2

What are the causes and mechanisms involved in flushing?

a. Fever-associated with increased temperature and sweating (on NSAIDs)

b. Alcohol
   1. Due to the main metabolite (acetaldehyde) which is a very potent vasodilator
   2. Alcohol dehydrogenase 2 is the enzyme that metabolises aldehyde. There can be a congenital or acquired deficiency of this enzyme resulting in the build up of acetaldehyde resulting in vasodilatation.
      - *Congenital deficiency:* In Asian people
      - *Acquired deficiency:* In Hodgkin's lymphoma, hypereosinophilic syndrome. Drug induced (with alcohol): Disulfiram; chlorpropamide; metronidazol.
        Local application of tacrolymus (on face) for acne/rosacea

c. *Benign cutaneous flushing:* Increased temperature (other than fever); emotional disturbance, exercise. May mimic idiopathic anaphylaxis, carcinoid, mastocytosis spicy capsaicin-foods in red pepper.
   Monosodium glutamate—facial flushing, constriction in the chest—"Chinese restaurant syndrome".
   Nitrites: Flushing + headache
   Sulfites (potassium metabisulfite): Flushing + wheezing
   Gustatory flushing: Flushing, salivation, sweating, nasal secretion
   Histamine fish poisoning—flushing, tachycardia, urticaria, palpitations—mimics allergy and responds to antihistamincs
   Ciguatoxin (of ciguatera fish poisoning): Flushing +vomiting, diarrhea, abdominal pain, pruritus, dysaesthesias (of tongue, teeth and gingival) myalgia, weakness, ataxia. This self limiting syndrome may last for years. Toxin is not destroyed by cooking.

d. *Menopause:* Mechanisms
   Estrogen deficiency—responds to HRT
   Role for alpha adrenergic pathways—clonidine (alpha 2 blockers help)
   Role for opioid pathways—naloxone helps

e. *Carcinoid:* Flushing, cramps, diarrhea, right sideded cardiac valvular lesions, bronchospasm. carcinoid syndrome is seen in 10% cases of carcinoid tumor (containing malignant enterochromaffin/Kulchitsky cells derived from neuroendocrine lineage.

CS associated with GI tumores—colon appendix, rectum

Non-GI tumors—ovarian teratoma, glomus jugulare tumor, thyroid tumors

Females: Lung and stomach; males: Small intestine and rectum

Mechanism of flushing in CS

Food triggers via gut hormone release foods—sherry, beer, fermented foods

Drug triggers—NE, E, dopamine—blocked by alpha blockers, pentagastrin, isoprenaline but NOT by beta blockers

Any stimuli increasing adrenergic activity—pain, anger, exertion, excitement

Likelyhood of flushing depends on vasoactive mediators—serotonin (5HT), kallikrein, prostaglandin and others extent of liver mets (substances derived from liver mets not inactivated by liver)

Diagnosis—5HIAA in urine, serum chromatogranin A, neuron specific enolase

Treatment: Octreotide, lantreotide (long acting form of octreotide), combination of H1 and H2 receptor blockers; ketanserin (5HT antagonist).

Surgical options: Total ablation (when feasible), tumor load reduction (partial hepatectomy), interferon alpha.

f. *Pheochromocytoma:* Chromaffin tumor from chromaffin cells of adrenal medulla. Chromaffin cells produce, store and release catecholamin paroxysms of palpitations, pressure (BP) increase, perspiration, pain in the chest and head, precipitated by powerful (deep) palpation of the abdomen, pallor/flushing.

Mechanism of facial flushing induced by pheohromocytoma

Less responsiveness of facial vessels to VC (E) resulting in overall increase in VD > VC

Other mediators: Calcitonin gene related peptide, VIP, adrenomedullin

Diagnosis—by measuring urinary levels of fractionated metanephrines (NE/E) and their metabolites

CT abdomen and pelvis for abdominal pheochromocytoma; abdominal aortography, nuclear scintigraphy using radioactive iodine for extra-abdominal pheochromocytoma

Preparation for surgery—alpha blockers first and then beta blockers when the alpha blockade is complete (unopposed beta blockade may lead to paradoxical increase in BP)

g. *Mastocytosis:* Flushing with hypotension, abdominal cramps, fatigue, nalaise.

Due to tissue unfiltration by the mast cells. Children > adults. Darier sign—pruritus on stroking the skin (children)

TMEP (telangiectasia muscularis eruptive perstans (adults) bone marrow and splenic involvement in adults;

Mechanism of flushing—histamine, prostaglandin D2, TNF alpha, vascular growth factors; any agent capable of precipitating anaphylaxis can produce these effects

Co-existing allergy—life threatening combination

Osteoporosis—common

Diagnosis: Flushing + hypotension + anaphylaxis + urticaria pigmentosa

Diagnosis proved by estimation of incereased urinary excretion of histamine, PG D2 metabolites (1, 4 methylimidazole acetic acid—metabolite of histamine)

Serum tryptas—normal in localized mastocytosis; elevated in systemic mastocytosis

Histopath analysis—presence of large number of mast cells + molecular diagnosis by detection of mutations in C KIT gene (CD 117)

Types of mastocytosis:

- Type I: (a) Indolent disease; (b) Indolent disease with systemic disease
- Type II: Mastocytosis + hematological disorder—myeloproliferative disease/myelodysplasia
- Type III: Lymphadenopathic mastocytosis + eosinophilia
- Type IV: Mast cell leukemia

Special points:

In adults—bone marrow involvement in 90%

Disappearance of the persistent skin lesions is associated with visceral spread

Treatment: Currently no cure

Features can be reversed by epinephrine IV

Combined H1 and H2 blockade

Others: Cromolyn, oral steroids

Localosed disease in adults—PUVA for urticaria pigmentosa, LASER for TMEP

Systemic disease: Imatinib—c-kit tyrosine kinase inhibitor

h. *Anaphylaxis:* Flushing + urticaria + hypotension + pulmonary symptoms + GI symptoms (due to IgE mediated anaphylaxis); angioedema (due to C1 esterase inhibitor deficiency)

Differential diagnosis histamine induced symptoms—CS, mastocytosis, anaphylaxis.

Elevated histamine and serum tryptase levels in anaphylaxis and mastocytosis during attacks; Serum tryptase levels are elevated inbetween attacks only in mastocytosis.

Treatment—epinephrine IV/IM 0.3 to 0.5 mg; CST (systemic) to prevent relapse

i. Medullary carcinoma thyroid: Malignant tumor of parafollicular cells protracted flushing of faced and extrimities. Cells are derived from the neural crest and they secrete calcitonin, histamine, PG, substance P, etc.

Flushing + sweating

Inheritance—sporadic/AD (MEN-MCT, pheo, hyper PTH)—mutations in RET proto-oncogene

Diagnosis—serum calcitonin levels (radioimmune assay after IV calcitonin and pentagastrin—more sensitive).

Treatment:

For MCT—total thyroidectomy + LN removal from the central zone

Pheochromocytoma (if coexists)—should be removed before thyroidectomy

j. Pancreatic islet cell tumor (Vipoma)

Verner-Morrison syndrome: WDHA—watery diarrhea, hypokelemia, alkalosis

Derived from non-beta cells with neuroendocrine lineage associated with MEN-secrete VIP, GIP, PG, PP.

C/F-WDHA + flushing (rare) + IGT (50%) + abdominal cramps

Diagnosis—high plasma VIP level + stool volume > 1 litre/day

Abdominal US, CT, autography—to localize the disease and mets

Treatment: Surgery

Medical: 5 FU, streptozocin—to reduce tumor mass and reduce stool volume

k. Renal cell carcinoma

Classic triad (10%): Hematuria, flank pain, abdominal mass

Mechanism of flushing—PGs, pituitary down regulation of gonadotrophin secretion

l. *Neurologic disease*

   Causes: Parkinsonism, dysautonomia, orthostatic hypotension, migraines, MS, epilepsy, brain tumors, spinal cord lesions that produce autonomic hyperreflexia.

   1. Damage to V nerve → antodromic sensory neural flushing;
   2. "Facial migraine"—episodic flushing, facial neuralgia, lacrimation
   3. "Horner's syndrome"—triad of ptosis, meiosis, anhydrosis + contralateral flushing (unaffected side)—due to sympathetic vasodilatation (reduced sympathetic activity on the side of Horner's syndrome causes vasoconstriction on that side)
   4. Frey's syndrome—auriculotemporal flushing—unilateral flushing + heat + sweating due to misdirected regeneration od PS fibers after injury to the parotid gland in adults.
   5. Diencephalic epilepsy (autonomic epilepsy) can present with seizures, loss of consciousness + paroxysmal flushing, tachycardia, hypertension, dilated pupils. Probably due to acutely dilated ventricles.

      Treatment: Flushing-clonidine; seizures-carbamazepine.
   6. Autonomic hyperrelexia—triad of flushing + headache + sweating. Also seen in hypertension/postural hypotension, painful flexor spasms of extrimities, hyperreflexia. Seen in transverse spinal cord lesions (85%) and severe spinal cord injuries at the thoracic level and lesions at the cervical and thoracic levels.
   7. Flushing is due to neurogenic hypertension which activates the vasomotor reflexes via the pressor receptors in the carotid sinus, aortic arch and cerebral vessels.
   8. Streeten syndrome—orthostatic hypotension itself can cause flushing due to hyper-bradykininism;

      Flushung and hypotension are prominent in recumbent position; purple discoloration of legs in upright position.

m. *Drugs*

   1. Vasodilators: Nitroglycerine, sildenafil
   2. Calcium channel blockers: Nifedipine, verapamil
   3. Vancomycin
   4. Contrast media
   5. Industrial solvents combined with alcohol: Trichloroethylene vapor; butyraldoxime (printing)
   6. Medications combined with alcohol—flushing + light headedness + dizziness

      Disulfiram, fungus caprinus atramentarius (disulfiram like substance), chlorpropamide, metronidazol, ketokonazole, griseofulvin, tacrolimus (topical)

      OHA related—flushing starts in 3 to 10 mins after alcohol and reaches maximum intensity in 15 mins, lasts for 1 hour. No hypertension, hypotension, diarrhea, syncope.

      Tacrolimus induced flushing may be inhibited by aspirin.

n. *Rare causes*

   1. Sarcoidosis—lupus pernio overlying a dilated vessel
   2. Mitral stenosis—flushing + cyanosis
   3. "Dumping syndrome" following gastrectomy after ingestion of foods containing hypertonic glucose
   4. Androgen deficiency—after orchidectomy
   5. POEMS syndrome—polyneuropathy, organomegaly, endocrinopathy, monoclonal proteins, skin changes.

6. Basophilic histiocytic leukaemia (via histamine) flushing + urticaria + pruritus.
7. Leigh's syndrome-subacute necrotizing encephalomyelopathy—due to elevated endorphin levels in CSF.
8. Rovsing syndrome—flushing + nausea in patients with polycystic kidney relieved by anti-flexed position.
9. Homocystinuria.

48. Horner's Syndrome

OBSERVATION

1. Ptosis: Unilateral—left side due to loss of innervations to superior tarsal muscle/Müller's muscle
2. Meiosis: Smaller (constricted) pupil on the same side
3. Anhidrosis

These 3 features form the main triad.
Other features include:
4. Enophthalmos
5. Loss of ciliospinal reflex
6. Blood shot conjunctiva
7. Sometimes there can be inverted ptosis—lower eyelid going up

Syndromes where Horner's syndrome forms a component
1. Lateral medullary syndrome
2. Mackenzie syndrome: Retroparotid space tumor = IX, X, XI, XII + Horner's syndrome.

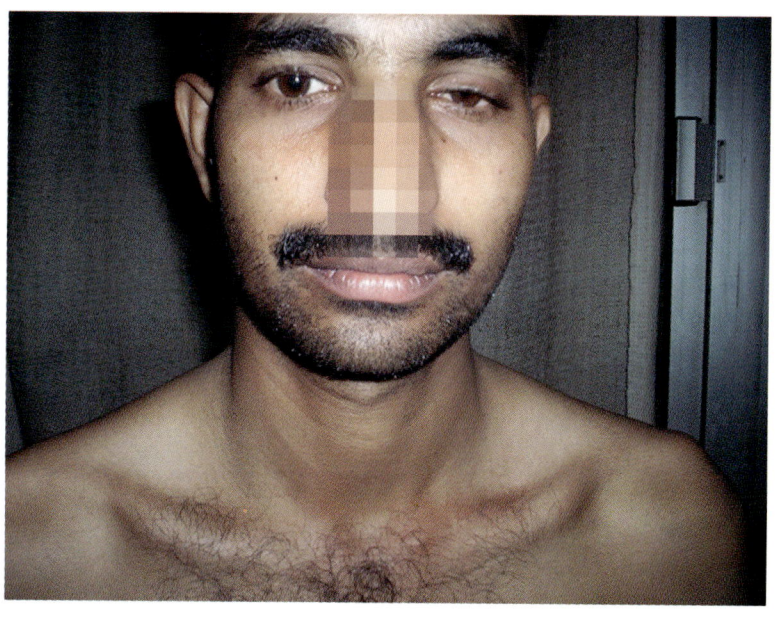

3. Wallenberg syndrome
4. Pancoast tumor: Malignant tumor of the superior fissure in the apex of the lung

What is Horner's syndrome?

A classic triad of ptosis, meiosis, anhydrosis due to interruption of the sympathetic supply.
Pharmacologic tests to localize the lesion in Horner's syndrome.

1. Cocaine drops fail to dilate the pupil as is normally expected (by preventing the reuptake of neurotransmitter NE)
2. If amphetamine dilates the pupil (as expected, the lesion can be localized in the 3rd order neurons (representing the phenomenon of denervation hypersensitivity). Failure to dilate the pupil localizes the lesion to 1st or 2nd order neurons.

Differential diagnosis: Unilateral ptosis + pupillary involvement

1. Unilateral ptosis + eyeball looks down and out (weak and restricted adduction + vertical eye movements) on an attempt to look straight ahead (revealed better on elevation of the ptosis eyelid) + pupil diated and fixed not reacting to light = 3rd nerve (oculomotor nerve) lesion.
2. Similar to 1 + papillary sparing + small vessel disease due to diabetes/hypertension.
3. Ptosis + constricted pupil + normal reaction to light + full range of extraocular movements.

Attempting to localize the lesion with associated features:
Basically localization becomes difficult due to long and tortuous course of the sympathetic.

1. Loss of corneal reflex on the same side = Orbital/Retro-orbital lesion
2. Weakness of muscles + loss of reflexes in the ipsilateral arm = Avulsion injury to brachial plexus/Pancoast tumor of the apex of the lung.
3. Pain and temperature lost on the face on the same side and on the body on the opposite side = Brainstem lesion.

Related Syndrome

1. Heterochromia—due to lack of sympathetic stimulation, melanin pigmentation of the melanocytes in the superficial stroma of iris seen in long standing Horner's syndrome.
2. Harlequin syndrome—asymmetric flushing on the upper thorax, neck and face due to lesion to the sympathetic nerves.
   Harlequin sign—unilateral sweating and flushing due to exposure to heat/on strenuous exertion.
   Syndrome so named because of the resemblance of the half flushed faces to the colorful Harlequin masks.

49. Ecchymotic Patch Seen on the Right Foot with Evidence of Active and Recent Bleeding on the Right Leg

OBSERVATION

Clinical picture suggestive of coagulation problem.

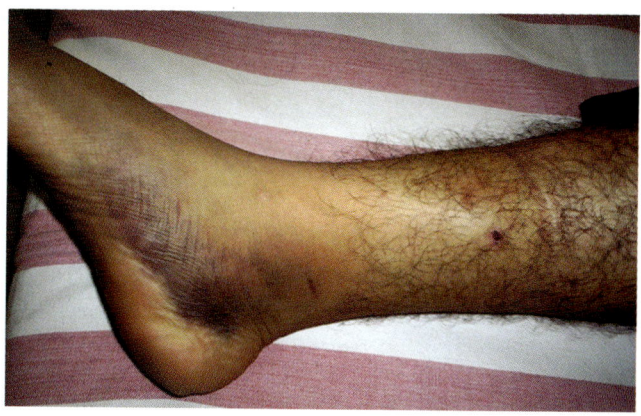

Quiz 1

What are the examples of acquired coagulation disorders?

Examples of acquired coagulation problems

1. Acute liver failure: Loss of synthesis of protein faction synthesized by the liver' coagulopathy-exacerbated by thrombocytopenia.
2. Anticoagulant overdose/toxicity.
3. DIC: Pathological stimulus to coagulation (sepsis) diffuse intravascular coagulation, deficiency (due to excessive consumption) of coagulation factors, platelets and stimulated fibrinolysis resulting in bleeding.
4. Vit K deficiency—coagulation failure due to deficiency of gamma carboxylate factors II, VII, IX, X.
5. Renal diseases.
6. Special situations—pregnancy, newborn.
7. DIC

Quiz 2

What are the various mechanisms?

a. *Liver disease*

   1. Reduced synthesis of coagulation, fibrinolytic, and coagulation inhibitory proteins.
   2. Impaired clearance of activated hemostatic components

b. *Vitamin K deficiency*

   Factors II, VII, IX, X require vit K for post-translational modification (activation). Deficiency of Vit K or the presence of antagonists of Vit K interfere with the activation (carboxylation) of these coagulation factors and proteins C and S. Deficiency results in prolonged PT, APTT.

Vitamin K itself is stored in the liver and the stores get depleted in 2–3 days if storage is interfred with.

c. Warfarin because of its structural similarity to Vit K can act as an anticoagulant. Warfarin therapy is monitored by PT INR. Warfarin overdose can produce similar changes.

d. *Renal diseases*

Multifactorial:

1. Thrombocytopenia
2. Associated Vit K deficiency—due to associated malnutrition and hepatic disorders
3. Loss in urine of factors IX and XII in nephrotic syndrome

These patients can have prolonged PT, prolonged APTT, thrombocytopenia, anaemia, prplonged BT.

e. *DIC:* Multifactorial

Characterised by extensive generalized hemorrhage/microvascular thrombosis-Multisystem organ dysfunction + limb necrosis

Triggers: Systemic inflammation—extrinsic coagulation pathway, IL 6. Causes include medical (inflammation, shock, infection, hemolysis); Surgical (trauma, fractures, vascular abnormalities); obstretic (amniotic fluid embolism)

Lab findings include: Prolonged PT, prolonged aPTT, increased D dimer, increased FDP, thrombocytopenias.

f. *Immunoglobulin mediated factor deficeincy*

1. Acquired factor VIII deficiency—bleeding following minor trauma + prolonged aPTT + normal PT can be idiopathic (50%), associated with SLE and other autoimmune disorders, lymphoid tumors, malignancies, penicillin treatment postpartum state.

   Treatment: DDAVP (mild bleeds); favtor VIII/VIIa concentrates (severe bleeds); immuno-suppressive therapy, immunoglobulin, rituximab

2. Other acquired coagulation factor deficiencies
   - Hemodilution—massive transfusion
   - Heparin therapy
   - Plasma cell dyscrasias
   - Hyperfibrinolysis due to thrombolytic treatments, liver diseases, cardiopulmonary bypass, malignancy
   - Snake venoms due to bite by venomous snakes.

Quiz 3

What are prothrombotic coagulation disorders?

1. *HIT:* Heparin induced thrombocytopenia—due to IgG antibodies *vs* platelet factor 4 and heparin. Clinical features start in 5 to 10 days

   C/F venous thrombosis: DVT, PE

   Arterial thrombosis: Stroke, AMI, limb thrombosis

   Adenocarcinoma associated chronic DIC—large vesssels involved. *Tretment*: Heparin.

   APLA: Due to antibodies to beta 2 glycoproteins, prothrombin.

   C/F: Intermittent thrombosis. May be due to lupus anticoagulant, anti-cardiolipin antibody

   Treatment: Need for long-term anticoagulant.

Quiz 4

What are the other conditions associated with microvascular thrombosis?

TTP, coumarin induced venous limb necrosis and gangrene, coumarin induced skin necrosis, purpura fulminans.

Quiz 5

What are the questions asked to evaluate the patient?

In such a patient, ask for and look for—past history of bleeds, joint bleeds, postsurgical bleeds, excessive bleeding following dental extraction and during the menstruation.

Look for bleeding at other sites—cannula sites, site of drawing blood, trauma, joint bleeds, intramuscular hematomas. Look for tachycardia, hypotension, shock.

Quiz 6

How do you clinically assess blood loss at the bedside?

"Tilt sign" positive, if substantial blood loss has been there.

Quiz 7

What does the preliminary lab screening involved?

Platelet count

P. smear

PT

aPTT

TCT: Thrombin clotting time

FDPs: Fibrin degradation products

D Dimer: Cross linked fibrin assay

Protamine sulfate paracoagulation assay

Assessment of fibrinogen

BT: Now sparingly used

CBC + PS

In patients with predisposition to thrombosis—look for natural anticoagulants—antithrombin III, protein C, protein S.

Quiz 8

What are the substances used in the control of bleeding?

a. Platelets

b. FFP

c. Vit K—For post-translational modification of factors II, VII, IX, X, protein C and protein S

d. Cryoprecipitate—for the treatment of hypofibrinogenemia

e. Specific factor concentrates used in specific deficiencies VII, IX, VIIa

f. Antifibrinolytic agents—EACA, tranexamic acid

g. Desmopressin—increases factor VIII and von Willebrand factor.

50. Bilateral Exophthalmos

OBSERVATION

1. Prominent, bilateral, symmetrical protruding eyeballs with lid retraction. A clear rim of sclera is seen all-round the cornea—exophthalmos.
2. Observe the goiter.

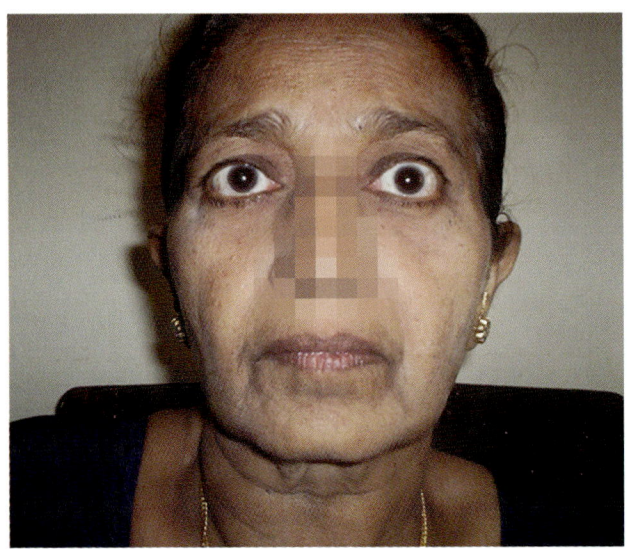

Quiz 1

What is the most probable diagnosis?
The most probable diagnosis is thyrotoxicosis.

Quiz 2

What are the mechanisms of exophthalmos?
Mechanism of exophthalmos:
1. Enlargement of the muscles
2. Increased fat within the orbit
3. Mucopolysaccharide infiltration

Quiz 3

What are the cardinal signs of Graves' disease?
The cardinal signs of Graves' disease include:
1. Diffuse goiter with a bruit
2. Pretibial myxoedema with thyroid acropachy—edema of the nail folds mimicking clubbing
3. Bounding pulse with tachycardia
4. Lid lag, chemosis, periorbital puffiness, ophthalmoplegia, papilloedema.

Quiz 4

What are the eponyms for Graves' disease.

1. Basedow's disease
2. Flajani's disease
3. Flajani-Basedow syndrome
4. Marsh's disease
5. Parry's disease

Quiz 5

What is apathetic thyrotoxicosis?

Apathetic/masked thyrotoxicosis is a state of thyrotoxicosis mainly characterised by
1. Absent eye signs
2. Presence of—atrial fibrillation, heart failure, weight loss.

51. Goiter

OBSERVATION

Note an asymmetric enlargement of the thyroid—goiter with a nodule seen on the left side.

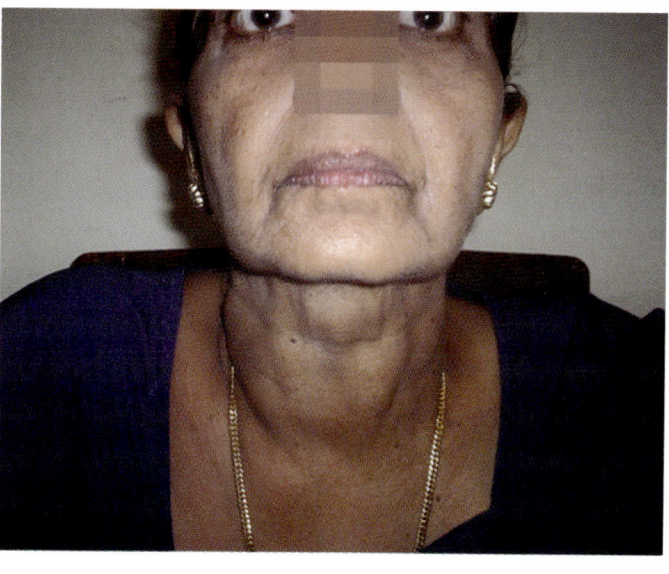

Quiz 1

What is the approach to a patient with goiter?

1. Age and sex: Men—older age; women—younger age
2. Symptoms
    • Swelling in front of the neck
    • Cough; coughing out blood

- Hoarseness—involvement of the recurrent laryngeal nerve
- Breathlessness
- Bone pain—secondaries
- Weight loss, heat intolerance, sweating, tremors, insomnia, diarrhea, = hyperthyroid
- Weight gain, cold intolerance, constipation, depression, muscle cramps.
- Higher risk of cancer if: History of radiation during childhood, family history of thyroid cancer/colon polyp/parathyroid or adrenal tumors.
- Thyroid is examined initially from behind with the patient sitting on the stool and the doctor standing.

3. *Signs*

Inspection
- Swelling-infront of the neck
- Movement with deglutition—goiter moves with deglutition; Thyroglossal cyst moves with protrusion of the tongue.

Palpation
- Surface-nodularity—nodules (solitary/multinodular), consistency (hard/cystic), is it fixed?
- LN, carotid pulsations (Berry's sign—inability to palpate the carotid pulsations due to malignant infiltration of the carotid sheath), position of trachea, can you get below the swelling?

Percussion
- Dull note over the sternum + inability to get under the swelling = Retrosternal extension

Auscultation
- For bruit over the thyroid—in toxic goiter.

Quiz 2

What is the importance of systemic examination in a patient with goiter?

Pulse: Irregular (atrial fibrillation)—toxic goiter; bradycardia—hypothyroid

Hands: Dry, cool carpal tunnel syndrome = Hypothyroid

Sweaty, tremors + tremors + thyroid acropachy = Hyperthyroidism

Face: Madarosis (loss of lateral 1/3 of eyebrows), xanthelasma, arcus, puffy face, thinning of hair (women) = Hypothyroid

Exophthalmos, lid lag, ophthalmoplegia = Thyrotoxicosis

CNS: Reflexes—Brisk in hyperthyroid/delayed relaxation in hypothyroid (pseudomyotonic reflexes)

Pseudomyotonic reflexes

Thyrotoxic myopathy: Weakness of muscles involving the limbs and trunk speech and swallowing.

52. Anatomical Snuffbox

OBSERVATION

An anatomic space at the base of the thumb.

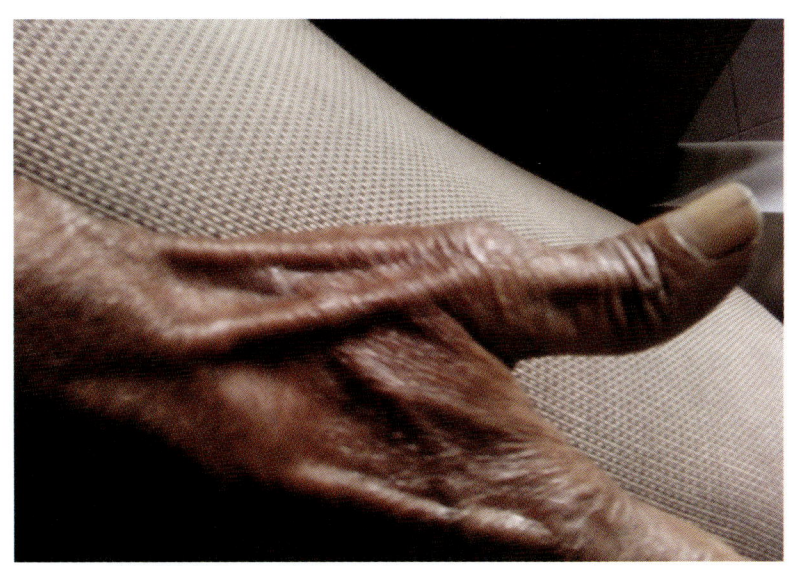

Quiz 1

Why is it called so?

That is the space where the snuff (sniffing tobacco) used to be kept before sniffing. Hence the name.

Quiz 2

What are the boundaries?

Boundaries:
Anterior: Abductor pollicis longus, extensor pollicis brevis
Posterior: Extensor pollicis longus
Proximal: Styloid process—radius
Distal: Apex of the isosceles triangle
Floor: Trapezium and scaphoid

Quiz 3

What are the contents?

- Trapezium
- Scaphoid
- Radial artery
- Cephalic vein

53. Lymphedema

OBSERVATION

Unilateral selling of the right leg which is visibly bigger than the left.

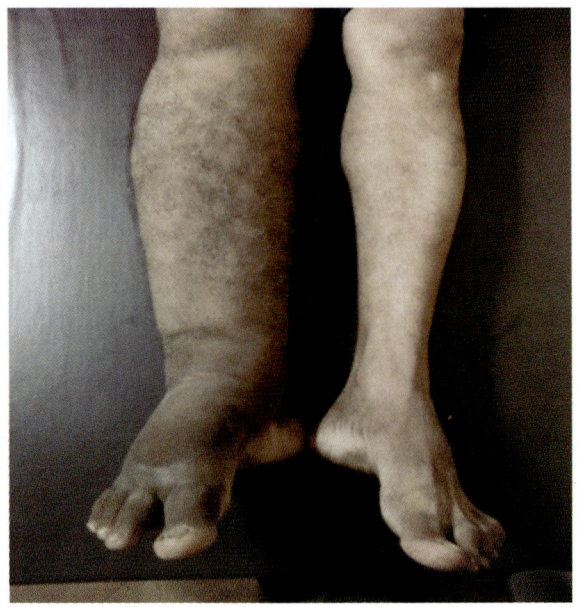

Quiz 1

What is elephantiasis?

Elephantiasis is the extreme form of lymphedema.

Quiz 2

What are the components of lymphedema?

Components:

1. Edema—non-pitting (except in very early stages).
2. Increased limb girth.
3. Thickening of skin and subcutaneous tissues.
4. Ulceration, nodules if any.
5. Usually indicates a chronic disease state.
6. Parts that can be involved—limbs, breasts, vulva, scrotum, penis.

Quiz 3

What are the causes of lymphedema?

1. Commonest cause—bilatrial—adult worm blocking the L.N.
2. Other causes—silica dust, radical dissection of LN, radiation, malignant infiltration—rarer

Quiz 4

What are the complications of elephantiasis (lymphedema)?
Complications
- Ulceration,
- Secondary infection—cellulitis, lymphangitis, lymphadenitis
- Lymphedema
- Lymphangiosarcoma: Stewart-Treves syndrome—lymphedema associated lymphangiosarcoma.
- After long standing lymphedema—0.45% after radical mastectomy.
- Retiform hemangioendothelioma—a low grade angiosarcoma.

Quiz 5

What are the features of acute lymphangitis?
Acute lymphangitis:
1. Acute attack of fever with rigors
2. Pain in the part involved—commonest-legs
3. Red streaks—inflamed lymphatics seen running on the surface of the skin with pain and itching
4. Enlarged tender regional (popliteal, inguinal, epitrochlear) LN

Quiz 6

What are the features of acute lymphadenitis?
Acute lymphadenitis:
1. Enlarged, tender regional LN
   Upper limb: Epitrochlear, axillary
   Lower limb: Popliteal, inguinal
   Breast: Axillary, cervical
   Genitalia: Inguinal, iliac
2. Features of lymphangitis may coexist

Quiz 7

Is lymphedema pitting? Why?
In the initial stages, yes, lymphedema is a pitting edema. This is because the lymph escapes out of the blocked/inflamed lymph vessel into the interstitium and being rich in proteins, attracts fluid. Hence, early lymphedema is indeed pitting.

Later stages, however, the lymphedema gets organized, produces permanent changes in the lymph vessels.

54. Exanthema and Enanthema

OBSERVATION

Exanthemata—on the skin of face, neck and chest.
Enanthemata—on the mucous membrane of lips and tongue.

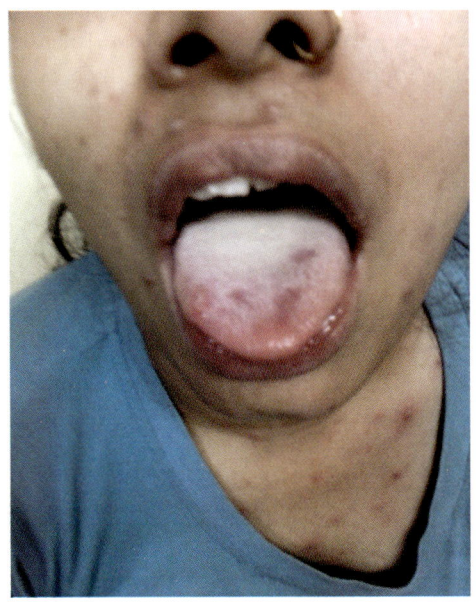

Quiz 1

What are exanthema?

Exanthema are skin eruptions as a manifestation of viral/bacterial disease.

Quiz 2

Give examples of exanthema and other skin manifestations of acute febrile illnesses?

Exanthema and other skin manifestatons of febrile illnesses:

1. *Haemorrhagic dengue:*
   Fever (biphasic) + Arthralgia + rashes (macular, maculopapular) + Petichiae with islands of sparing "white islands in the sea of red". Tourniquet test positive.
2. *Chikungunya*: Flushing erythema + joint pains + conjunctival injection + IgM positive.
3. *Scarlet fever:* Fever + pharyngitis + abdominal pain + rashes—sandpaper, pinpoint papules on erythematous background + Pastia's lines (linear petechiae) + palm and soles spared + Elevated ASO Titre and ESR.
4. *Kawasaki disease:* High fever + irritability + strawberry tongue + LN + coronary artery aneurysms + elevated ESR + thrombocytosis.
5. *Toxic shock syndrome:* Sudden fever + erythroderma (scarlatiniform rash) + hypotension + renal involvement + elevated CPK.

6. Erythema infectiosum (5th disease) parvovirus B19; slapped cheek appearance + lacy rash + Aplastic crisis (women arthritis, spontaneous abortions).
7. *Measles:* Erythematous macules later confluent, papules + Koplik's spots + leukopenia + low ESR + IgM positive.
8. *German measles:* Erythematous pinpoint maculopapular rash face and trunk + arthralgia + tender cervical LN + nasal culture of virus + antibody titres.
9. *Roseola:* Exanthema sabitum HHV 6 + pale pink macules trunk and neck, proximal limbs + leukocytosis followed by leucopenia.
10. *Infectious mononucleosis:* Fever + Malaise + polymorphic, urticarial generalized rash + LN + pinhead petechiae at the junction of soft and hard palate (Forchheimer spots) + leukocytosis + elevated atypical lymphocytes + elevated transaminases and bilirubin + serology for heterophil antibodies positive.
11. *Secondary syphilis:* Fever + pharyngitis + non-prurutic rashes + moth eaten alopecia + LN + condyloma lata + positive VDRL.
12. *Typhoid fever:* Fever + headache + rose spots + generalised erythema (erythema typhosum) + rose spot cultures Salmonella positive.

Quiz 3

What are enanthema?

Enanthema: Eruption in the mucous membrane usually associated with exanthema.

Note the enanthemata in the mucous memebrane on the inner aspect of the mouth, lips, tongue, etc.

This patient had chikenpox.

55. Exanthema on the Face and Enanthema on the Lips of the Same Patient who had Chickenpox

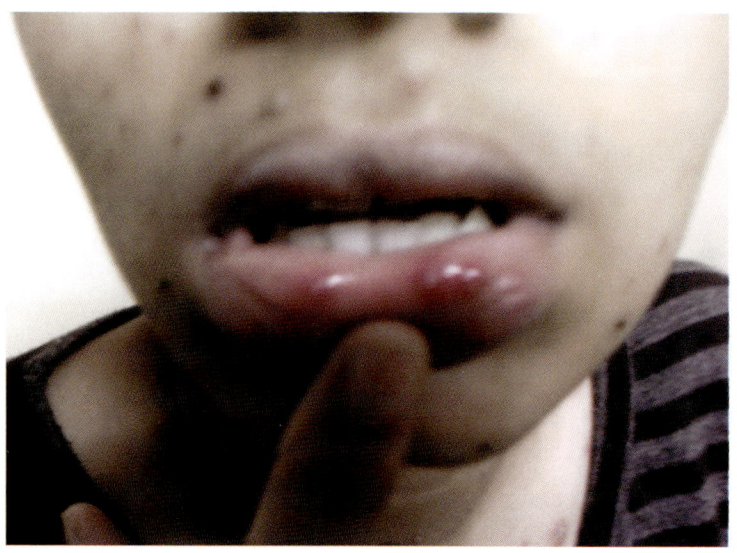

56. Hand Deformities

OBSERVATION

1. Long transverse palmar crease—on both sides reaching up to the ulnar margin of the palm.
2. Single palmar crease on the right side
3. Short 5th and 4th metacarpals on right side.
4. Very small and thin but completely formed little finger on the right side
5. Absence of distal phalanges in left index, middle fingers
6. Thin, long little finger on the left side

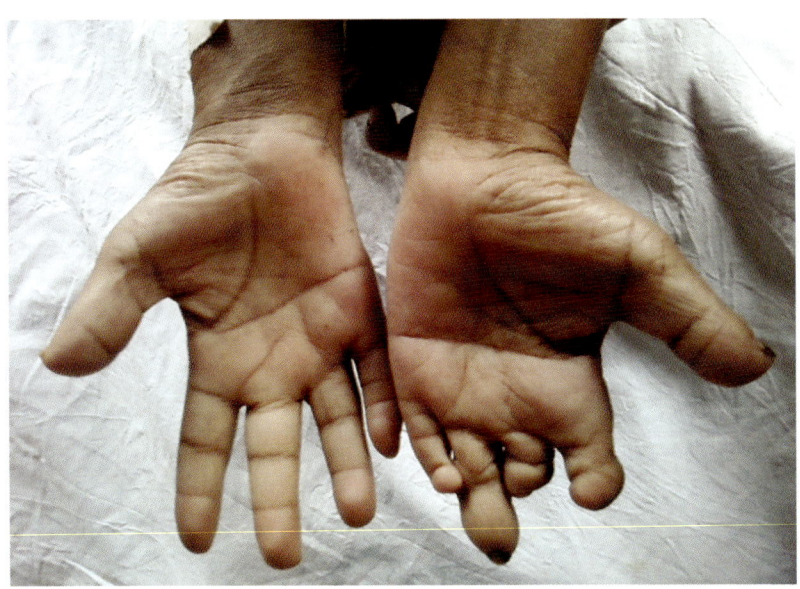

57. Deformities of the Feet

OBSERVATION

Congenitally deformed limbs.

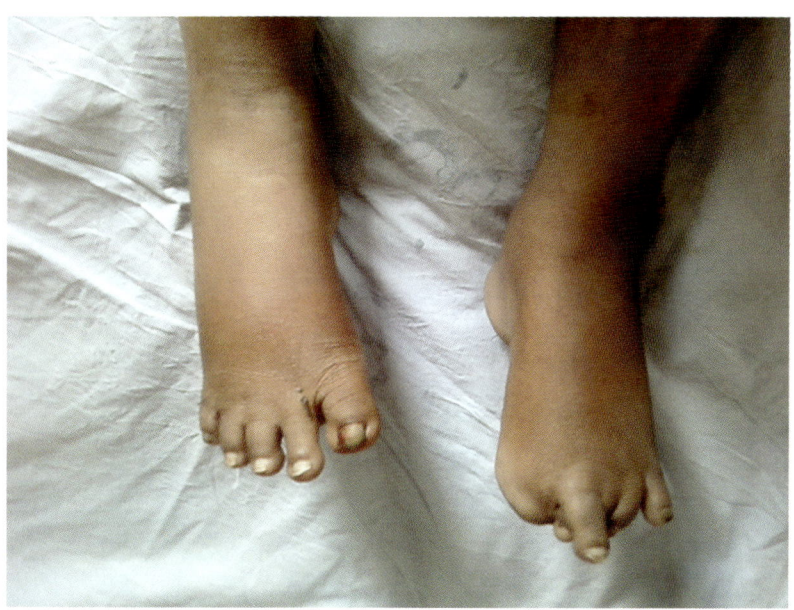

Quiz 1

What are trhe abnormalities seen?

1. Short 5th metatarsal—right side
2. Short 1st metatarsal—right side
3. Increased interdigital space between right great toe and 2nd toe
4. Deformities of multiple toes on the left side
5. Phalages of the left great toe are not formed
6. Left two-toe long—in fact, the longest toe on the left foot
7. Remaining toes on the left foot are small.

Quiz 2

What are the technical terms used to denote these abnormalities and what are their meanings?

1. Ateliosis—Incomplete/imperfect development—many digits.
2. Brachybasophalangia—short proximal phalanx—right thumb and little finger; left index, middle and little finger.
3. Brachydactyly—short fingers.
4. Brachymegalodactyly—short broad digit—stub thumb-bilatral.
5. Brachymesophalangia—left middle finger.

6. Brachymetapodia—short metacarpals and metatarsals.
7. Dystelephalangia—deformed terminal phalanx—left middle finger.
8. Ecterophalangia—terminal absence of one or more phalanges—left great toe.
9. Hyperphalangia—presence of more than the normal number of phanlanges in the tranverse direction.
10. Macrodactyly—excessive size of the limb or a part—distal phalanx of left middle finger.

Quiz 3

Which are the other parts of the body to be studied in this situation?
Other parts to be examined in this situation:
As these are birth defects, it is mandatory to examine other structures developing at the same time—ear lobes, eyes, heart, lungs.

Quiz 4

Give a brief outline of the development of the upper limb.

Days	Development
33–36	Hand plate
41–43	Digital ray; auricular hillock
44–46	Elbow regions
52–53	Fingers free; toes webbed
52	Separation

Quiz 5

Give a brief outline of the development of the lower limb

Days	Development
37–40	Foot plate
44–46	Digital ray; eye lid; nipple
49	Notch
52	Web
56	Separation of toes; external genitalia sexless apearence
	Tail disappears

Quiz 6

Give examples of some muscle disorders?
a. Some muscles can be absent—pectoralis major (sternocostal head); palmaris longis; trapezeus; serrratus anterior; quadratus femoris = Poland's syndrome
b. Palmaris longus (sternocostal head absent) + syndactyly
c. Congenital absence of diaphragm—associated with pulmonary atelectasis
d. Sternomastoid involvement at birth—torticollis
e. Accessory muscle—soleus

Quiz 7

Give some examples of finger anomalies?
a. *Brachydactyly:* Short fingers; reduced length of metacarpals; AD.
b. *Polydactyly:* Hand—extra digit, medial; foot—extra digit, lateral; AD.
c. *Syndactyly:* Simple webbing—cutaneous syndactyly; osseous syndactyly.
d. *Amelia:* Complete absence of the limb.
e. *Meromelia:* Partial absence of the limb.
f. *Ectrodactyly:* Absence of central digits—"Lobster claw" hand.
g. *Hemivertebra* = ½ body + 1 pedicle + 1 lamina—scoliosis.
h. *Craniostenosis:* Premature closure of 1 or more cerebral sutures.
i. *Klippel:* Feil-Short neck + low hairline + fewer cervical vertebrae + restricted neck movement.
j. *Absence of the sternal part of sternomastoid:* Nipple placed lower than on the other side.
k. *Prominent:* Sternomastoid on 1 side—wry neck/torticollis—head pulled to 1 side.

58. Fine Horizontal Scar in the Neck

OBSERVATION

A fine horizontal linear scar in front of the neck.

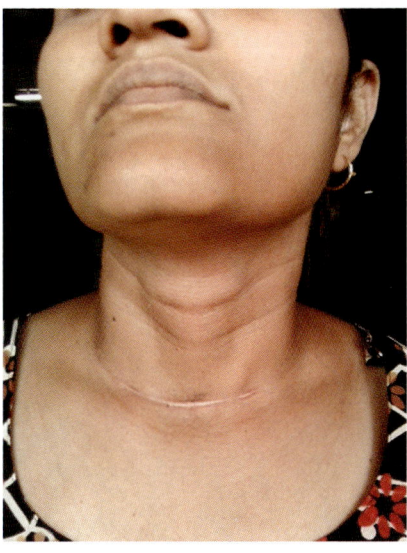

Quiz 1

What is the most likely cause for this scar?
Most likely a thyroid surgery.

Quiz 2

What do you look for when you examine those patient?
Look for features of hypothyroidism: Hypocalcemia (hypoparathyroidism).

59. Adenoma Sebaceum

OBSERVATION

Reddish raised angiofibromas on nose and cheek (butterfly distribution on face) associated with tuberous sclerosis.

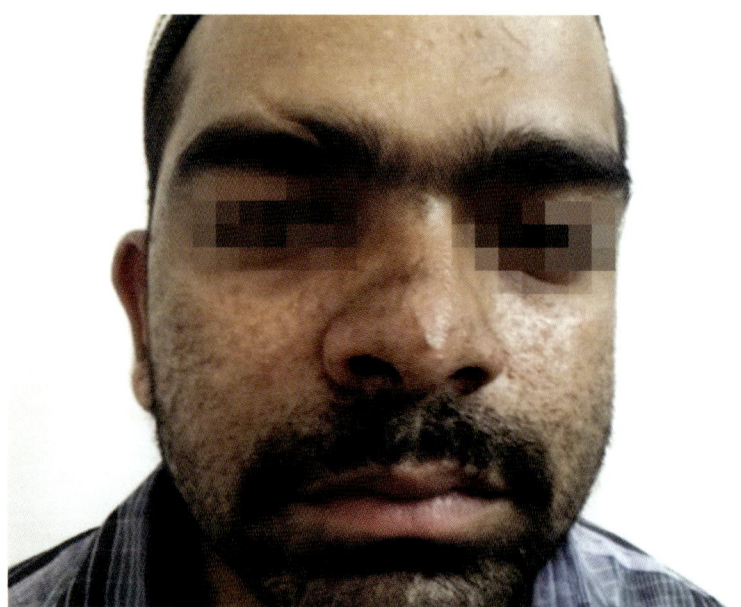

Quiz 1

What are adenoma sebaceum?

These are raised, reddish lesions on the "butterfly area" of the face (over the cheek and the nose) seen in tuberous sclerosis.

Quiz 2

What are they made of?

They consist of blood vessels and fibrous tissue.

Quiz 3

They are seen in which conditions?

Tuberous sclerosis (Bourneville's disease).

Quiz 4

Which lesions do they resemble?

Acne.

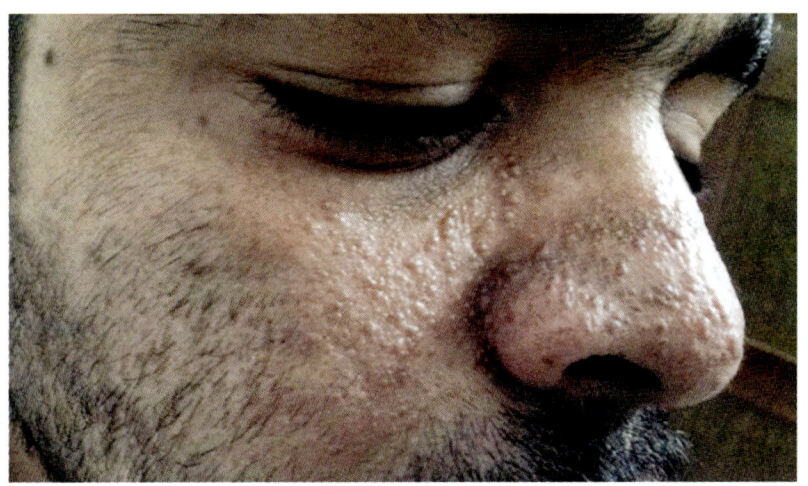

Quiz 5

Which are the other associated lesions in tuberous sclerosis?

a. *Skin*
1. Periungual fibromas—Koenen's tumors.
2. Ash leaf spots/macules—lack of melanin; may be present at birth; examination with Wood's lamp may help.
3. Shagreen patches—leathery, elevated, arrange peel like pigmented skinlesions—at nape of the neck/trunk/thighs—frequency of lesions increases with age.
4. Café au lait spots.

b. *Eyes*
1. Retinal—phakomas—astrocytic hamartomas
2. Non-retinal—coloboma, papilloedema, angiofibromas of lids

c. *CNS*
1. Learning disability, autism, self injurious behavior
2. Brain tumors—giant cell astrocytomas, cortical tumors, sub-ependymal nodules

d. *Kidneys*
Angiolipomas, APUDs, RCC, oncocytomas

e. *Lungs*
Lymphangiomyomatosis

f. *Heart*
Rhabdomyomas—arrhythmia, murmur

Quiz 6

What is the genetics?
AD inheritance
2 Genetic loci: TCS 1, TCS 2—tumor suppressor genes that work according to Knudson's "two hit" hypothesis.

60. Ash Leaf Macule

OBSERVATION

A hypopigmented lesion on forearm.

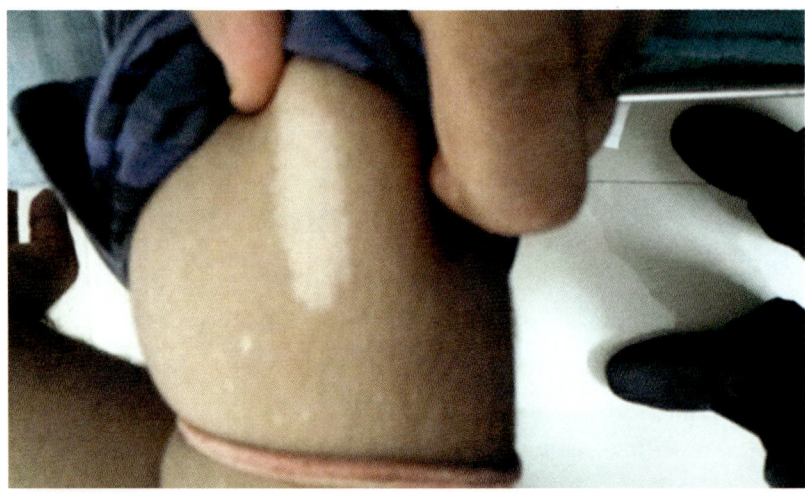

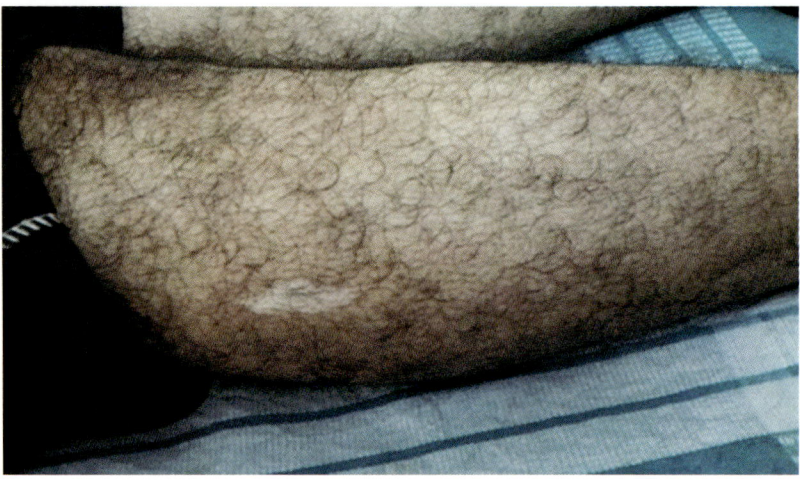

Quiz 1

What is an ash leaf macule?

A hypopigmented lesion seen on the body (trunk > limbs, face)
Oval at one end, pointed at the other end.

Quiz 2

What is its significance?
- Associated with tuberous sclerosis
- Can be present at birth
- Usually the first cutaneous sign of TS
- TS is strongly suspected if there are > 3 ash leaf patches.

Quiz 3

How can it be detected if inconspicuous?
Using Wood's light for examination.

Quiz 4

What are the synonyms for TS?
Borneville's disease
Epiloia

Quiz 5

What are the genetic facts?
Chromosome 9 9q34 TSC 1—gene product—hamartin tumor suppressor.
Chromosome 16 16p13 TSC2—gene product—tuberin.
Tuberin and hamartin heterodemerise and inhibit mTOR the mammalian target of rapamycin-thereby resulting in tumor lysis/shrinkage.

Quiz 6

What are the other associated lesions?
1. Forehead plaque—facial angiofibromas—pink, macules on butterfly region of face including nasolabial folds, cheek and chin.
2. Dysplastic periungual fibromas—"Koenen tumors"—skin coloured papules emerging from nailfolds.
3. Shagreen patch (connective tissue naevus)—soft papules in the lumbosacral area—with pebbly surface and prominent follicular openings.
4. Cortical tuber
5. Subependymal nodule
6. Subependymal astrocytoma
7. Cardiac rhabdomyoma
8. Lymphangiomyomatosis
9. Renal angiolipoma

61. Periungual Fibroma

OBSERVATION

Periungual fibroma

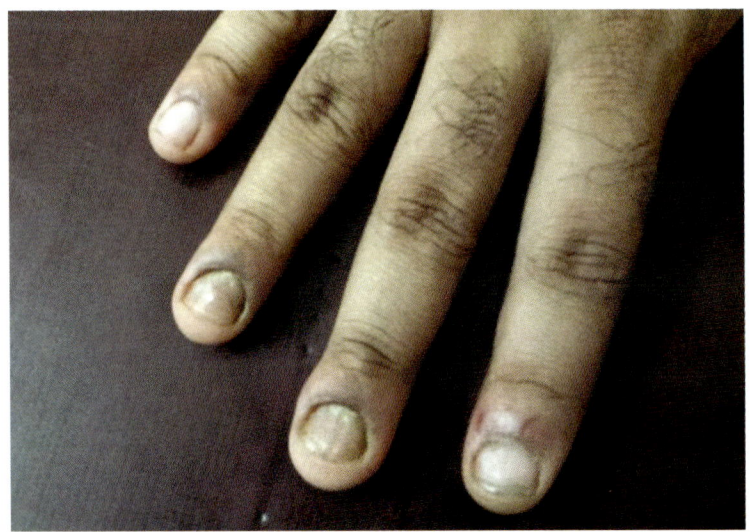

Quiz 1

What is the eponym?
Koenen's tumor.

Quiz 2

What is the significance?
Association with TS.

Quiz 3

What is subungual fibroma?
Fibroma arising below the nail.

Cases in Medicine

62. Elephantiasis

OBSERVATION

1. Increased limb girth
2. Thickening of the skin
3. Nodules on the skin
4. Pigmentation of the foot and toes

These changes indicate chronicity of the lesion

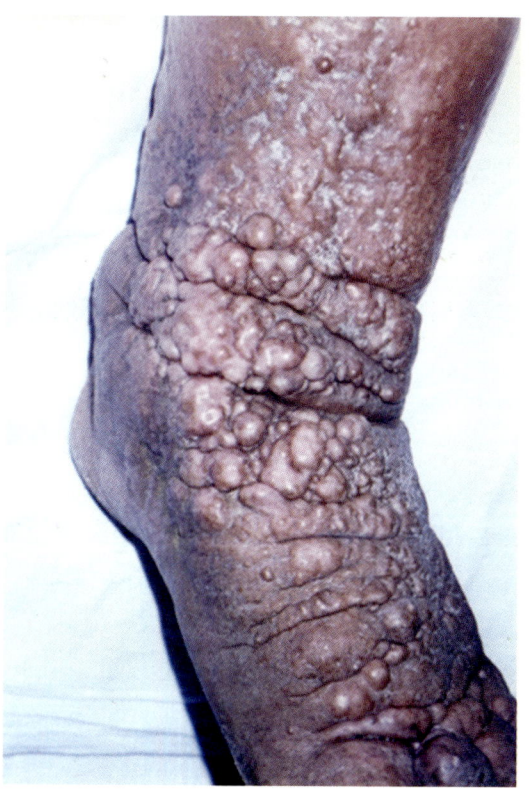

Quiz 1

What is elephantiasis?

Condition characterised by swelling of limbs, increase in the thickness of skin and soft tissues. Initially the edema is pitting the chronic stage, the edema will be non-pitting.

Quiz 2

What are the parts involved?

Limbs, genitalia (scrotum, penis vulva), breasts.
Extreme swellings are sometimes seen.

Quiz 3

What is the mechanism of elephantiasis?
1. Blockade of the lymphatics by the filarial worm—*Wuchereria bancrofti, Brugia malayi*
2. Pococoniosis—non-filarial elephantiasis.

Quiz 4

Filarial elephantiasis
Comlex interplay of various factors:
The filarial parasite (*W. bancrofti, B. malayi*);
The Wolbachia bacteria in the worm which live in symbiosis
Immunity of the body
Opportunistic infections complicating the elephantiasis.

Quiz 5

What is the medical treatment of filarial elephantiasis?
1. DEC for the microfilariae
2. Albendazole + ivermectin for the adult worms
3. Doxycycline to eliminate Wolbachia bacteria without which the worms.

Quiz 6

What is the role of surgery?
1. For hydrocele—useful
2. For elephantiasis of the limbs—may not help

Quiz 7

What is podoconiosis?
Podoconiosis is non-filarial elephantiasis (non-parasitic elephantiasis)

Quiz 8

What causes podoconiosis?
Podoconiosis is due to contact with irritant soils—reds clay rich in alkali metals—sodium, potassium associated with volcanic activity.

63. Left Renal Angle Fullness

OBSERVATION

Left sided renal angle fullness.

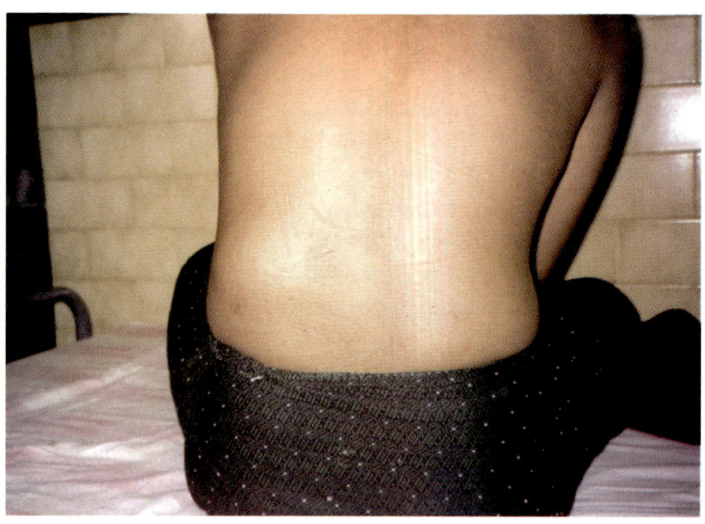

Quiz 1

What is the renal angle?

Angle formed by the inferior border of the 12th rib and the lateral border of erector spinae muscle on the back is known as the renal angle.

Quiz 2

What is its importance?

Fullness indicates a mass arising from the kidney.

Tenderness indicates possibly infective or inflammatory etiology.

Quiz 3

What are the physical signs of an enlarged kidney?

  1. Location—in the paracolic gutter

Inspection

  2. Direction of enlargement directly downwards towards the iliac fossa.
    Renal mass can result in a fullness in the loin, lower part of hypochondrium, iliac fossa.
    Kidney must enlarge at least two times before the mass becomes visible.

  3. Shape—reniform.

Palpation

  4. Palpable bimanually in the loin

  5. Can be pushed and coaxed back into the loin

6. Moves with respiration—but to a lesser extent than the liver/gall bladder. As it comes down in deep inspiration, it can be held fown bimanually
7. Pressure exereted over the renal angle with the thumb can produce tenderness—Murphy's Renal punch—indicator of deep seated sepsis. Compare on the other side.
8. Ballotable
9. Gap exists between the lump and the costal margin and hence the finger can be insinuated.

Percussion

10. Band of colonic resonance in front of the kidney may be present.
    If not found, Baldwin's method can be used where a plastic tube inserted rectally is inflated to insufflate the colon and the band of resonance may be found anterior to the mass.
11. Percussion outside the erector spinae is normally resonant—due to the presence of colon. This resonance is list as the colon is displaced.
12. Dullness elicited over the mass by percussion is NOT continuous with liver/splenic dullness as a zone of resonance exists between the mass and the liver/spleen.

64. Left Renal Mass

OBSERVATION

Fullness and bulge in the left renal angle.

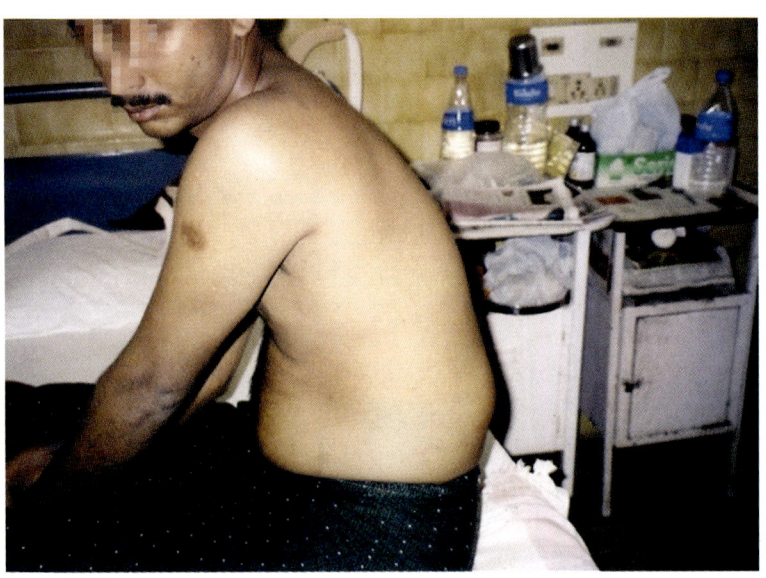

Quiz 1

What is the most likely diagnosis?

Renal mass

Quiz 2

What are the causes of a "Renal Mass"?

SOLID—compensatory hypertrophy, neoplasm, advanced TB
CYSTIC—hydronephrosis, pyonephrosis, solitary cust, polycystic kidney.

Quiz 3

What are the common causes for the enlargement of the kidney/kidneys?

1. Hydronephrosis—unilateral > bilateral (if the obstruction is distal to the bladder neck)
   Pyonephrosis—containing pus
2. Perinephric abscess
3. Renal malignancy
4. Renal cyst—APKD > solitary cyst.

Quiz 4

What is bimanual palpation?

Patient lies in the supine position:

- One hand on the renal angle—lifts the kidney.
- One hand on the front of the abdomen just below the costal margin.

Quiz 5

What is "Murphy's renal punch"?/renal angle test?

- Palpation with pressure on the renal angle using thumb.
- Tenderness indicates deep seated renal infection/sepsis.

Quiz 6

What is ballottement?

With the patient in a supine position, one hand over the renal angle and the other placed anteriorly just below the costal margin, short sharp thrusts are given by the posterior (displacing) hand (thereby displacing the kidney) while the impact is felt by the anterior (watching) hand. This is possible in a renal mass as the kidney is surrounded by a perinephric pad of fat which is fluid at body temperature.

Cases in Medicine

65. Hepatomegaly with Gallbladder Enlargement

OBSERVATION

Hepatomegaly + gallbladder enlargement.

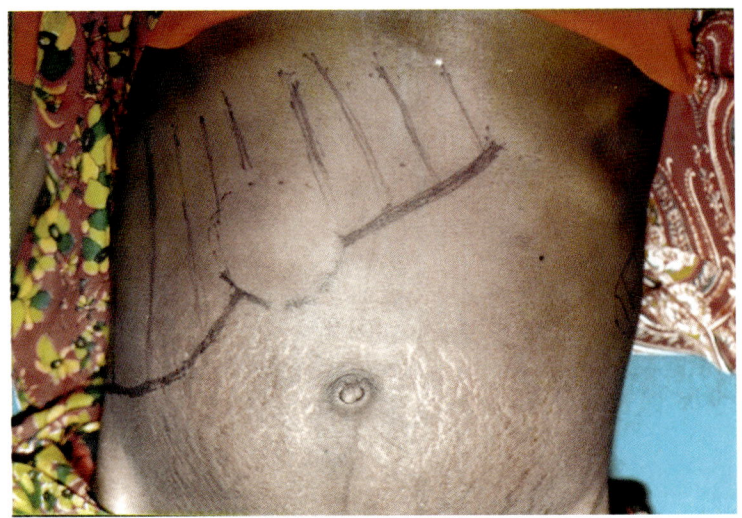

Quiz 1

What are the physical signs of an enlarged liver?
1. Descends below the right costal margin and the costal angle.
2. Moves freely with respiration.
3. Movement is only possible downwards and not sideways.
4. Margin of the enlarged liver is parallel to the right costal margin. Lateral margin of the index finger rides over the free margin of the palpable liver.
5. Cannot insinuate the finger between the enlarged liver and the costal margin.
6. Edge sharp/rounded; surface–smooth/irregular.
7. Percussion note is dull and the dullness continues with the known liver dullness up to the 8th rib in the mid axillary line. No colonic resonance anterior to it.

Quiz 2

How do you determine the upper border of the liver?
Percuss over the right midaxillary line commencing from the 4th IC space. Resonance will be replaced by dullness if the liver is enlarged upwards.

Quiz 3

What are the causes of upward enlargement of the liver?
Amoebic liver abscess—soft, very tender, IC tenderness
Hydatid cyst

Quiz 4

What are the differential diagnosis for upward enlargement of the liver?
- Pleural effusion
- Basal pneumonia
- Subdiaphragmatic effusion/abscess

Quiz 5

What are the features of the enlarged liver?
a. Extent below the costal margin—size in cms; liver span
b. Surface—smooth/irregular/nodular—with or without umbilication
c. Consistancy—soft/firm/stony hard
d. Tenderness/no tenderness
e. Border/margin—sharp/rounded
f. Movement with respiration, tidal percussion
g. IC tenderness
h. Upward enlargement of the liver.

Quiz 6

Can a normal liver be palpable?
a. In deep inspiration—sometimes.
b. Anatomic variation—Riedel's lobe; pectus excavatum; narrow costal angles; flared costal margin.
   Reidel's lobe: A downward extension of the right lobe of the liver below the right costal margin along the anterior axillary line.
c. *"Pushed down" liver:* Emphysema (flattened diaphragm); pneumothorax; pleural effusion.
d. *"Apparent hepatomegaly":* Perihepatic disease; retroperitoneal mass; COPD.
   Therefore, "all palpable livers are not necessarily enlarged livers".

Quiz 7

What is the liver span?
The distance between the lower border of the liver in the midclavicular line (obtained by palpation) and the upper border of the upper border of the liver in the midclavicular line (obtained by percussion).
A liver span of >15 cm is abnormal and indicates liver enlargement.

Exceptions:
a. A normal liver span + abnormal liver—cirrhosis
b. An apparently increased liver span + normal liver
   Subpulmonic effusion; subphrenic abscess + thickened diaphragm; basal pneumonia

Quiz 8

What are the mechanisms of hepatomegaly?
a. Intrinsic liver disease—inflammation, infiltration, congestion.
b. Due to a systemic disease.

Quiz 9

What are the examples?

Inflammation: Hepatitis—viral (A to G); toxic—INH, alcohol

Infiltration: Malignancy (primary/secondary); steatosis—obesity, DM, alcohol, malnutrition, hyperalimentation; storage disorders—alpha 1 antitrypsin deficiency, hemochromatosis, amyloidosis; metabolic—Niemann-Pick and Gaucher.

Congestion—vascular congestion—CCF, cor pulmonale; constrictive pericarditis; tricuspid regurgitation; portal hypertension.

Liver involvement in systemic disease: Bacterial—TB, syphilis; viral—infectious mononucleosis; Parasitic—schistosoma, amoebiasis, hydatid cyst; leptospirosis; septicemia.

Quiz 10

What is the differential diagnosis for tender hepatomegaly?

a. Tender hepatomegaly + jaundice—hepatitis (viral, drugs), leptospirosis, amebic liver abscess, RVF

   Non-tender/tender hepatomegaly + jaundice—biliary tract obstruction (stones, carcinoma head of the pancreas); cholangitis, portal pyemia.

b. Tender hepatomegaly + no jaundice—RVF, amoebic hepatitis.

   tender/non-tender hepatomegaly + no jaundice—cirrhosis, reticulosis, Budd-Chiari syndrome (hepatic vein obstruction).

c. Asymmetrically enlarged tender hepatomegaly—abscess, bacterial, parasitic.

d. Diffuse tenderness due to rapid capsular distension CCF, vascular tumor.

e. *Focal tenderness:* Infected cyst, infarcted focal nodule, regenerative nodule.

f. *Soft hepatomegaly:* Steatosis, CHF, hepatitis.

g. *Firm hepatomegaly:* Cirrhosis (nodular); granulomatous—TB, sarcoid, histoplasma; congestive (sometimes)

h. *Nodular hepatomegaly:* Hepatoma; secondaries; cirrhosis; polycystic liver disease

i. *Pulsatile hepatomegaly:* Tricuspid regurgitation, tricuspid stenosis

j. *Liver failure + No jaundice:* Reye's syndrome

k. Drug induced vascular disease of the liver with/without hepatomegaly—

   • *Vinyl chloride:* Hepatic angiosarcoma

   • *Androgen therapy:* Peliosis hepatitis

   • *OCs:* Focal nodular hyperplasia

l. *Sources of metastasis to the liver with or without hepatomegaly:* Lung, breast (above the diaphragm); Pancreas, colon (below the diaphragm)

m. *Diffuse infiltration of the liver:* Leukemia (acute/chronic); myeloma; histocytosis syndromes

n. *Hepatomegaly + rock hard liver:* Malignancy

o. *Endocrine causes of hepatomegaly:* Hypothyroidism, acromegaly

p. *Tropical diseases causing hepatomegaly:* Viral hepatitis, protozoa, helminthic disorders

q. Example of benign sol (with/without enlargement)—polycystic liver disease

r. Storage disorders in adults + what is store

   Alpha 1 antitrypsin deficiency—fructose deficient glycoprotein is stored in hepatocytes

   Hemochromatosis (primary/secondary)—iron stored in Kupffer cells.

Amyloidosis—fragments of IGG polypeptides (light chains) deposited in connective tissue and the parenchyma of the liver.

s. What is the "congestive syndrome of the biliary tract"?

Hepatomegaly resulting from extrahepatic cholestasis due to large bile duct obstruction (stricture/tumor/stone). To be differentiated from the hepatomegaly die to intrahepatic cholestasis.

t. *Localised hepatomegaly:* Reidel's lobe (mistaken for hepatomegaly); hepatoma; secondaries; liver abscess; hydatid cyst.

Quiz 11

What is the surface marking of the gallbladder?

Where the costal margin meets the outer border of the rectus muscle.

In case of an enlarged liver—where the border of the enlarged liver meets the outer border of the rectus muscle.

Quiz 12

What is Courvoisier's law/Courvoisier's sign?

In a case of obstructive jaundice, painless enlargement of the gallbladder is likely to result from the carcinoma of the head of the pancreas and not from stone in CBD (as the wall of the gallbladder is scarred in the latter situation and is therefore unlikely to distend.

Quiz 13

What are the exceptions to the Courvoisier's law?

a. Double impaction—one stone in cystic duct + one stone in CBD
b. Pancreatic calculi obstructing the ampulla of Vater
c. Mucocele of the gallbladder due to a stone in the cystic duct
d. Oriental cholangiohepatitis—seen in East Asian people with recurrent bouts of cholangitis with intrahepatic pigment stones and intrahepatic biliary obstruction. Due to high incidence of *E. coli* infection in the bile (also *Chlonorchis sinensis*, ascaris lumbricoides). Complicating sepsis may prove fatal in the acute phase.

Quiz 14

What are the causes of a palpable HARD gallbladder?

Cancer of GB.

Cases in Medicine

66. Spider Nevi

Synonym: Nevus araneus

OBSERVATION

Spider nevi + Gynecomastia

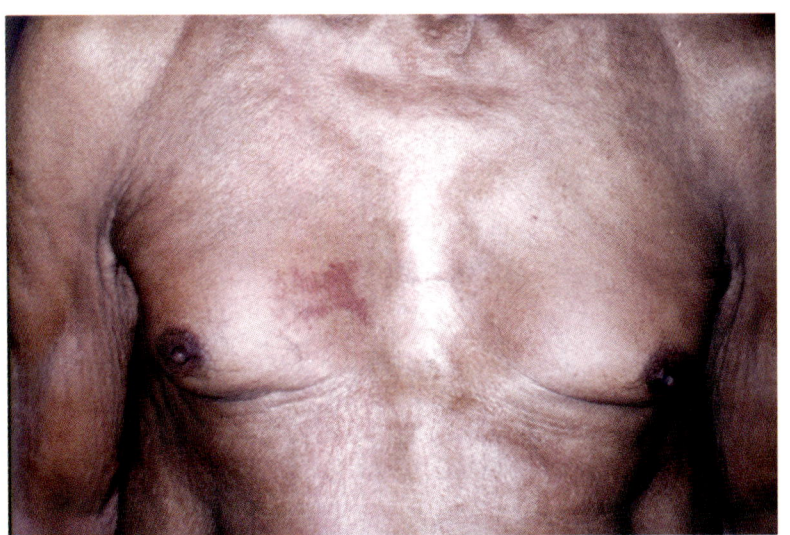

Quiz 1

What are the synonyms?
Vascular spiders

Quiz 2

What is it?
Vascular skin lesion—supplied by a central arteriole—surrounded by smaller thin branches which resemble the legs of the spider.

Quiz 3

What is the mechanism?
Endocrine (increased estrogen)—manifestation.
Other endocrine manifestations of cirrhosis include—gynecomastia, testicular atrophy, loss of secondary sexual characteristics (including testicular atrophy), plamar erythema.

Quiz 4

What are the properties of spider nevi?
a. *Location:* In exposed areas in the distribution of the SVC—chest above nipples, face, arms hands.

b. Pulsation may be observed in the larger spider nevi
c. May be surrounded by pale white areas known as white spots. Careful observation refveals white spot in the lower portion in this picture
d. May be occasionally seen in normal people—pregnancy, childhood
e. Pathological spider nevi
  • Appear later years
  • Increase in size and numbers
  • Associsated with diseases known.
f. Blanch when occluded with a pinhead; refill on removing the pinhead.

Quiz 5

What are the situations associated with pathological spider nevi?
Cirrhosis of the liver, chronic active hepatitis, hyperthyroidism, pregnancy (3rd trimester), Cushing's, 2% of normal population.

Quiz 6

What are the differential diagnosis for the spider nevi?
a. Campbell de Morgan spots:
  • Bright red discrete punctuate spots; 1–2 mm diameter; located on the chest and abdomen
  • Seen at advanced age; no clinical significance
b. Telangiectasia
c. Insect bites.
d. Osler-Weber-Rendu syndrome.

Quiz 7

What are white spots?
• Spots seen on arms, buttocks, legs of patients with chronic liver disease.
• Seen on the areas where the skin is cold.
• An arteriole is present in the centre of the white spot which later develops into a spider nevus
• Seen in cirrhosis, chronic active hepatitis, pregnancy.

Quiz 8

What are the cutaneous (skin) manifestations of cirrhosis of the liver/chronic liver disease?
a. Spider nevi
b. White spots
c. *Paper money skin:* Thread like vessels seen in the skin resembling the threads in the American dollar bills—can be seen in alcoholic hepatitis, chronic active hepatitis, cirrhosis.
d. *Palmar erythema:* Exaggerated flushing of palms (thenar eminence, hypothenar eminence, bases of fingers) fading on pressure
   Seen in chronic liver disease, pregnancy, thyrotoxicosis, carcinoma bronchus
e. *Central cyanosis:* AV shunts in the lungs causing vasodilatation—seen in decompensated cirrhosis.
   May be associated with hepatopulmonary syndrome—characterized by orthodeoxia (desaturation and cyanosis in the sitting up position). May also be associated with clubbing

f. Red soles may be associated with plmar erythema
g. *Leukonychia/white nails:* May be seen in cirrhosis. Tip may remain pink.
  - Lunula may disappear
  - Clubbing may co-exist—in cholestasis
h. *Gynecomastia*
  - Enlargement of breasts seen in the males with cirrhosis, chronic active hepatitis
  - Palpable breast tissue must be present—may be tender.
  - Areola may be pigmented
  - Associated with reduced libido, testicular atrophy.
  - May be due to drugs—spironolactone
  - In women—breast atrophy + amenorrhea may be seen
i. Bruising on the skin; ecchymoses
  - Bleeding from venepuncture sites
  - Massive extravasation from site of arterial puncture—in fulminant hepatitis
  - May be associated with prolonged PT
j. *Hyperpigmentation:* Hemochromatosis, primary biliary cirrhosis.

67. Dilated Tortuous Veins on the Chest Wall

OBSERVATION

Dilated veins mainly on the arm, neck and upper chest.

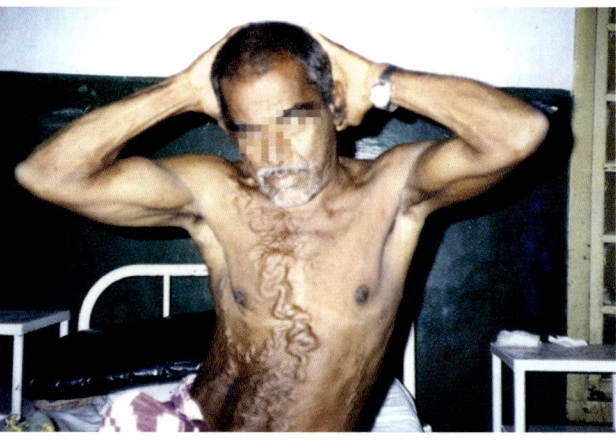

Quiz 1

What is the likely cause, if only veins on upper limb and neck are involved?

Highly suggestive of innominate vein obstruction particularly if the piture is unilateral—dilated veins on the arms + dilated external jugular vein.

Innominate vein (brachiocephalic vein) is formed by the subclavian vein and the internal jugular vein on the same side.

SVC is formed by the two innominate veins (brachiocephalic veins).

What are the possibilities if the findings are bilateral?
Bilateral innominate vein obstruction/SVC obstructions.

68. Dilated Veins

OBSERVATION

Dilated veins on the chest wall and the abdominal wall.

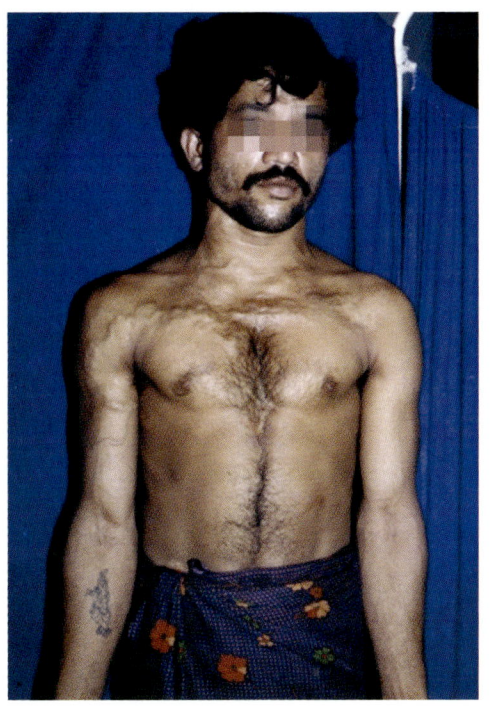

Quiz 1

What is the most likely cause for this?
SVC obstruction.

Quiz 2

What are the mechanisms and causes of SVC obstruction?
a. Pressure from outside
   Solid structures
   Malignant: Lymphomas—Ca bronchus, breast, thyroid; lymphomas—Hodgkin's, non-Hodgkin's
   Rare: Thymomas; germ cell tumors
   Benign: Aortic aneurysm; retrosternal goiter.

Cases in Medicine

b. Obsriction from within the lumen
- Thrombosis of SVC/tributeries
- Thrombophlebitis
- "Dramatic" rupture of thew aortic aneurysm.

c. *Causes in the wall*
Fibrosing diseases involving the wall fibrosing mediastinitis.

Quiz 3

What are the benign causes of SVC obstruction?

a. SVC/branch thrombosis
b. Fibrosing mediastinitis
c. Mediastinal granulomatous diseases—TB, histoplasmosis
d. Idiopathic mediastinal fibrositis
e. Mediastinal goiter
f. Bronchogenic cyst
g. Teratoma
h. Pleural calcification
i. Thoracic aortic aneurysm
j. SVC obstruction due to indwelling catheters

Quiz 4

What are the causes in childhood?

a. Following cardiac surgery
b. Mediastinal neoplasms—non-Hodgkin's lymphoma
c. VA shunts
d. Mediastinal fibrosis

Quiz 5

What are the described alternate collateral channels?

a. Azygos system
b. Lateral thoracic vein
c. Internal mammary vein
d. Vertebral plexus
e. Esophageal plexus

a. *Azygos system*
- Drains to IVC through lumbar veins
- Symptoms mild if this system is patent
- But it is frequently involved in the disease process

b. *Lateral thoracic vein*
Drains to femoral vein through connections with
- Thoracoepigastric vein
- Superficial epigastric vein
- Superficial circumflex vein

c. *Internal thoacic veins to iliac veins*
   - Superior epigastric vein and inferior epigastric vein
d. *Vertebral plexus*
e. *Oesophageal plexus*
   - Retrograde drainage to portal vein.

Quiz 6

What is the direction of blood flow?

a. *Normal:* Away from the umbilicus
b. SVC obstruction above the entry of the azygos vein into the SVC
   - Collaterals drain into the azygos vein and then into the unobstructed part of the SVC
   - Direction of flow is normal.
c. Obstruction at/below the entry of the azygos vein into the SVC

   Principle—blood cannot enter the right heart via SVC; so it has to enter the right heart using IVC blood from arms + upper part of the body flows through lateral thoracic, thoracoepigastric, superficial epigastric and superficial circumflex veins into long saphenous and femoral veins and then to IVC—right heart.

Some observations
a. Direction of flow in the distended veins—reversed
b. Inspiratory filling of neck veins may be present
c. Hepatojugular reflux—present

Quiz 7

What are the symptoms and signs of SVC obstruction?

They are mainly due to venous hypertension: 300–500 ml saline

Symptoms: Devolopment of distended veins; recurrent infections—facial carbuncles; Aggravation on bending forwards; epistaxis; cerebral symptoms; facial puffiness/swelling; dyspnoea; nasal stuffiness; increasing collar size; hoarseness; stridor; dizziness; tongue swelling; headache; somnolence; visual distortion; syncope; vertigo; convulsions.

Signs: Facial edema; neck vein distension; upper extremity edema; upper extremity venous distension; cyanosis, plethora; mental aberrations; laryngeal edema; conjunctival suffusion; stupor; coma; pleural effusion (chylothorax); "Wet brain syndrome"—cerebral edema.

Quiz 8

What are the differential diagnosis for SVC obstruction?

a. Mandor's disease

   Thrombophlebitis of the superficial veins of the breast and the anterior heat wall; can also affect the arm. Examination reveals indurated subcutaneous thrombophlebitic cord.
b. May mimc right heart failure and constrictive pericarditis—if the clinical picture shows predominantly edema.
c. Innominate vein obstruction if swelling involves only 1 arm + ipsilateral external jugular vein dilatation.
d. Subclavian vein obstruction—swelling of 1 arm only

69. Noonan's Syndrome

OBSERVATION

- Low posterior hairline
- Low set ears
- Wooly hair

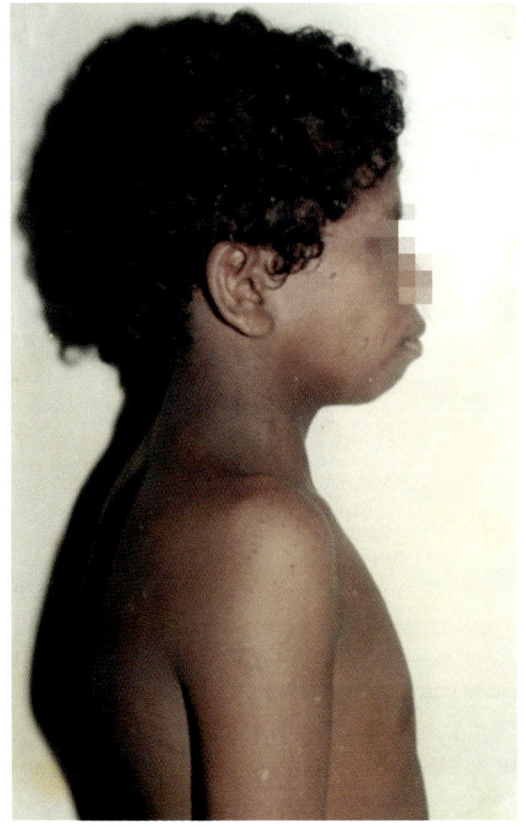

Quiz 1

What is the likely diagnosis?
Noonan's syndrome

Quiz 2

What are the components?
a. General
- Short stature
- Low hair line

- Triangular face
- Low set ears
- Wooly hair
- Absence of axillary and pubic hair

b. Eye
- Hypertelorism
- Coloboma of iris (right side)

c. Neck
- Webbed neck

d. Shield like chest
- Widely spaced nipples
- Pectus excavatum

e. CVS
- Right sided congenital HD
- PS—due to dysplastic pulmonary valve, ASD, HOCM

Quiz 3

What are the differential diagnosis?

XO/XY mosaicism
Fetal hydantoin syndrome
Fetal alcohol syndrome

Quiz 4

What is the genetics of Noonan's syndrome?

- Mutations in the 3 genes—PTPN11, SOSI, RAFI
- AD inheritance

Quiz 5

What are the synonyms?

- Familial Turner syndrome
- Female pseudo Turner syndrome
- Male Turner
- Turner phenotype
- Ullrich-Noonan syndrome.

OBSERVATION

- Wooly hair
- Webbed neck
- Scoliosis with convexity to right

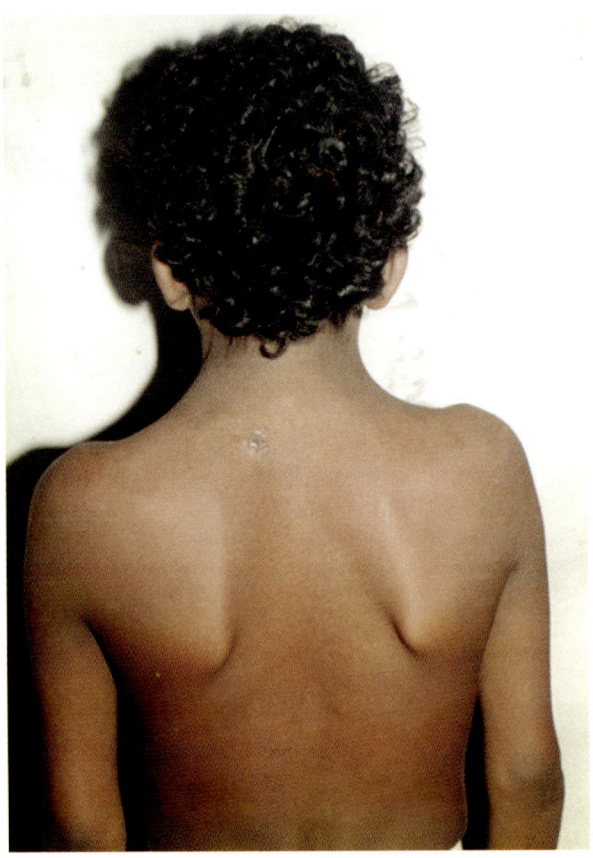

OBSERVATION

- Short stature
- Shield like chest
- Widely spaced nipples
- Absence of pubic hair
- Hypertelorism
- Flat bridge of the nose

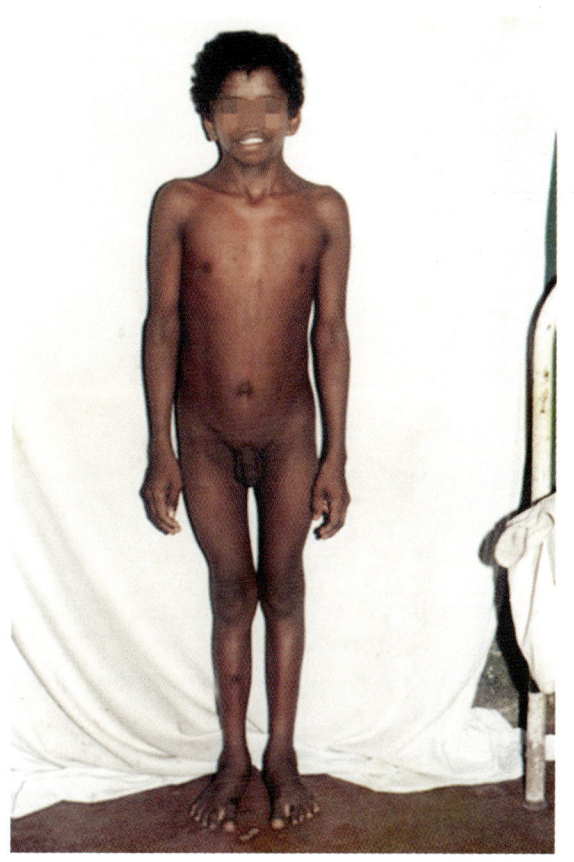

70. Ichthyosis

OBSERVATION

Dry, scaly skin.

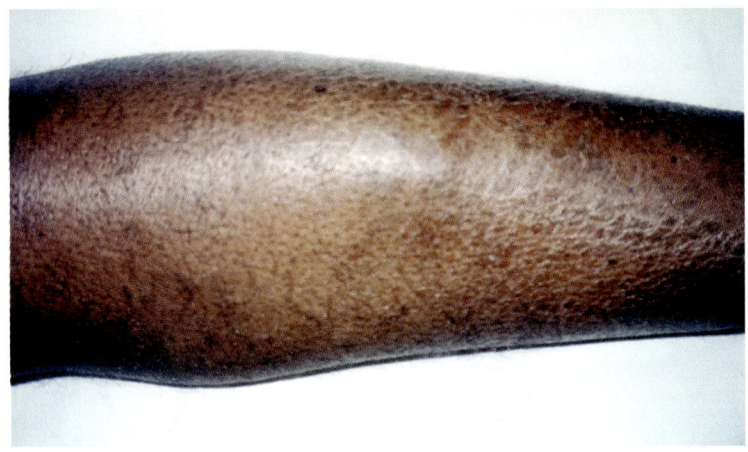

Quiz 1

What is ichthyosis?

Ichthyosis is the dry scaly skin with appearance of a fish.

Quiz 2

What is the cause?

Genetic. Varying degrees of severity are seen with the involvement of the same gene. Some genetic associations are better documented.

a. X-linked ichthyosis associated with Kallmann's syndrome—close to KAL1 gene.

b. Ichthyosis vulgaris-FLG gene—filaggrin protein

c. Harlequin type ichthyosis—ATP binding cassette transporter 12

d. Lamellar ichthyosis, type 1—transglutaminase 1

e. Ichthyosis en confetti—congenital ichthyosis—mutation in KRT10 gene.

Quiz 3

What are the conditions associated with acquired ichthyosis acquisita?

Tuberculosis; leprosy; AIDS; Hodgkin's disease; mycosis fungoides; typhoid fever; Kaposi's sarcoma; visceral carcinoma.

Drugs; autoimmune conditions; endocrine disorders; metabolic diseases.

71. Café au lait Spots

OBSERVATION

Café au lait spot.

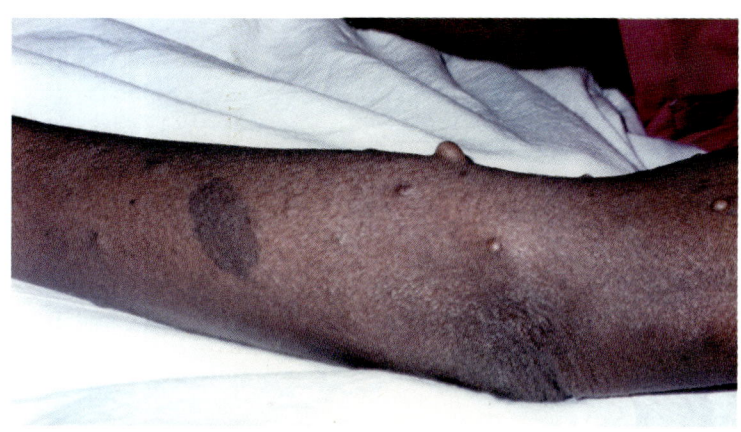

Quiz 1

What are café au lait spots?
They are pigmented birthmarks—"coffee with milk"

Quiz 2

What are the synonyms?
Coast of maine spots; giraffe's spots

Quiz 3

How many spots are significant?
- 6 spots of >5 cm before puberty
- 6 spots of >15 cm after puberty

Quiz 4

What are the conditions where the café au lait spots can be seen?
- von Recklinghausen's disease—neurofibromatosis type 1 (NF 1)
- McCune-Albright syndrome
- Tuberous sclerosis
- Ataxia telangiectasia
- Hunter's syndrome
- Multiple mucosal neuroma syndrome
- Noonan syndrome
- Russell-Silver syndrome
- Wiskott-Aldrich syndrome

What are the features of neurofibromatosis 1?

Syn: Peripheral neurofibromatosis; von Recklinghausen's disease.

Neurofibroma 1 (NF 1) = (>2) or plexiform neurofibroma (>1); axillary/inguinal freckles; Lesch nodules;

Bone lesions (sphenoidal dysplasia, tibial pseudoarthrosis); hyperplastic gums; phakomas; 1st degee relatives with NF 1.

Quiz 6

What are the features of neurofibromatosis 2?

Neurofibroma 2 (NF 2): Few or no skin lesions; bilateral acoustic neuromas; cerebral and optic nerved gliomas; meningiomas; spinal neurofibromas.

72. Marfan's Syndrome—Arachnodactyly

OBSERVATION

Arachnodactyly
IC tube for (recurrent) pneumothorax

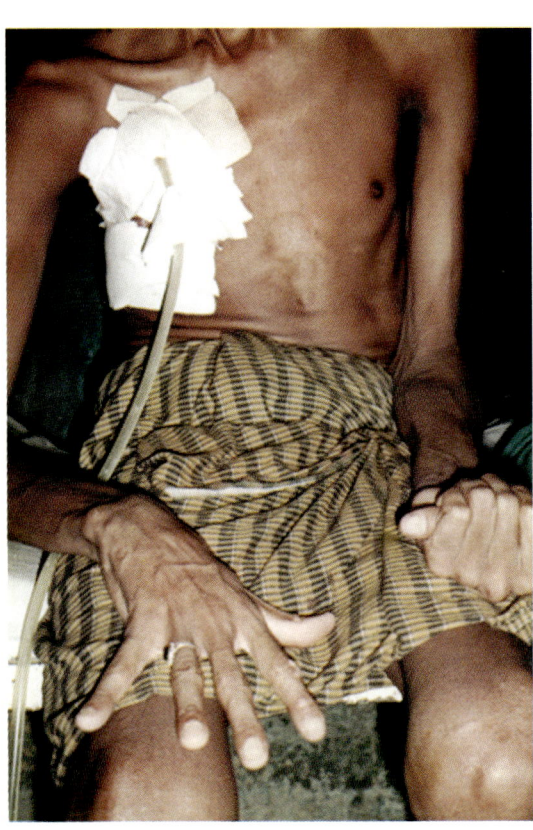

Quiz 1

What is the diagnosis?

With the available clues, one has to consider the possibility of Marfan's syndrome.

Quiz 2

What is Marfan's syndrome?

Marfan's syndrome is an inherited disorder of the connective tissue, in which the most pronounced abnormalities occur in the musculoskeletal, cardiovascular and ocular systems. Aortic dilatation and dissection are the major causes of mortality and morbidity.

Quiz 3

What are the components of Marfan's syndrome?

a. *Skeletal:*
  - Arm span > height
  - Lower segment > upper segment
  - Arachnodactyly—long, spidery fingers
  - Tall stature
  - Joint hypermobility
  - Sternum depressed—pectus excavatum. Sometimes severe pectus carinatum
  - High arched palate
  - Genu recurvatum

b. *Cardiovascular:*
  - Aortic root dilatation, aortic incompetence
  - Aortic dissection (ascending aorta)
  - MVP (elongation of chordate tendinnae)
  - MR, TR (myxomatous degeneration of valve leaflets)

c. *Ocular*:
  - Upward dislocation of the lens
  - Flat cornea
  - Increasaed axial length of the globe
  - Redued meiosis

d. *Pulmonary*:
  - Apical blebs (may be visible on CXR)
  - Complicating pneumothorax (may be recurrent)

e. *Skin*:
  - Striae atrophicae
  - Recurrent incisional hernia

73. Marfan's Syndrome

OBSERVATION

- Tall stature
- Long, slender limbs—dolichostenomelia
- IC tube for pneumothorax
- Arachnodactyly

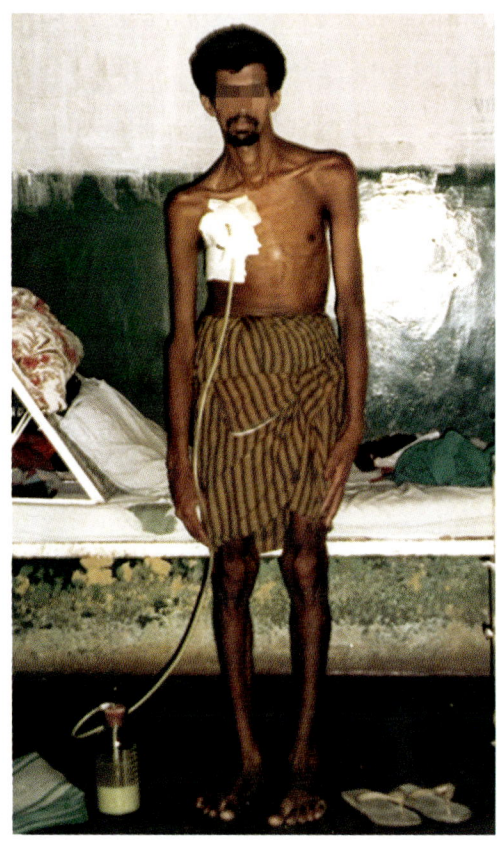

Quiz 1

What is the genetics of Marfan's syndrome?

Mutations on FBN1 gene of chromosome 15 which encodes glycoprotein fibrillin 1 which results in weak elastin fibres found in and, therefore, weaken connective tissue—joint ligaments, fasciae, etc. resulting in dislocations, subluxations, hernia.

TGF beta (transforming growth factor beta) also plays an important role—in the slow degradation of elastic fibres and other components of the extracellular matrix. Also has a role in Loeys-Dietz syndrome, involving TGF beta R2 gene on chromosome no. 3, a receptor protein for TGF beta. Because of similar pathologies, can be confused with Marfan's syndrome.

Quiz 2

What are the differential diagnosis for Marfan's syndrome?

1. Homocystinuria
2. Congenital contractural arachnodactyly (CCA)/Beals syndrome
3. Ehlers-Danlos syndrome
4. Loeys-Dietz syndrome
5. Mass phenotype
6. Shprintzen-Goldberg syndrome
7. Stickler syndrome
8. Men type B

Criteria	Marfan's	Homocysteinuria	CCA
Dislocation of lens	+ (Upward)	+ (Downward)	–
Mental deficiency	–	+ (Variable)	–
Aortic dilatation	+	–	–
MVP	+	–	–
Thrombosis (arterial)	–	+	–
Arachnodactyly	+	+	+
Scoliosis	+	+	+
Osteoporosis	–	+	+
Contractures	Rare	–	Always
Inheritance	Dominant	Recessive	Dominant
Homocystinuria	–	+	–
Increased hydroxyproline in urine	+ (Sometimes)	–	–
Others	–	Flair hair Malar flush	Abnormal Helix/ear

Quiz 3

What is Ehlers-Danlos syndrome? (Cutis hyperelastica)?

Defective synthesis of collagen (due to mutations in COL 3A and COL 5A genes) results in excessive elastin production resulting in hypermobility of joints. A Marfanoid syndrome characterised by arachnodactyly, tall stature, long skinny arms and legs, high arched palate.

Mencke's kinky hair disease mimics it.

Quiz 4

What is Loeys-Dietz syndrome?

AD syndrome caused by mutations in TGFβ1/2 receptors.

Characterised by—bifdid uvula/cleft lip; hypertelorism; corkscrew arteries (aortic and arterial aneurysms and dissections with tortuosity); pectus excavatum/carinatum; campylodactyly (contractures of fingers and toes); joint hypermobility; craniostenosis; CHD (PDA/ASD); Arnold-Chiari malformation; bicuspid aortic valve; increased risk of aortic root dilatation and dissection.

Quiz 5

What is mass phenotype?

MVP; aortic root at upper limits of normal; strech marks; skeletal conditions resembling Marfan's.

Quiz 6

What is Shprintzen-Goldberg syndrome?

Craniostenosis; multiple abdominal hernias; cognitive impairment; skeletal malformations.

Quiz 7

What is Stickler syndrome?

A genetic collagenopathy involving collagen types II and XI, characterised by distinctive facial abnormalities; ocular problems; hearing loss; joint problems.

Quiz 8

What are the features of MEN type 2B?

Synonyms: William Pollock syndrome; Gorlin-Vickers syndrome;

Due to variation in RET proto-oncogene.

Genetic disorder characterised by multiple tumors in mouth, eyes and endocrine glands. Patients are tall and lanky with elongated face, protruding blubbery lips; benign tumors of mouth, eyes, submucosa; endocrine neoplasia (medullary carcinoma of thyroid, malignant pheochromocytoma).

Diagnosis with calcitonin (elevated) and DNA testing 9 variation in RET porto-oncogene. A variant known as "multiple mucosal neuroma syndrome" has been described without variation in RET and no malignancies.

74. Cardiomegaly

OBSERVATION

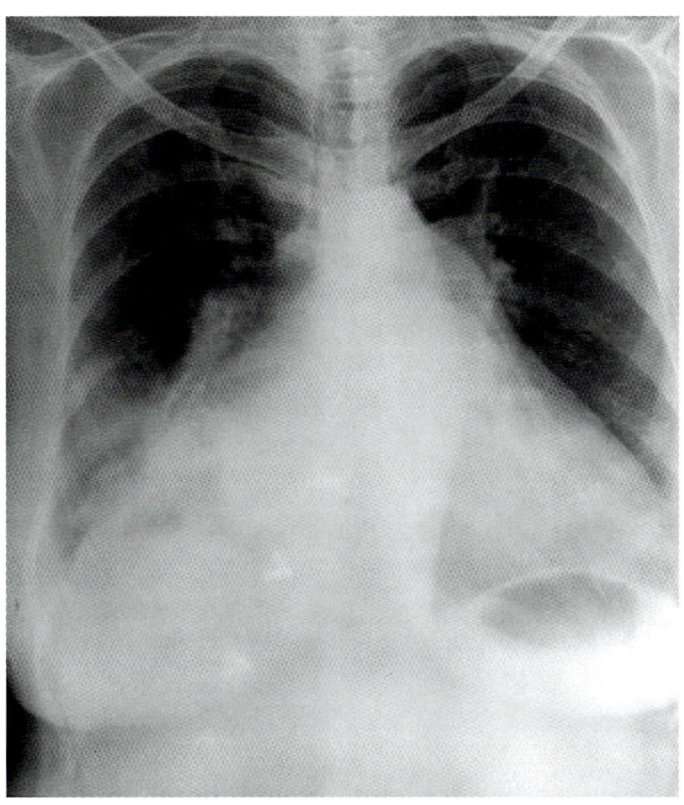

Quiz 1

What are the evidences of LA enlargement in this CXR?

a. Double atrial shadow on the right side—inner shadow is occupying the upper portion parallel to the outer shadow—indicating enlargement of the body of the left atrium.

b. Splaying of the carina at the cost of left main bronchus—also indicating the enlargement of the body of the left atrium.

c. "Straightening of the left heart border"—aortic knuckle, enlarged PA, enlarged LA (filling up the concavity between the PA and—the ventricle), and the enlarged ventricle. The part of the enlarged LA filling up the concavity is the appendage of the LA.

75. Walking Man Sign

OBSERVATION

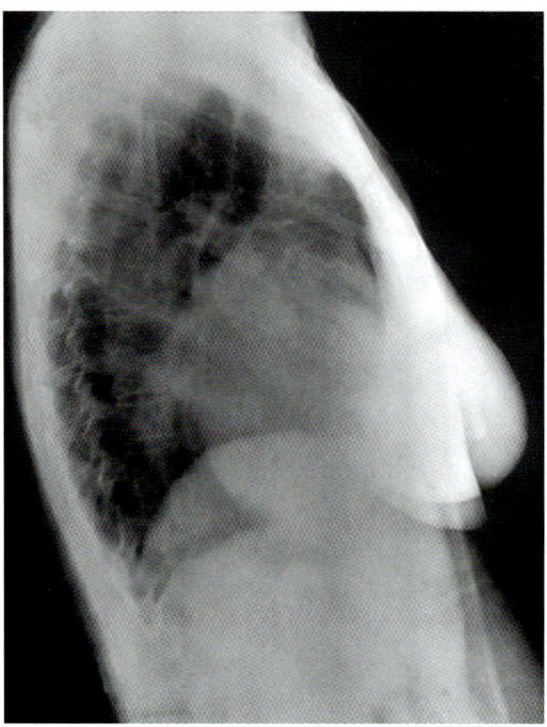

Walking man sign—the lower (left) main bronchus has been moved upwards and posteriorly compared to the upper (right) main bronchus which has remained where it was—as if the man has walked by moving his left leg.

The circular opening seen just below the tracheal air column is the right main bronchus.

The circular opening seen below that is the left main bronchus.

Quiz 1

What is the normal relationship of the right and the left main bronchi?

The upper circular shadow below the tracheal air column is due to the right main bronchus and the lower circular shadow is due to the left main bronchus—these should usually be in one vertically straight line—akin to a person standing with his two legs right and left, close together.

Quiz 2

What happens in LA enlargement?

The direction of the enlargement of the LA is posterosuperior, and the enlarged lA shifts the left main bronchus upwards and posteriorly (so the the right and the left main bronchi are no longer on one straight line). The left main bronchus instead of being alined vertically close

126

any is shifted posteriorly and superiorly as if the man standing with his right and left legs closeby has wolked moving his left leg. This is known as the walking man's sign.

The walking man's sign is positive in this patient indicating the presence of LAE.

Quiz 3

Where do you find the larger LA?

In MR > MS. This is because the MR produces both volume and pressure overload. The largest LA are seen in MR1"Giant LA".

76. Normal Vertical Alignment of the Right (Superior) and the Left (Inferior) Bronchi. No Walking Man's Sign

OBSERVATION

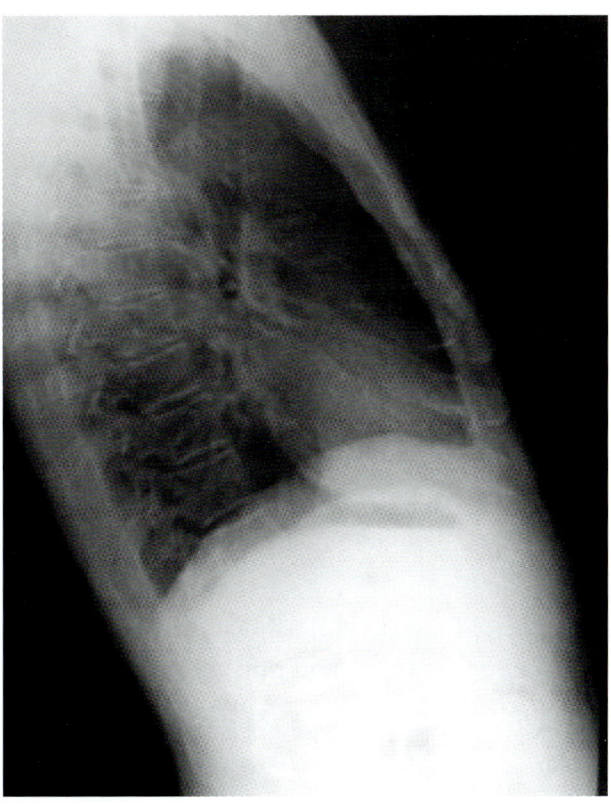

The upper circular opening seen just below the tracheal air column is the right main bronchus The lower circular opening below that is the left main bronchus.

In this lateral view, the two are normaly vertically alingned—that is to say the lower one lies just beneath the upper one in one vertical line. This is a normal lateral view. Patient does not have LA enlargement. There is no walking man's sign.

77. Gum Hyperplasia

OBSERVATION

Hyperplasia of the gums

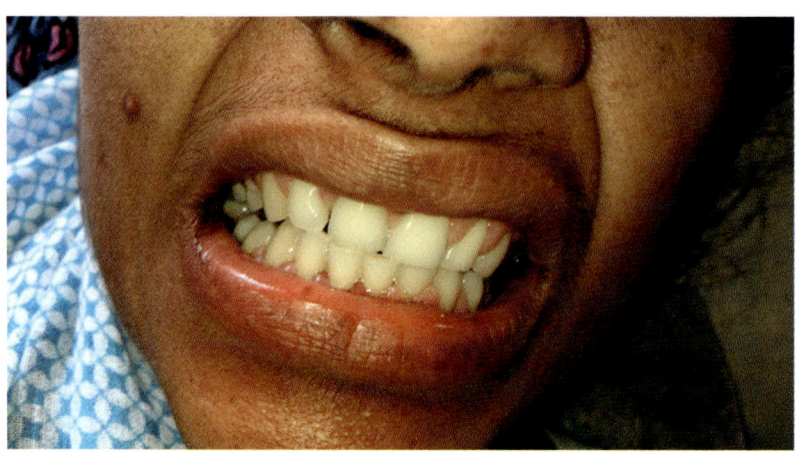

Quiz 1

What are the common causes for the hyperplasia of the gums?

a. Inflammatory
b. Drug induced
c. Systemic disorders

Quiz 2

What are the inflammatory causes?

Periodontal inflammation due to bacterial plaques which inturn is due to poor oral hygiene.

Quiz 3

Which drugs can cause it?

Anticonvulsants—phenytoin, barbiturates, ethosuximide, primidone, opiramate
Calcium channel blockers—nifedipine > amlodipine, verapamil.
Cyclosporine (tacrolimus has less gingival hypertrophy but is equally nephrotoxic)
However, the commonest drugs include—phenytoin (50%), nifidipine (30%), cyclosporine (20%).

Quiz 4

What are the systemic causes?

- Pregnancy, puberty
- Vitamin C deficiency
- Leukemias
- Granulomas—Wegener's granuloma, sarcoid, giant cell granuloma

78. Chipmunk Facies in Thalassemia

OBSERVATION

- Prominent facial bones—maxillary hypertrophy
- Prominent forehead—frontal bossing
- Depressed nasal bridge
- Malocclusion of teeth
- Mild jaundice
- "Chipmunk facies"—due to bone marrow hyperplasia

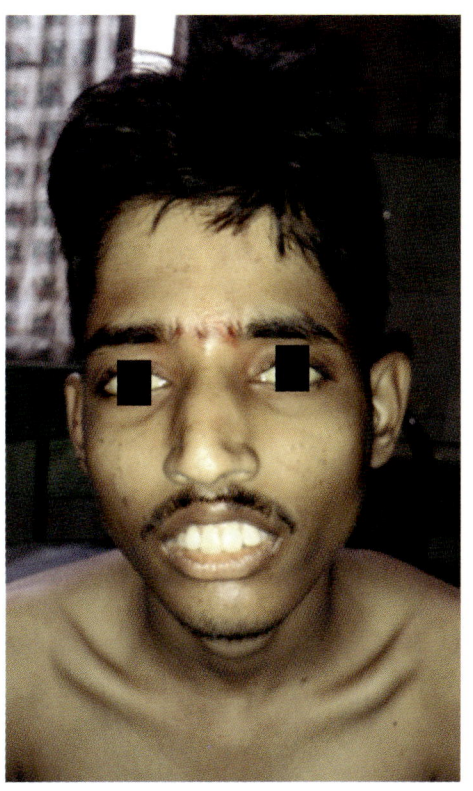

Quiz 1

What is the diagnosis?

Thalassemia

Quiz 2

What are the features?

- Anemia, failure to thrive.
- Growth retardation

- Jaundice
- Hepatosplenomegaly—extramedullary erythropoiesis
- Chipmunk facies—bone marrow hyperplasia
- Pathological fractures—cortical thinning
- Sinus and middle ear infection—due to ineffective drainage
- Folate deficiency—due to increased RBC turnover
- Hypermetabolic state—fever and wasting
- Increased absorption of iron from intestine.

Quiz 3

What are the mechanisms of these findings?

Hepatomegaly: Extramedullary erythropoiesis; hemosiderosis; hemochromatosis; transfusion related infections—hepatitis B, C, HIV; chronic active hepatitis.

Splenomegaly: Extramedullary erythropoisis; work hypertrophy (due to constant hemolysis); hypersplenism (progressive splenomegaly).

Jaundice: Hemolysis (unconjugated hyperbilirubinemia); hepatitis, transfusion, hemochromatosis; gallstones (obstructive jaundice); cholangitis.

Infections: Increased incidence—poor nutrition; increased iron stores; blocked macrophage monocyte system; hypersplenism—leukopenia; transfusion related infections.

Hemochromatosis: Pituitary deposition (short stature, delayed puberty; poor secondary sexual characters); liver cirrhosis; cardiomyopathy (cardiac hemosiderosis), CCF, sterile pericarditis, arrhythmias, heart block; pancreatic deposition' diabetes mellitus; lung—restrictive lung disease; adrenal insufficiency; hypothyroidism; hypoparathyroidism; increased susceptibility to infections (particularly Yersinia).

Bony changes: Chipmunk facies; cortical thinning; delayed pneumatization of sinuses; premature fusion of epiphyses—short stature.

Quiz 4

What are the complications?
- Growth retardation, short stature
- Delayed menarche, poor secondary sexual characters
- CCF, pericarditis
- Gallstones
- Infections
- Hypersplenism
- Cirrhosis of the liver
- Diabetes, hypoadrenalism, hypogonadism hypopituitarism; hypothyroidism
- Paraparesis (compression from paravertebral masses due to extramedullary erythropoiesis.

Quiz 5

What are the peripheral smear changes of thalassemia?
- RBC—microcytic hypochromic RBCs with anisocytosis and poikilocytosis; target cells; nucleated RBCs; leptocytes; basophilic stippling; tear drop cells.

- Cytoplasmic inclusion bodies in alpha thalssemia
- Post-splenectomy—Howell Jolly bodies, Heinz bodies
- Increased reticulocyte count (up to 10%).

Quiz 6

What are the features of thalassemia minor?
- Asymptomatic
- Resemble iron deficiency anemia not responding well to iron therapy
- No skeletal abnormalities, no splenomegaly
- Normal life expectancy

Quiz 7

What are the lab tests in thalassemia?
- Serum bilirubin—increase in total and indirect bilirubin
- Haptoglobin and hemopexin—depleted
- Increased serum iron, ferritin; transferrin—saturated
- Bone marrow—hyperplastic erythropoiesis
- RBC folate—decreased; Free RBC porphyrin—normal
- Serum uric acid—raised
- Urine—hemosiderinuria

Quiz 8

What is the type of hemoglobin in thalassemia?
- Major—mainly Hb F; no Hb A; variable Hb A2
- Minor—mainly Hb A; Hb <10%; Hb F variable

Quiz 9

What are the radiological clues?
Earliest changes: Small bones of hand—rectangular appearance = cortical thinning + medullary expansion.
Skull: Hair on end appearance/crew cut appearence = widened diploid spaces + increased porosity.
Maxilla overgrown with prominent malar eminences = delayed pneumatization of sinuses.

Quiz 10

How do you assess iron overload?
Serum ferritin; urinary iron excretion
Liver biopsy; tissue iron estimation
Biopsies: Liver/endomyocardium
ECHO, myocardial MRI

Quiz 11

What are the principles of management of thalassemia?
a. *Blood transfusions:* Hb to be maintained. 10 (hypertransfusion); >12 (supertransfusion); If transfusions are given regularly—no splenomegaly, no facial changes

b. *Neocytes transfusion:* Mean cell age 30 days; more expensive (X2 to X4)

c. *Iron chelation therapy:* Desferrioxamine 30–60 mg/kg/day—IV/SC infusion pum pover 12 hours/day for 5–6 days/week; start when ferritin >1000 ng/week; best > 5 years; Vit C 200 mg on the day of chelation to increase DFO induced urinary excretion of iron.

Quiz 12

What are the adverse effects of iron chelation therapy—desferrixamine?

Heart—arrhythmias; Ears—SM hearing loss; Eyes—cataract; bone dysplasia—growth retardation; Rapid infusion—histamine related reaction (hypotension, erythema, pruritus); infection, sepsis.

Quiz 13

Is oral chelation therapy available?

Oral chelator: Deferiprone has been used. %0–100 mg/kg/day; Patient >2-year-old
Adverse effects: Reversible arthropathy, drug induced lupus, agranulocytosis
Other oral chelators
Desferrithiocine; pyridoxine hydrazine; ICL 670—removes iron from myocardial cells.

Quiz 14

What are the indications for splenectomy?

Massive splenomegaly
Progressively increasing transfusion requirements of paced PBCs (>180–200 ml/kg/yr)

Quiz 15

Any modality of therapy with a cure in mind?

Bone marrow transplantation—hepatomegaly (>2 cm; portal fibrosis; iron overload; older age)

Quiz 16

Add a note on newer therapies

a. Gene manipulation and replacement:
   Remove beta gene and replace gamma gene
   Increase gamma gene synthesis with 5-azacytidine
b. Hb F augmentation
   Hydeoxyurea; myeleran; butyrate derivatives; erythropoietin in thalassemia intermedia.

Quiz 17

What is the role of supportive therapies?

1. Tea—thebaine, tannins—Chelate iron
2. Vit C—increases iron excretion
3. Reduce oral intake of iron—reduce meat, liver, spinach
4. Folate supplementation—1 mg/day
5. Psychological support; gentic counselling
6. Hormones used—GH, estrogen, progesterone; levothyroxine
7. CCF treatment.

79. Bilateral Ptosis with Dysphagia

ANATOMY OF PTOSIS

Elevation of upper eyelid is facilitated by muscles levator palpebrae superioris (supplied by III nerve) and Müller's muscle (supplied by the sympathetic). LPS helps in opening the upper eyelid and Müller's muscle helps in overelevation in the excited patient.

OBSERVATION

1. Bilateral ptosis
2. Ryle's tube in place suggesting dysphagia

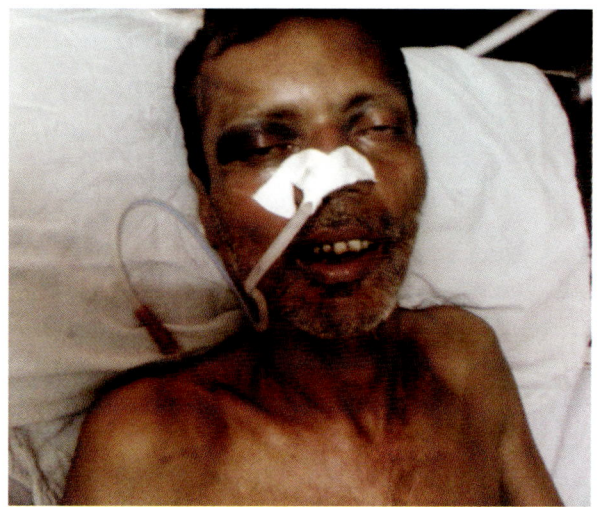

80. Differential Diagnosis of Bilateral Ptosis with Dysphagia

1. Botulism
2. OPMD—oculopharyngeal muscular dystrophy
3. Myotonic dystrophy
4. Mitochondrial myopathies—Kearns-Sayre (chronic progressive external ophthalmoplegia) with MNGIE syndrome—mitochondrial myopathy + PN + GI disease + encephalopathy.
5. Myasthenia gravis—dysphagia seen in elderly patients.

81. Appraoch to Bilateral Acquired Ptosis

1. RRF on biopsy + chronic progressive ophthalmoplegia + retinitis pigmentosa + cardiac defects → Kearns-Sayre's syndrome (mitochondrial myopathy).

2. Cataract + frontal balding → myotonic dystrophy.
3. Tongue atrophy + neurologic dystrophy → oculopharyngeal muscular dystrophy.
4. History of eating pre-cooked food + vomiting + dysphagia + muscle weakness + diplopia—botulism.

82. Bell's Phenomenon

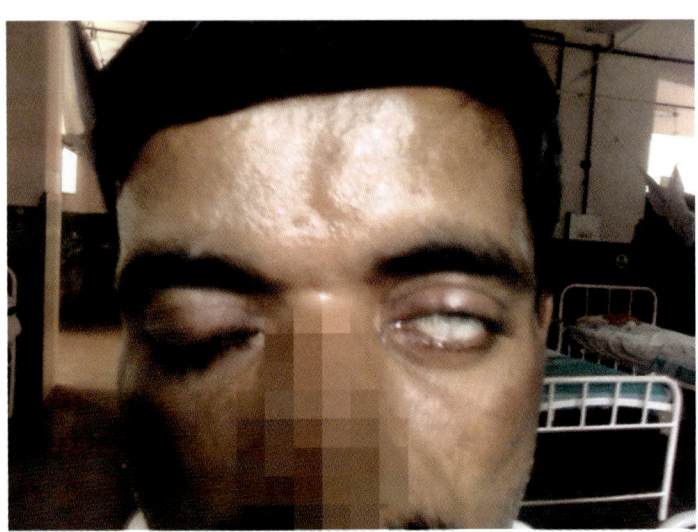

Quiz 1

What is Bell's phenomenon?

Voluntary attempt to close the eye is associated with upward and outward movement of the eyeball.

This is a palpebral—oculogyric reflex.

Quiz 2

Whom is it named after?

Anatomist and physiologist Charles Bell.

Quiz 3

What is it?

A defensive mechanism while blinking or when threatened—an attempt to touch the person's cornea. This defense reflex is seen in 75% people.

Quiz 4

When is it observed?

It becomes visible when there is weakness of orbicularis oculi—usually due to facial nerve palsy.

Quiz 5

What are the details of Bell's phenomenon?

Three stages of eye movements (in voluntary eye closure—Hiraoka):

a. Initial phase—eye moves upwards and inwards.
b. Static phase—eye remains upwards and inwards for a few seconds and is abducted in tight lid closure.
c. Final phase—eye moves down from its upwards and inwards position.

Quiz 6

What are the diagnostic uses of Bell's phenomenon in diagnosis and management of systemic and ocular disorders?

a. Supranuclear palsy (Steel-Richardson syndrome, Parinaud's syndrome and double elevator palsy)—voluntary elevation of eyes not possible but can do so on attempting the Bell's phenomenon. In nuclear and infranuclear gaze palsies, the Bell's phenomenon is normal.
b. To distinguish inferior rectus infiltration (no upward eye movement is possible in attempted Bell's phenomenon due to tethering of the inferior rectus) in thyroid eye disease from a supranuclear palsy (upward movement is possible).
c. To demonstrate superior rectus weakness in myasthenia gravis
d. Myotonia of the Bell's phenomenon in myotonia dystrophica.
e. It may be the only demonstrable abnormality in some neurologic conditions—some cases of idiopathic epilepsy, tuberous sclerosis, Sturge-Weber syndrome.

Quiz 7

What is the mechanism of the Bell's phenomenon?

- It involves the brainstem pathways between the 7th nerve nucleus in the pons and the third nerve nuclear complex in the rostral midbrain.
- Intact Bell's phenomenon indicates normal functioning of brainstem pathways, nuclear cell complex for upward gaze, associated motor pathways and extraocular muscles.
- Upward gaze palsy is usually due to a supranuclear defect.

Quiz 8

What is exaggerated Bell's phenomenon?

Synonyms: Inverse jaw winking, ocular stammer, Marcus-Gunn phenomenon
Involuntary drooping of the eyelid while eating (and sometimes while talking).
May indicate a survival of associated movement in fishes.

83. Brachydactyly of 4th Toe Bilateral

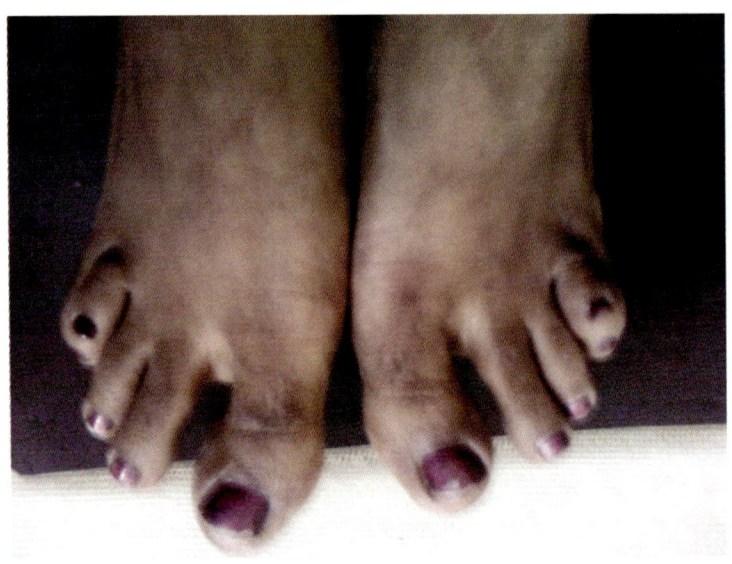

Quiz 1

What is the observation?

Isolated short 4th metatarsal resulting in short 4th toe.

Quiz 2

What type of brachydactyly is it?

Type E

It resembles pseudopseudohypoparathyroidism (PPHP) but lacks some features—no mental retardation, no cataracts, no ectopic calcification. However, it is indistinguishable for PHP-PPHP.

Quiz 3

How do you diagnose it at the bedside?

By a positive metacarpal sign—when a pencil is used to connect the heads of 3rd and 5th metatarsals the 4th metatarsal seems to recede (this test is basically described for the metacarpals using a closed fist).

AD inderitance.

Quiz 4

What is brachymetatarsus IV?

Unilateral or bilateral short metatarsals resulting in unilateral or bilateral short 4th toe—seen in northern India. AD inheritance.

Quiz 5

What is Kirner deformity?

Deformed little toe.

Quiz 6

What is Sugarman deformity?

Defromed non-articulating great toe with small other toe.

Quiz 7

Mention some other syndromes with brachydactyly

a. Rainbow syndrome—with hypogenitalism (mesomelia, gingival hyperplasia)
b. Rubinstein-Taybi syndrome—short broad thumbs
c. Du Pan syndrome complex brachydactyly
d. Temtamy preaxial brachydactyly syndrome—preaxial brachydactyly (hands and feet) with hyperphalangism.

Quiz 8

Give list of conditions causing brachydactyly finger/toewise

a. Great toe/thumb—Rubinstein-Taybi syndrome
b. 4th digit—brachydactyly E (E1) syndrome, brachymetatarsus IV syndrome
c. 4th and 5th metatarsals—PHP (pseudohypoparathyroidism), PPHP (pseudopseudohypo-parathyroidism)
d. Non-articulating great toe, all metatarsals short—Sugarman brachydactyly
e. Brachydactyly, absent fibula—Du Pan syndrome.

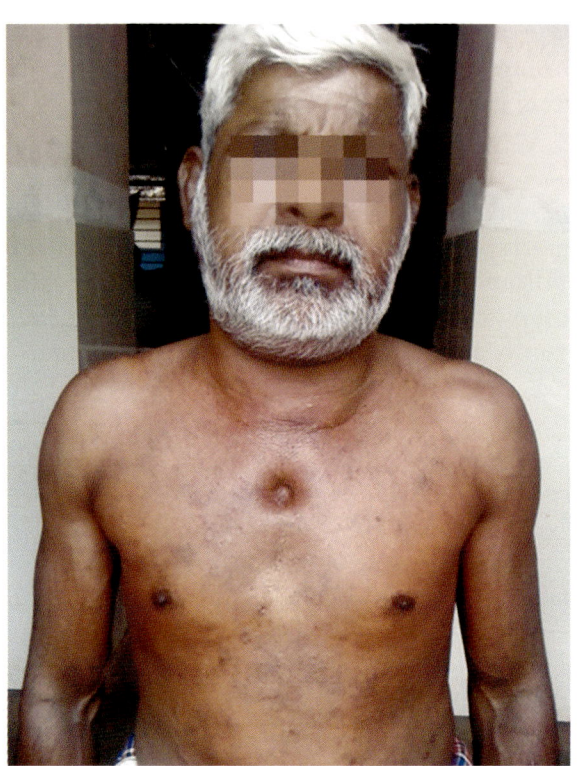

Quiz 1

What is the observation?

A depressed lesion on the sternum.

Quiz 2

What are the possible causes?

a. Infections—Staph, Pseudomonas

b. Osteomyelitis—sterna lesion and collection around it

c. TB—sternal lesion in the middle and collection around it.

d. Syphilitic gumma

e. Tumors—chondrosarcoma, mets (breast, lung ca) plasmacytoma, lymphoma

f. Congenital deformities—pectus excavatum—much larger depression

g. Poland's syndrome—sternal deformity, absence of pectoral muscles (pectoralis major and minor). Malformed ribs (2nd to 5th).

h. FB granuloma—infected mesh or wire.

85. Autoamputation of Fingers

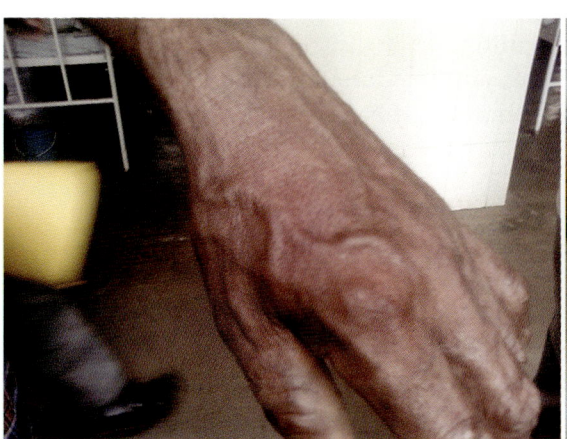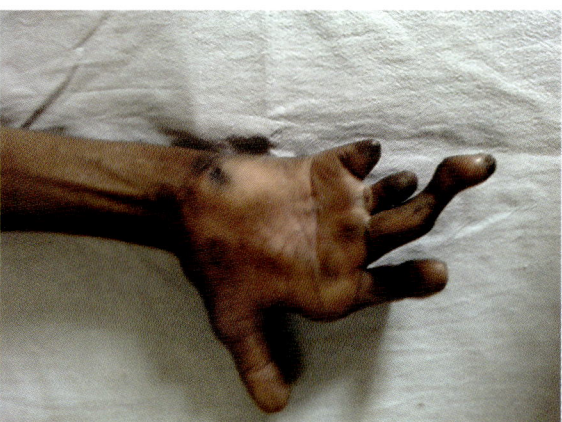

Quiz 1

What are your observations?

Autoamputation of fingers

Wasting of thenar, hypothenar and intrinsic muscles of the hand

Deformities of fingers

Trophic ulers.

Quiz 2

What are the differential diagnosis for autoamputation of fingers?

a. Vascular—vasculitis, cryoglobulinemias, peripheral vascular diseases, Kawasaki disease

b. Neurologic—leprosy, syringomyelia

c. Traumatic.

Quiz 3

What are the differential diagnosis for trophic ulcers?

a. Ischemic—arterial

b. Neuropathic

c. Vasculitis.

Quiz 4

What are the distinguishing features of the trophic ulcers due to various causes?

a. Ischemic history of intermittent claudication;

Hair loss, trophic changes in the nails, reduced local temperature; pallor, elevation pallor dependent rubor, absent pulses;

Ulcer—irregular edge, necrotic base, punched out with sharp demarcation.

b. Neuropathic ulcers history of numbness, pallor, burning, loss of sensation in the foot, DM; Evidence of neuropathy, may be associated with underlying bone involvement (osteomyelitis). Ulcers on pressure points—plantar aspects of 1st and 5th metatarsals. Punched out edge, tendon, fascia, joint capsule or bone may be involved.

c. Vasculitis—history of CTD
  • Associated with fat necrosis, chronic panniculitis
  • More likely to have ulcers in the pretibial area and the dorsum of the foot
  • Multiple, extremely painful ulcers, inflamed indurated base (pathergy phenomenon).

Quiz 5

What are the differential diagnosis of wasting of small muscles of the hand?
Classification:

a. Due to lesions involving the AH cells at T1 level
  • Cord compression, polio, meningovascular syphilis,
  • MND, Charcot-Marie-Tooth disease; syringomyelia, Friedrich's ataxia
b. T1 root lesions: Cervical spondylosis, Dumb bell neurofibroma
c. Brachial plexus (lower cord): Cervical rib, Pancoast's tumor, Klumpke's paralysis
d. Peripheral nerve lesions: Median nerve lesions, ulnar nerve lesions
e. Others: RA.

86. Depigmentation of the Tongue

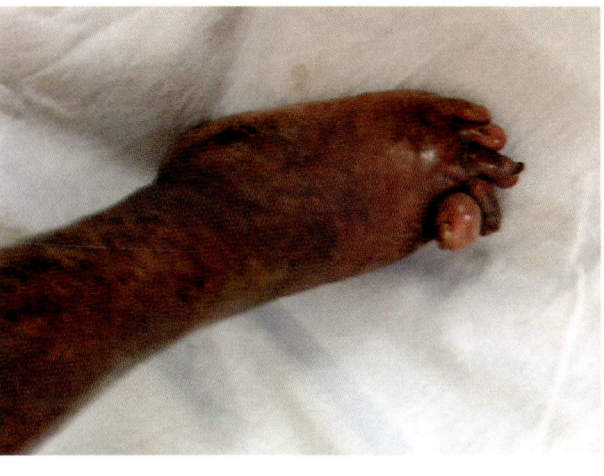 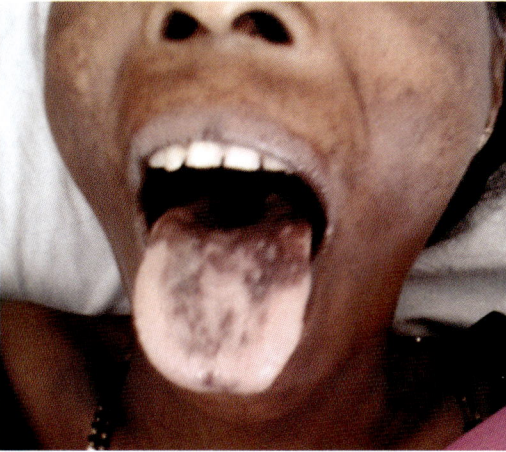

Quiz 1

What is the observation?
Patchy depigmentation of the tongue.

Quiz 2

What are the differential diagnoses?
a. Vitiligo.

b. Candidiasis—temperory white lesions seen on tongue/throat which bleed on attempted removal; seen in immunosuppressed (DM, cancer, anticancer chemotherapy, corticosteroid therapy, HIV, malnutrition) individuals.
c. Tertiary syphilis.
d. Hairy leukoplakia—EB virus associated; may antedate HIV/AIDS.
e. Leukoplakia—premalignant—white patches not removable by scraping.

Quiz 3

Name various lesions producing variously coloured tongue
a. Black hairy tongue—ovewrgrowth of filiform papillae + black colour due to tobacco/chromogenic bacteria/aspergillus niger.
   Associated factors—tobacco, smoking/chewing
   Amphotericin B may help in aspergillus niger infection
b. Blue tongue in central cyanosis
   5 gm/dl of recuced haemoglobin is required in blood to produce cyanosis.
c. Blue tongue in methaemoglobinaemia—acquired due to exposure to drugs (phenacetin), aromatic amino/nitro-compounds; aniline dyes (laundry marks, waxed crayons).
   1.2–2 gm/dl of methaemoglobin in blood is required to produce the blue color.
d. Pale tongue—in anemia.
   May be associated with hemangioma on tongue/lips in Sturge-Weber syndrome.
e. Red colored tongue—geographical tongue/erythema migrans.
   Clean and smooth tongue with loss of papillae which regrow again and therefore appear to migrate. Also called erythema migrans.
f. Magenta colored tongue/glossitis—vitamin B_2 deficiency—riboflavin deficiency.
g. Telangiectasia of the tongue—Sturge-Weber syndrome.

87. Single Transverse Palmar Crease

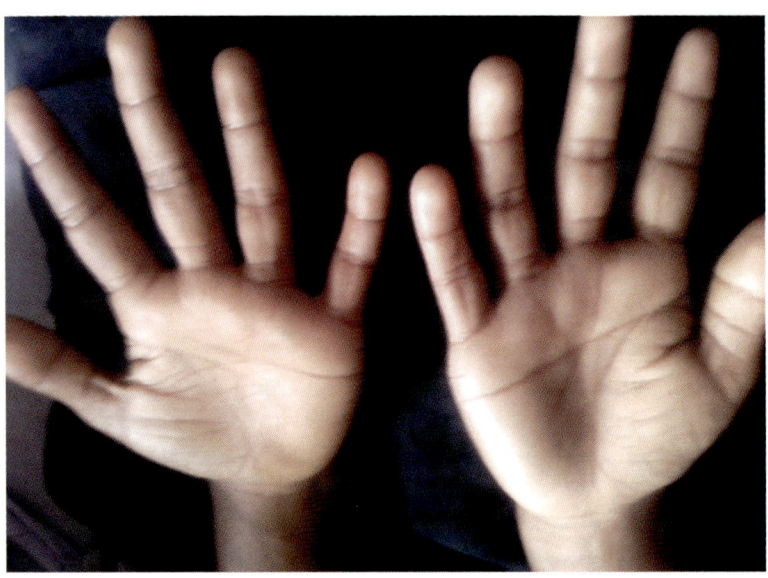

Quiz 1

What is your observation?

A single palmar transverse crease extending from the radial to the ulnar side better seen on the right palm.

Quiz 2

What are the conditions associated with single palmar crease?

a. Genetic/chromosomal abnormalities—Down syndrome (Chr 21), cri du chat syndrome (Chr 5), Noonan (Chr 12), Patau (13), Edwards 18), Aarskog-Scott syndrome (X linked R), aberrations on Chr 9.
b. Fetal alcohol syndrome.

Quiz 3

What is the difference between Simian crease and Sydney line?

- Simian crease—an extended proximal palmar crease—a single crease formed by complete fusion of 2 creases. Proximal transverse crease is long and distal transverse crease is absent.
- Sydney line/Sydney crease—A Sydney line exists when a proximal transverse crease extends beyond the middle axis of the 5th finger towards the ulnar border of the palm (Purvis-Smith, 1972)—2 palmar creases still exist separately but the proximal crease is extraordinarily long.
- Suwon crease—partial fusion of two creases (unlike the simian crease where the fusion is complete).

Quiz 4

What are the chromosomal abnormalities encountered in Down syndrome?
a. Trisomy 21 (47, +21) 94%; seen with increasing maternal age
b. Robertsonian translocation involving chromosome 21. 3–4%. Not related to the maternal age.
c. Trisomy 21 mosaicism-2–3%.

Quiz 5

What are the hand changes in Down syndrome?
a. Short broad hands
b. Cleinodactyly of the 5th finger
c. Single transverse palmar crease
d. Increased gap between the great and the second toes
e. Hyperflexibility of joints.

Quiz 6

What are the hematologic disorders seen in Down syndrome?
Increased risk of leukemia—ALL, AML, transient leukemia (exclusively involving NB with spontaneous resolution in 3 monthes. Polycythemia with hypoglycemia in the newborn.

Quiz 7

What are the endocrine disorders in Down syndrome?
Hypothyroidism, type I DM, infertility (in males only related to impaired spermatogenesis, obesity.

Quiz 8

What are the Hall criteria for diagnosis?
Flat face, upward slanting of palpebral fissures, small dysplastic ears, joint hyperflexibility, short neck with redundant skin, short 5th digit with cleinodactyly, single transverse palmar crease, pelvic dysplasia, hypotonia.

Quiz 9

What are the cuases for death?
a. Congenital HD
b. Leukemia
c. Dementia (Alzheimer)
d. Hypothyroidism
e. Infections—pneumonia
Survival is better for males and blacks.

88. Depigmentation of Lips, Nose, Face

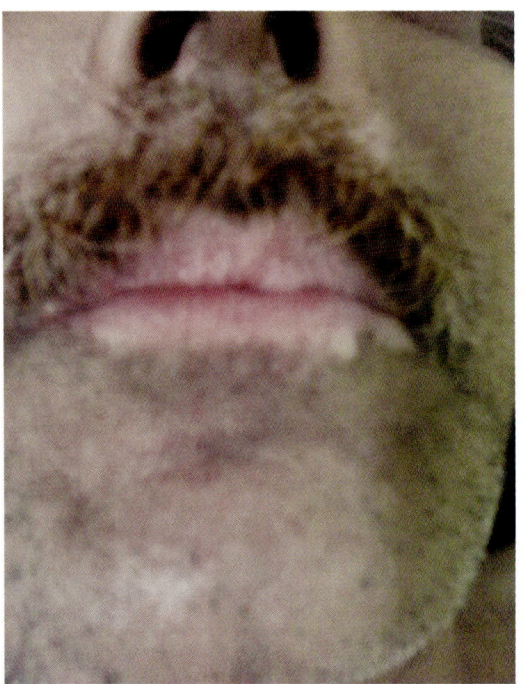

Quiz 1

What are the observations?

Depigmentation of lips, mouth, nose chin facial hair.

Quiz 2

What are the differential diagnoses?

a. Those due to retarded formation of melanin
   Vitiligo, oculocutaneous albinism, pityriasis alba, nevus depigmentosus

b. Those due to complete absence of melanin due to absence of melanocytes, piebaldism, leukoderma of SLE, vitiligo.

Quiz 3

What are the mechanisms of destruction of melanocytes in vitiligo?

a. The patients inherit a set of 3 vitiligo genes.

b. Melanocytes are abnormal and have fastidious growth characteristics and undergo apoptosis easily.

c. The environmental factors that affect the melanocytes and enhance the process of destruction of the susceptible melanocytes.

Quiz 4

What is the concept of cutaneous troika?

Epidermis consists of 3 main cells—epidermal cells, Langerhans' cells and melanocytes that work in unison like a troika, hence the name. If some function of troika is missing, depigmentation of skin can result.

Quiz 5

What are the conditions associated with vitiligo?

a. Endocrine
b. Polyendocrine deficiency syndrome—type 2 Schmidt's syndrome vitiligo + hypothyroidism, diabetes, hypogonadism. (Type 1—no vitiligo—hypoparathyroidism, hypogonadism, pernicious anemia, chronic candidiasis, chronic active hepatitis, alopecia.)
c. Autoimmune—vitiligo associated with Graves' disease, Hashimoto's thyroiditis, RA, chronic urticaria.
d. Rare syndromes associated with vitiligo
    Allezzandrini syndrome—vitiligo, poliosis, unilateral pigmentary retinitis, hyperacusis.
    Vogt-Koyanagi-Harada syndrome—idiopathic bilateral anterior uveitis, dysacusis, poliosis, alopecia.

APS—autoimmune polyglandular syndrome

APS 3—autoimmune thyroiditis + another autoimmune disease

APS 3B + C—thyroiditis, vitiligo, autoimmune gastritis

APS 3C—autoimmune thyroiditis, vitiligo, alopecia.

Quiz 6

What conditions resemble vitiligo?

a. Pityriasis alba
b. Eczema (in young)
c. Tenia versicolor.

Quiz 7

What is poliosis?

Decrease or absence of melanin in head hair, eyebrows, eyelashes.

89. Vitiligo Involving the Hand

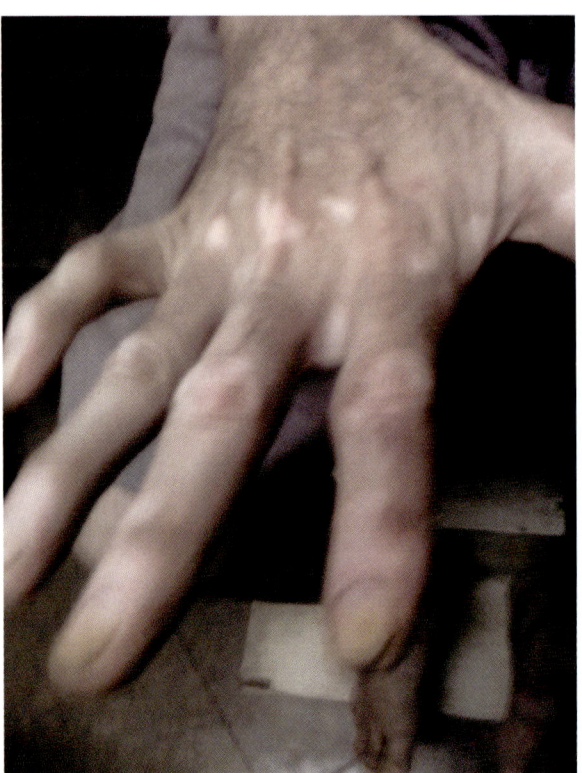

Quiz 1

What are the types of vitiligo?

Non-segmental vitiligo (NSV)—symmetrical patches of depigmentation

a. Generalized-wide and randomly distributed
b. Universal—depigmentation involving most of the body
c. Focal—scattered—seen in children
d. Acrofacial—fingers and periorificial
e. Mucosal—involving the mucus membranes

Segmental—unilateral—involves the skin associated with the dorsal roots of the spine. Static in course. Not associated with autoimmune diseases. Highly amenable to treatment—topical steroids.

90. Ascites with Gynecomastia and Spider Nevus

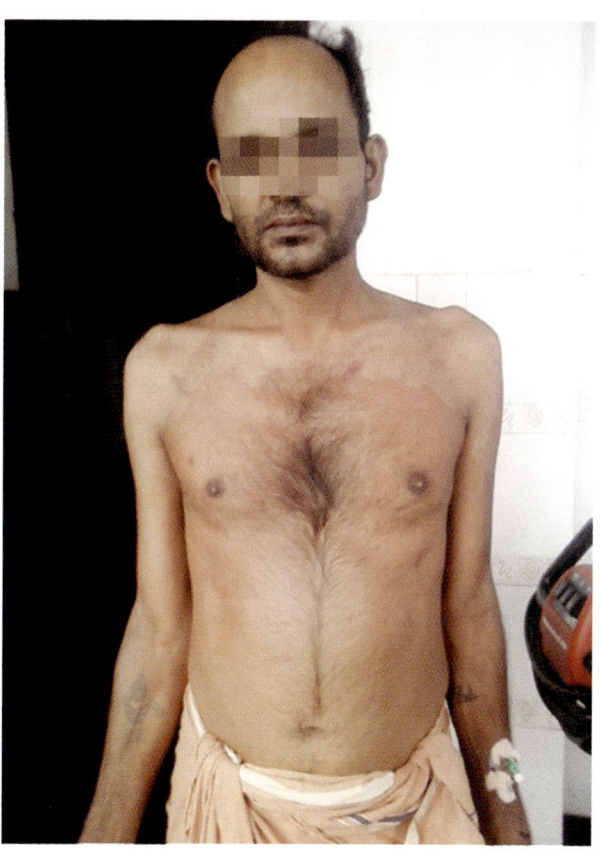

Quiz 1

What is the most likely cause of ascites in this patient?

Liver involvement—observe gynecomastia and spider nevus and a tattoo on the right forearm.

Quiz 2

Ascites can result from involvement of which organs?

a. Liver—chronic disease-cirrhosis; acute disease—alcoholic hepatitis, fulminent hepatitis; hepatoma

b. Lung—cor pulmonale

c. Kidney—nephrotic syndrome, nephritis

d. Heart—CCF, pericarditis

e. Peritoneum—peritonitis, tuberculosis, malignancy

f. Pancreas—pancreatitis (increased serum amylase).

Quiz 3

What are the causes of ascites based on peritoneal involvement?

a. Diseases involving the peritoneum
   Infections: Bacterial, fungal, parasitic
   - Neoplasms
   - Vasculitis
   - Familial Mediterranean fever
   - Endometriosis
   - "Starch peritonitis"
   - Whipple's disease

b. Diseases not involving the peritoneum
   - Cirrhosis of the liver
   - CHF
   - Budd-Chiari syndrome
   - Neoplasms
   - Protein losing enteropathy
   - Myxedema
   - Ovarian diseases
   - Pancreatic diseases
   - Chylous effusion.

Quiz 4

How do you classify ascites based on the nature of fluid?

a. Exudate (cloudy fluid, protein >2.5, SG >1020)
   - Infection including peritonitis
   - Vasculitis
   - Neoplasms

b. Transudate (clear fluid, protein <2.5)
   - Cirrhosis
   - Nephrotic syndrome
   - Hypoproteinemia (hypoalbuminemia).

Quiz 5

What is ascites albumin gradient (SAAG)?

SAAG + (albumin concentration in serum)—(albumin concentration in ascitic fluid)

a. High = High gradient >1.1
   - Due to portal hypertension ' Increased hydrostatic pressure
   - CCF
   - Budd-Chiari syndrome

b. Low = Low gradient <1.1
   - TB
   - Pancreatitis
   - Nephrotic syndrome
   - Neoplasm
   - Vasculitis.

Quiz 6

What are the causes of abdominal distension?

a. **6 Fs** of abdominal distension—Fat, Fluid, Flatus, Feces, Fetus,"Fatal" tumors

b. Depending on location

Generalized—symmetric: 6 Fs

Asymmetric:

RUQ—liver, gallbladder

Epigastrium—stomach, liver (left lobe)

LUQ—spleen

Around umbilicus—SI obstruction

LLQ—colon

Lumbar—kidney

Pelvis—suprapubic—pregnancy, urinary bladder.

Quiz 7

What are the clues to identify the etiology of abdominal distension associated with ascites?

a. Generalized distension + flanks full + umbilicus everted = ascites

b. Generalized distension + generalized obesity + umbilicus inverted = obesity

c. Generalized abdominal distension + visible peristalsis = intestinal obstruction

d. Ascites, jaundice, spider naevi, gynecomastia, testicular atrophy, splenomegaly = cirrhosis
Dupuytren's contracture + parotid enlargement = alcoholic etiology

e. Ascites, breathlessness, edema, cardiomegaly, P. rub, arrhythmias, pulsatile liver, right sided pleural effusion = cardiac etiology

f. Ascites, anasarca, history of dialysis = renal cause

g. Ascites, abdominal pain, Cullen's sign, Grey-Turner's sign, Fox's sign = acute pancreatitis

h. Ascites, peritoneal involvement = TB peritonitis, carcinomatosis

i. Ascites, dilated veins, hum over the veins = Crueilhier-Baumgarten syndrome

j. Ascites, pelvic mass, altered menstrual cycles = ovarian tumor

k. Ascites, Virchow's lymph node = secondaries

l. Ascites, tenderness, rebound tenderness = peritonitis (spontaneous or secondary)/ hemoperitoneum.

m. Ascites, varicose veins on leg, varicose veins on back, dilated veins on the abdominal wall draining upwards = IVC obstruction.

n. Ascites, anasarca, poor muscles, Beau's lines on nails = hypoproteinemia.

o. Ascites out of proportion to peripheral edema = intra-abdominal cause—abdominal TB, malignancy, TB, CHF, cirrhosis, nephrotic syndrome, constrictive pericarditis, cor pulmonale.

91. Imminent Carpal Spasm in Left Hand

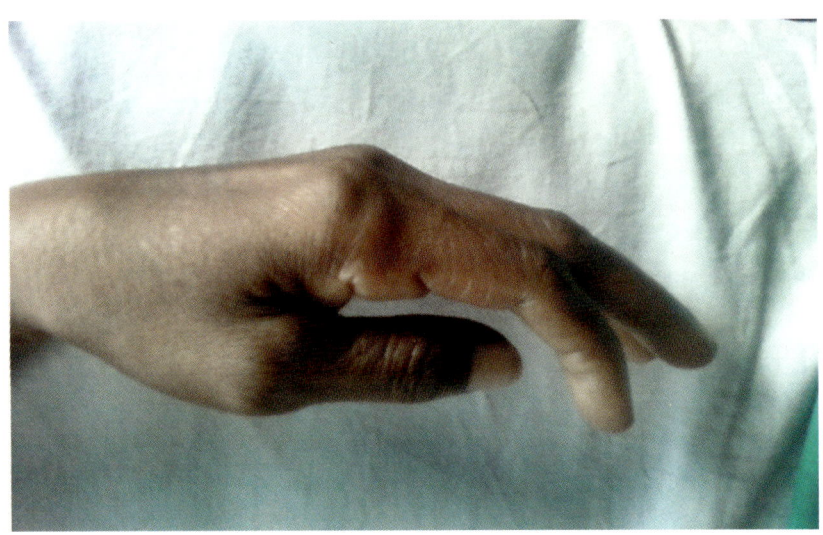

Quiz 1

What are the observations?

Imminent carpal spasm in the left hand—suggestive of tetany.

Quiz 2

What may be the other complaints?

Spasms and cramps of hands and feet.
Tingling of hands, face, and feet.

Quiz 3

What may be the lab findings?

a. Low serum calcium
b. High serum phosphorus
c. Low PTH
d. Prolongerd QT interval on ECG.

Quiz 4

What are the causes?

a. Neck surgery—particularly thyroid surgery
b. Radiation
c. Hemochromatosis
d. Repeated blood transfusions.

Quiz 5

What are the signs of latent tetany?

a. Tapping over the facial nerve anterior to the ear causes local muscle twitching—Chvostek's sign.

b. Insufflation of the sphygmomanometer over the forearm precipitates an intense carpal spasm—Trousseau's sign.

c. Tapping of the skin at the angle of the mouth produces protrusion of the lips—Escherich's sign.

d. Pressure on the inner aspect of biceps results in closure of hand—Hochsinger's sign.

e. Application of hot/cold irritants result in hyperaesthesia/spasm—Kashida's thermic sign.

f. Tapping of the peroneal nerve just below the head of the fibula results in dorsal flexion and abduction of the foot—peroneal sign.

g. Tapping of the tongue results in its depression with a concave dorsum—Schultze's sign.

Quiz 6

What are the causes of hypocalcemia?

Parathyroid removal, vitamin D deficiency, shock, sepsis, acute pancreatitis, hypomagnesemia, alkalosis, phosphate overload, CRF, hypoalbuminemia, tumor lysis syndrome drugs—dilantin, phenobarbitone, theophylline.

Quiz 7

What are the conditions seen in autoimmune polyglandular syndrome (APS) type I?

Chronic mucocutaneous candidiasis (80%), primary adrenal insufficiency, primary hypogonadism, DM1, autoimmune gastritis, alopecia, vitiligo, autoimmune hepatitis, thyroid diseasae, teeth enamel hypoplasia, nail dystrophy.

Hypoparathyroidism is not a feature of APS II and hence hypocalcemia does not occur. APS II consists of type I DM, autoimmune thyroid disease, pernicious anemia, primary gonadal failure, adrenal insufficiency.

APS type II without adrenal insufficiency is sometimes called type III APS, though some consider it as early type II APS.

Quiz 8

What are the differential diagnoses for APS?

Other conditions where autoimmune and non-immune endocrinopathies can exist together include:

a. POEMS syndrome: Polyneuropathy, organomegaly, endocrinopathy, M protein, skin changes.

b. Wolfram's syndrome

c. Kearns-Sayre syndrome

d. Chromosomal abnormalities—trisomy 21, Turner's syndrome

e. Thymomas.

92. Black Nail—Right Thumb

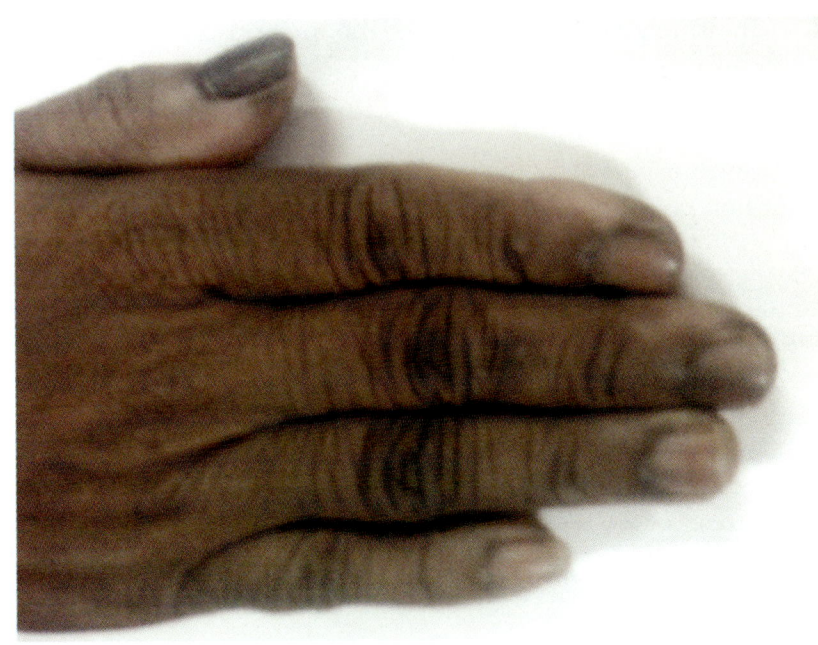

Quiz 1

What are your observations?

Nail of the right thumb is black.

Quiz 2

What are the causes?

- Trichophyton fungal infection
- Bleeding under the nail due to trauma.

93. Ascites with Umbilical Hernia

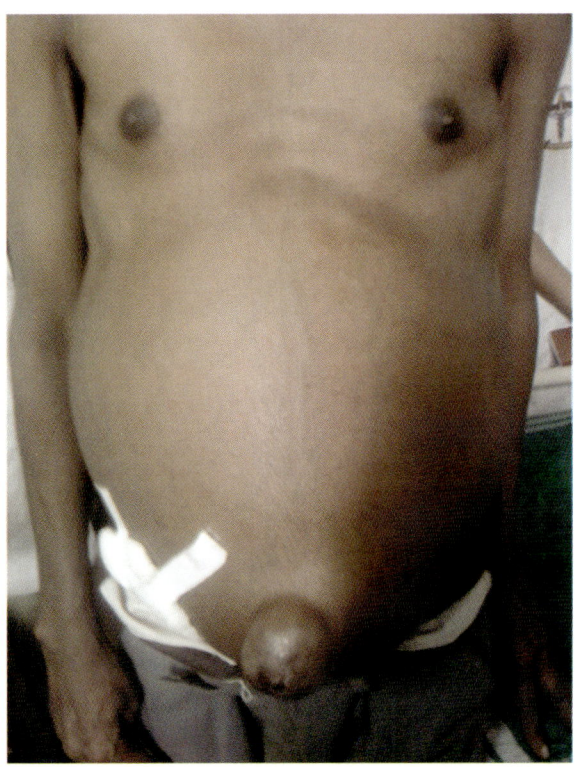

Quiz 1

What is ascites?

Ascites is abnormal accumulation of fluid in the peritoneal cavity—an intraperitoneal expansion of the increased extracellular fluid space.

Quiz 2

How do you suspect and diagnose ascites?

a. Distended abdomen
b. Full flanks
c. Everted umbilicus
   These are the hallmarks of ascites.
d. Puddle sign
e. Dipping sign
f. Fluid thrill
g. Shifting dullness
h. Percussion finding: Fluid thrill, shifting dullness, flank dullness.

Quiz 3

What is the minimum amount of fluid needed for these tests to be positive?

a. Fluid thrill—most reliable—2000 ml
b. Shifting dullness (must be bilateral)—1000 ml
c. Puddle sign—120 ml
d. Ultrasound 30—100 ml.

Quiz 4

What is the importance of percussion of central abdomen?

a. Dull note on both sides + resonant central percussion = Ascites
b. Dull note on both sides + Dull central abdomen = Tense ascites (large volume), organomegaly, short mesentery.

Quiz 5

What are the clinical features of ascites?

a. Asymptomatic—minimal fluid
b. Symptomatic—anorexia, nausea, early satiety, heartburn, abdominal pain, respiratory distress.
c. Associated features—penile edema, scrotal edema, vulval edema, pleural effusion.

Quiz 6

What are the complications of ascites?

a. Three hernias—inguinal, umbilical, diaphragmatic
b. Associated with cirrhosis—SBP—spontaneous/secondary bacterial peritonitis
   Hepatorenal syndrome, hepatopulmonary syndrome, varicial bleed, respiratory distress, IVC obstruction, renal failure.
c. Related to treatment—azotemia, hypokalemia, hepatic encephalopathy, shock—rapid tapping in the absence of peripheral edema.

Quiz 7

What is the approach to a patient with ascites?

a. Acute onset—Budd-Chiari syndrome, RHF, decompensted cirrhosis, panceatic ascites
b. Gradual onset—chronic Budd-Chiari, decompensated cirrhosis, TB, Ca, hypoalbuminemia, NS, RHF, hypothyroidism, constrictive pericarditis
c. Associated pedal edema-
   Abdominal distention precedes and is > pedal edema = Intra-abdominal cause—cirrhosis, NS, RF, RHF, constrictive pericarditis, cor pulmonale, abdominal TB, Budd-Chiari
   Pedal edema precedes and is > abdominal distension = General cause—hypoproteinemia.
d. Associarted with jaundice—Budd-Chiari, cirrhosis (decompensated, primary biliary), hepatoma, CHF.
e. Associated hematemesis/melana—portal hypertension
f. Associated fever
   Low grade—TB, Ca
   High grade—peritonitis—spontaneous/secondary bacterial peritonitis.

g. Associated abdominal pain

Diffuse, mild—peritonitis, TB

Right hypochondrium—RHF, hepatoma, Budd-Chiari

h. Associated facial puffiness, coarse hair, hoarse voice, cold intolerance, constipation—hypothyroidism

i. Associated puffiness of face, massive proteinuria—nephrotic syndrome

j. Associated ortopnoea—RHF

k. Associated orthodeoxia—hepatorenal syndrome

l. Associated fatigue—anemia, hypoproteinemia

m. Associated with wasting—cirrhosis, disseminated TB

n. Associated with elevated JVP-RHF (not in Budd-Chiari syndrome)

o. Associated non-pitting pedal edema—myxoedema

p. Associated Virchow's node—GI malignancy

q. Associated stigmata of chronic liver disease—cirrrhosis

r. Associated spider naevi, jaundice—hepatitis, cirrhosis

s. Associated cutaneous markers of internal malignancy.

94. Skin Lesions and Mucosal Lesions

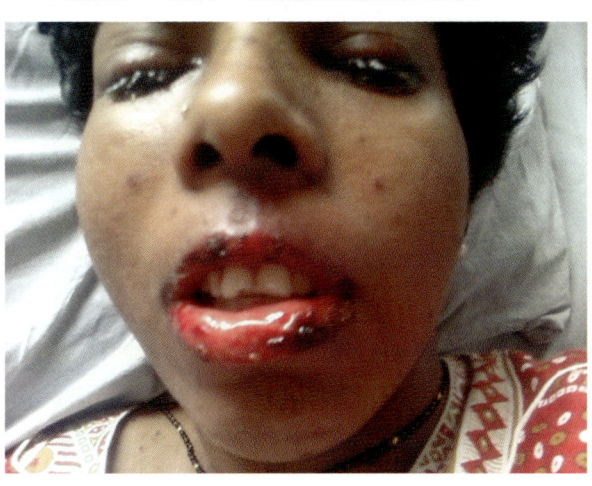

Quiz 1

What do you see?

Generalized erythema of the mucosa with enanthemata and exanthemata.

Quiz 2

What are the possibilities?

Differential diagnosis of lesions simultaneously involving the oral mucosa and the skin:

a. Intravascular blood lesions:

  • Varix-blue > red; blanch on pressure (except when thrombosed)

- Hemangioma—congenital, thickened
- Immunocompromiswd patient—purple, raised/flat.

b. Extravascular blood lesions: History of injury; do not blanch
- Hematoma—thickened, firm
- Echymoses—not thickened
- Petichiae—small pinpoint, multiple, not thickened.

c. Candidiasis: Diffuse mucosal erythema, painful ulcers, no LN, immunosuppression +

d. Autoimmune: Mucosal ulcers with submucosal erythema

e. Viral: Herpes simplex—oral vesicles with erythematous gingival, LN common

f. Erythema multiforme: Sudden onset of oral and labial mucosal lesions. Recurrence after varying periods of remission; iris/target lesions on palm/sole. LN rare.

95. Hemorrhagic Lesions on the Palm

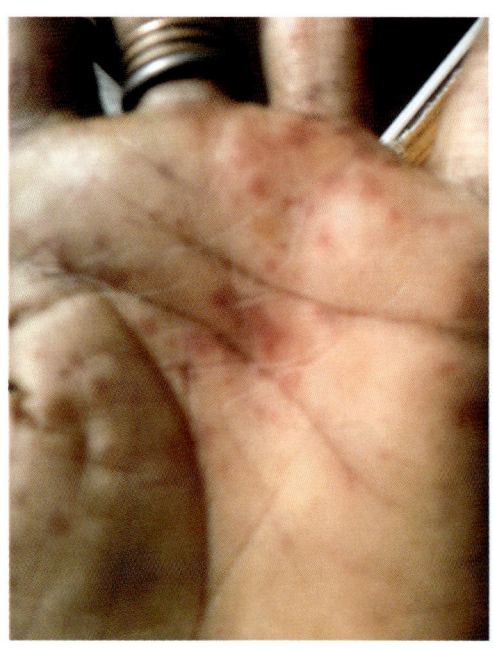

Quiz 1

What are the observations?

Hemorrhagic lesions on the palm. The patient also had hemorrhagic lesions on the sole.

Quiz 2

What are the conditions where these may be seen?

a. Hand-foot and mouth disease
- Usually seen in children <6 years—buccal and lip ulcers
- Caused by Coxsackie A and B viruses.

- Stomatitis + vesicular rash on hands, foot; nail dystrophy; onychomadesis (nail shedding).
- Caused by coxsackie A5, 6, 10, 16; B 5. Also by enterovirus 7.
- Chemotherapy induced HFM disease—fluorouracil, capecitabine, liposomal doxorubicin.
- Painful palms progressing to blistering desquamative ulcerations.
- Treated with pyridoxine 200 mg. OD, cool packs.

b. Janeway lesions—seen in infective endocarditis
- Hemorrhagic macular/nodular lesions—microabscesses in dermis (not epidermis)
- Embolic lesions—painless.
- So named after Prof. Theodore Caldwell Janeway.

c. Osler's nodes—painful, red lesions seen on hands and feet
- Seen in infective endocarditis.
- Immunologic in origin—resulting inflammatory response results in redness and pain
- So named after William Osler.

d. Henoch-Schönlein purpura (HSP)
- Palpable purpura, arthralgia/arthritis, abdominal pain, GI bleeds, nephritis.
- Ig A mediated small vessel vasculitis predominantly seen in children.

e. Drug reactions.

96. Hemorrhagic Lesions on Soles

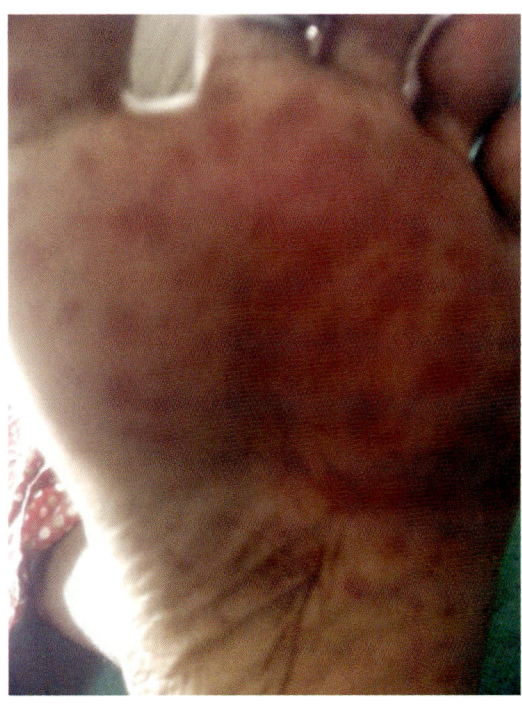

For further discussion and differential diagnosis refer above—hemorrhagic lesions on palms.

97. Polydactyly

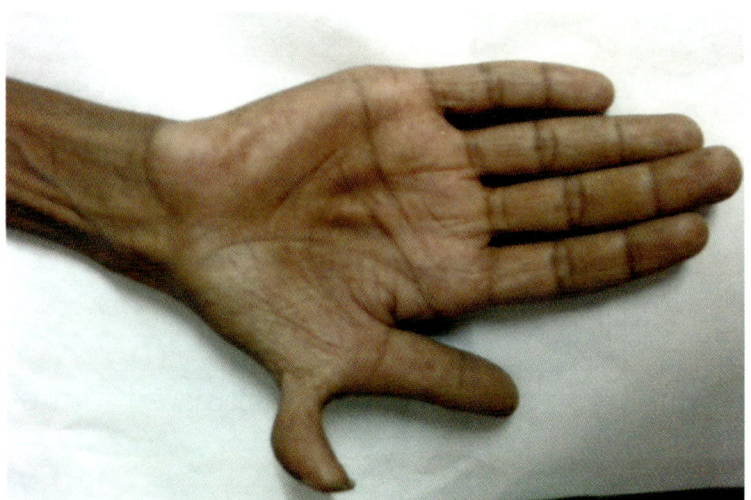

Quiz 1

What are the observations?
- Supernumerary thumb—preaxial polydactyly
- Supernumerary little finger—postaxial polydactyly
- Oligodactyly—fewer fingers or toes.

Quiz 2

Which is the commonest finger involved in plydactyly?
Little finger > thumb > middle fingers (very rare).

Quiz 3

What is preaxial polydactyly?
Radial polydactyly—extra digit (s) near the thumb.

Quiz 4

What is "triphalangeal thumb"?
- A finger liked first digit with 3 phalanges (instead of the normal 2).
- Thumb is apposable with a pincar like action in mammals.

Quiz 5

What are the types of TPT?
a. Apposable—sporadic inheritance; longer thumb; X-ray resembles 5 fingered hand.
b. Non-apposable—AD inheritance; shorter thumb; X-ray—intercalated 2nd phalanx, ulnar deviation of the distal phalanx.

Quiz 6

What are the conditions associated with polydactyly?

- Polydactyly + congenital HD
- Laurence moon biedl syndrome (AR)—obesity, mental retardation, retinitis pigmentosa, renal abnormalities.
- Ellis-van Crevelt syndrome (AR)
- Radial polydactyly
- Holt-Oram syndrome (AD) (*synonym*: Cardiomelic syndrome, hand heart syndrome); cardiac defects (OS ASD, PDA, VSD, transposition of great vessels;
- Limb disorders—UL only involed (LL never); right > left; thumb—absent/rudimentary/TPT
- Polydactyly syndactyly syndrome (AD)
- Carpenter syndrome
- Fanconi pancytopenia
- TPT + polydactyly can have "Delta phalanx"—Triangular shaped middle phalanx.
- Can also have polydactyly of foot
- Bilateral preaxial polydactyly can be associated with hypoplasia of sterna head of pectoralis major, winging of the scapula, pectus excavatum, pigmented nevi.

Quiz 7

What are the conditions associated with megalodactyly of thumb?

- Neurofibromatosis (AD)
- Hemangioma (sporadic)
- Isolated (sporadic).

Quiz 8

What are the conditions associated with the broad thumb?

- Alpert syndrome (AD)
- Pfeiffer syndrome (AD)
- Taybi syndrome (X linked)
- Rubinstein-Taybi syndrome (multifactorial).

Quiz 9

What are the conditions associated with short/hypoplastic thumb?

- Bracydactyly (types A and B—both AD)
- Holt-Oram syndrome (AD)
- Fanconi pancytopenia (AR)
- Cornelia de Lange syndrome (unknown)
- VATER syndrome (unknown)
- Aminopterin embryopathy.

Quiz 10

What are the conditions where the thumb is absent?

- Holt-Oram syndrome (AD)
- Fanconi pancytopenia (AR)

- Chromosomal abons—ring D, 13 q-, trisomy 18
- Thalidomide embryopathy.

Quiz 11

What are the conditions associated with TPT (tri-phalangeal thumb)?

- TPT + radial hypoplasia—Holt-Oram syndrome, Fanconi pancytopenia, sensorineural hearing impairent (all AR).
- Schmitt—TPT, radial hypoplasia, hypospadias, maxillary diastema.
- Weidmann—TPT, radial hypoplasia, recurrent bleeding (factor X def, N platelets), SN hearing loss
- TPT, radial hypoplasia, thrombocytopathy
- TPT + bone marrow dysfunction-Diamond-Blackfan syndrome (AR/AD); Fanconi pancytopenia (AR); Radial hypoplasia, thrombocytopenia, SN hearing impairment
- TPT + CHD—Aase syndrome (AR); Holt-Oram syndrome (AD).
- TPT + Agenesis of lung + CHD-
- Manouvrier—lung agenesis, CHD, hand abnormalities.
- Mardini, Nyhan—lung agnesis, CHD, TPT, polydactyly (pre-axial), hemivertebrae
- TPT + anorectal malformations
- Towen's syndrome—TPT, anorectal anomalies, abnormal auricles, urinary tract anomalies, anomalies of thumb, deafness.
- IVIC syndrome
- TPT + maternal teratogen exposure
- Phenytoin thalidomide, aminopterin
- TPT + onychodystrophy
- Goodman—osteodystrophy, missing phalanges, bulbous fingertips, deafness, dystrophic fingernails, AD
- Qazi—TPT, distal osteodystrophy, deafness, mental retardation, seizures.

Quiz 12

What is "Lobster clawfoot and -hand"?

"Split foot" deformity—associated with EEC syndrome—ectodermal dysplasia, cleft lip and palate.

Genesis of the Lobster claw deformity—Lobster clawhand/-foot, preaxial polydactyly, syndactyly share the common pathogenesis—failure of the apical ectodermal ridge to separate. (Apical epidermal ridge coordinates the proximal to distal sequence of limb development.)

Quiz 13

What are the rare conditions associated with TPT?

- TPT + absent pectoral muscles
- TPT + abnormal sternum.

- TPT (bilateral) hypomelanosis of ITO/Itos syndromes—Motlled skin hypopigmentation, mental retardation, seizures, microcephaly, cleinodactyly. Sporadic.
- TPT + Lacrimoauricular dento digital syndrome—Hollister-cleinodactyly. AD.
- TPT + Langer-Giedeon syndrome—trichorhinopharyngeal syndrome type 2
- TPT + Acrofacial dysostosis. AD
- Trisomy 13 associated with polydactyly with TPT.
- TPT + teratogen exposure
- Hydantoin—fetal hydantoin syndrome
- TPT, limb defects, cleft lip and palate, congenital HD, unusual facies, mental retardation. Limb defects—hypoplastic nails and distal phalanges, finger-like thumbs, increased fingertip arches, big toe.
- Thalidomide syndrome—seen in 1960–62 Sweden, Germany. Exposure to thalidomide in 4 to 6 weeks of pregnancy. Hypoplasia/aplasia of thumb; Amelia (one or more limbs—even tetra-amelia), hearing loss, blindness, hemangioma, duodenal stenosis, atresia.

Quiz 14

Why does thumb have only 2 phalanges while all the other fingers have 3?

a. Galen's theory—metacarpal bone of the thumb is actually the proximal phalanx (proposed in 2 nd century AD).
b. Alternate theory—the middle and distal phalanges arise separately from two different ossification centres which later fuse to form the distal phalanx. This theory probably explains the fact that the shortest digit has the longest distal phalanx. TPT indicates failure of fusion of the middle and distal phalanges to form a single distal phalanx.
c. Joachimsthal hypothesis—advanced in 1900, said that the absent thumb (in some cases where the thumb is absent) is replaced with an extra digit—clinically and radiologically resembling the little finger, which is mistaken for thumb with TPT.
d. TPT is the result of incomplete duplication of the thumb (Lapidus and Guidotti hypothesis).

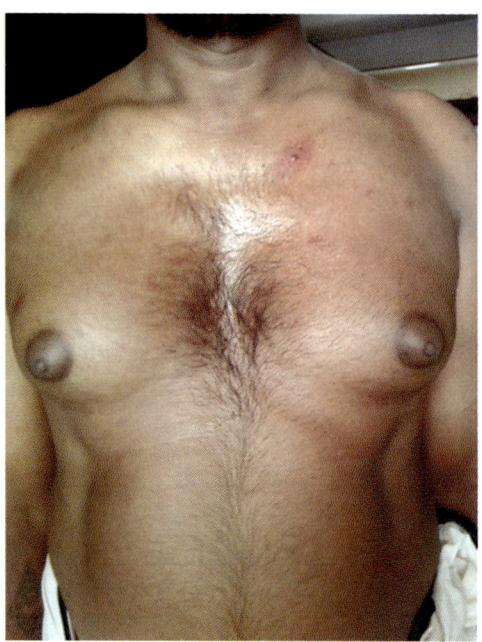

Quiz 1

What are your observations?
- Bilateral gynecomastia
- Spider nevi
- Reduced chest hair
- Abdominal distention possibly due to ascites
- Tattoo on the right forearm.

Quiz 2

How do you connect these findings?
- Tattooing done unhygienically could have resulted in viral hepatitis B/C. In due course, this could jave resulted in a complication—cirrhosis of the liver producing ascites and spider nevi.
- Apparently reduced chest hair is probably least significant as the glimpe of facial hair shows a good amount of it!

Quiz 3

What is gynecomastia? What are the physiological causes?
- Benign proliferation of male breast glandular tissue.
- Physiological asymptomatic gynecomastia has a trimodal age distribution—neonatal, pubertal, elderly males.

Cases in Medicine

Quiz 4

What is the commonest mechanism of gynecomastia?

Imbalance between estrogen action and androgen action at the level of breat tissue.

a. Elevated estrogen/HCG/estrogen precursors

Elevated estrogen/estrogen precursors secreted by certain tumors: Leydig cell tumors, Sertoli cell tumors

Extragonadal conversion of androgens to estrogen—obesity

HCG producing tumors

Estrogen precursor producing tumors—adrenal cortical tumors.

b. Reduced levels of testosterone

Gonadal failure

Primary: Klienfelter's, Mumps, orchitis, astration

Androgen resistance syndrome

Altered levels of sex hormone binding globulin—hyperthyroidism, chronic liver disease, medications—spironolactone

Faults in androgen receptors

Genetic defects

Blocked by medications—bicalutamide used in prostate cancer.

c. Activation of estrogen receptors by environmental exposure, e.g. puberty (with a normal estrogen—androgen ratio).

Quiz 5

What are the important points in the history?

a. Age of onset and duration

b. Local symptoms—mass/enlargement, tenderness, nipple discharge

c. Medications, supplements, illicit drugs, anabolic steroids

d. Stress/distress resulting in coping with it.

Quiz 6

What are the important points in the physical examination?

a. Height, weight

b. Signs of feminization—Tanner stage

c. Stigmata of liver disease

d. Breast, overlying skin

e. Regional lymph nodes

f. Thyroid

g. Scrotum—varicocele, testicular tumor

Quiz 7

Which drugs cause gynecomastia and how?

a. Hormones: Androgens, anabolic steroids, estrogens, estrgen agonists, hCG

b. Anti-androgens, inhibitors of androgen synthesis—bicalutamide, flutamide, cyproterone, GRH agonis (leuprolide, goserelin)

c. Antimicrobials—metronidazole, ketaconazole, INH, minocycline

d. Antiulcer medications—cimetidine, ranitidine, omeprazole

e. Chemotherapeutic agents—methotrexate, alkylating agents, vinca alkaloids

f. Cardiovascular drugs—digoxin, ACE inhibitors, spironolactone

g. Others—anti-retroviral therapy, metoclopramide, phenytoin.

Quiz 8

What are the systemic causes of gynecomastia?

a. Hypogonadism—Klinefelter's syndrome, hypopituitarism

b. Endocrine—Leydig/Sertoli cell tumor (Peutz-Jeghers syndrome)
  - Choriocardinoma secreting HCG, adrenocortical tumors
  - Prolactinomas (pituitary gland tumors)
  - Bronchogenic carcinoma with ectopic hormone secretion
  - Hyperthyroidism—influences sex hormone binding globulin

c. Kidney failure
  - Dialysis related hypogonadism
  - Uremia associated hypogonadism—testosterone is suppressed by elevated urea

d. Liver failure and cirrhosis
  - Reduced estrogen metabolism
  - Alcohol may hinder testosterone synthesis
  - Phytoestrogens present in alcohol may have a contributory role

e. Malnutrition
  - Hormonal imbalance leading to reduced testosterone levels (reduced secretion) and elevated estrogen (reduced degradation by the liver)
  - Malabsorption—cystic fibrosis, ulcerative colitis.

Quiz 9

What are the differential diagnosis for gynecomastia?

a. Pseudogynecomastia—only has breast prominence due to excessive adepose tissue (as against hypertrophy of breast glandular tissue, ches adipose tissue and skin in true gynecomastia)

b. Male breast cancer

c. Other conditions—mastitis, sebaceous cyst, sebaceous cyst, dermoid cyst, metastasis

d. Mimics—muscle hypertrophy of pectoralis.

Quiz 10

What are the investigations available for diagnosing the cause of gynecomastia?

a. Mammography—differential diagnosis bening from maligmancy

b. LFT—liver related causes

c. RFT—kidney related causes

d. Hormonal studies—testosterone, estrogen, prolactin, LH, hCG assays
  - Reduced testosterone + increased LH = Primary hypogonadism
  - Reduced testosterone + reduced LH = Secondary hypogonadism
  - Increased HCG + U/S showing testicular germ cell tumor
  - Increased hCG + normal scrotal U/S—extragonadal germ cell tumors—brochogenic, hepatogenic, renal; non-trophoblastic germ cell tumors.

- Increased prolactin +/− reduced testosterone, +/− reduced testosterone +/− normal or low LH-MRI may show → pituitary adenoma/empty sella/mass panhypopituitarism
- Increased estrogen + normal/low LH—testicular U/S-Mass—Sertoli ell/Leydig cell tumor
- Testicular U/S normal + abdominal CT abnormal—abdominal neoplasm
- Testicular U/S normal + abdominal CT normal → increased aromatase activity—obesity, adrenal or liver disese/thyrotoxicosis; exogenous estrogen intake.

99. Partial Hanging—Healing Stage

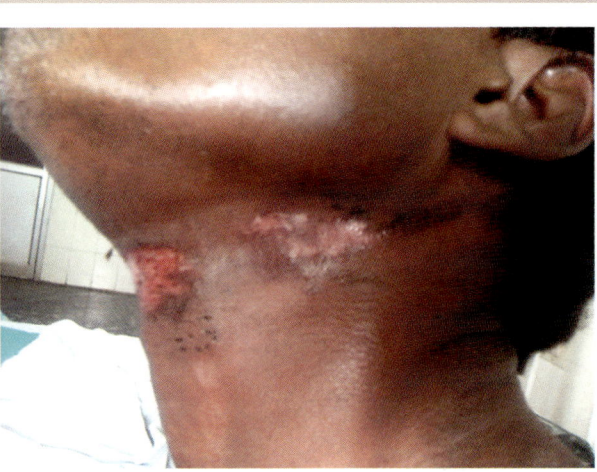 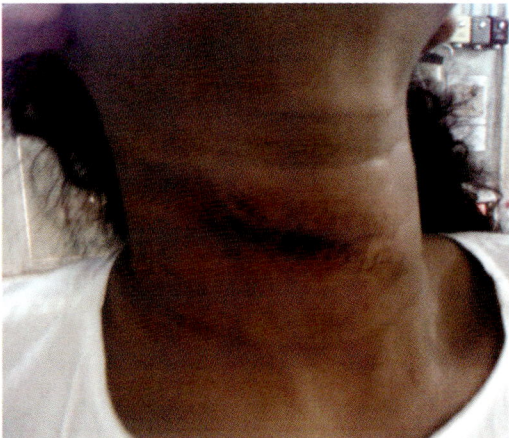

Quiz 1

What are the observations?

Ligature marks and evidence of partial hanging.

Quiz 2

What are the effets of hanging by the neck?

a. Carotid artery closure → cerebral ischemia
b. Jugular veins closure → congestion
c. Carotid sinus reflex mechanically stimulated → bradycardia, death
d. Cervical frature—breaking of the neck"Hangman's fracture—bilateral fractures of the pars interarticularis of the C2 vertebra → spinal cord injury, decapitation
e. Tardieu spots—petechiae—face and eyes
f. Caynosis
g. Protrusion of the tongue
h. Airway closure
i. Death erection
j. Hypoxia b, f, g are signs of hypoxia.
   Clenched teeth and protrusion of the tongue are indicate hanging but are not specific to it.

Quiz 3

What are the other types of hanging?

a. Inverted hanging—Jewish method—hanging by the legs

b. Hanaging by the ribs—hanged by hook and the chain till slow and painful death

Quiz 4

How do you distinguish suicidal from homicidal hanging?

Hyoid bone compassion indicates murder by choking.

Quiz 5

What is the importance of ligature mark and the knot?

Typical ligature mark is seen on the occipital region or the chin. Atypical knot mark can be seen left > right side.

Course if the ligature mark is decided by the knot. Interrupted ligature mark above the thyroid cartilage is diagnostic of hanging.

100. Botulism

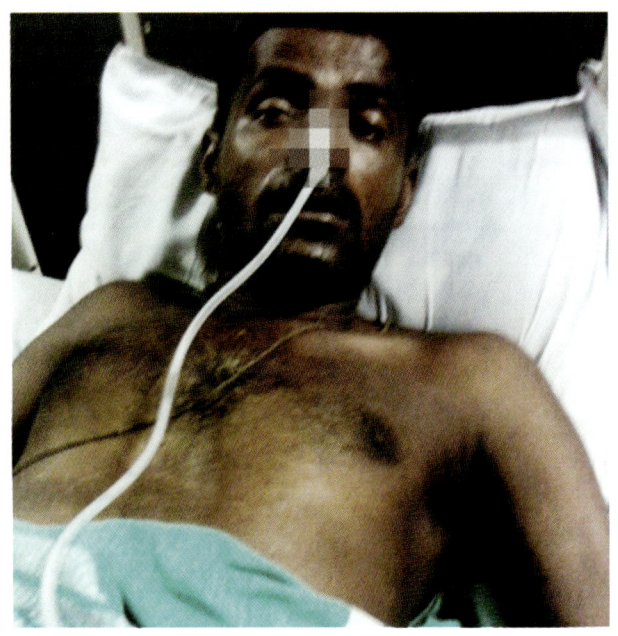

Quiz 1

What are the observations?

a. Patient looks ill

b. Ptosis—bilateral

c. Dysphagia/muscle weakness—indicated by the Ryle's tube.

Quiz 2

How do you distinguish weakness, fatigue and asthenia?
- Weakness of muscles is associated with some loss of function—proximal/distal.
- Fatigue indicates inability to continue performing a task after multiple repetitions.
- Asthenia is a sense of weakness or exhusion in the absence of muscle weakness.

Quiz 3

What are the possibilities?
Differential diagnosis muscle weakness + ptosis + dysphagia
a. Stroke
b. Myesthenia
c. Cobra bite-mimcs acute myasthenia; due to neurotoxin
d. Botulism—food poisoning with vomiting, proximal muscle weakness, diplopia, dysphagia
e. Dermatomyositis—proximal muscles involved, Gottron's papules, heliotrope rashes, ILD
f. PM—proximal muscles, elevated ANA, ILD
   Inclusion body myositis—distal muscles (forearm and hand), dysphagia—unlikely
g. Myotonic dystrophy—type 1—proximal muscles, baldness, cataract, MD
h. Infections—Lyme disease, rabies
i. Hyperthyroidism—proximal and bulbar muscles can be involved. Periodic paralysis may have a role.

Quiz 4

What is the mechanism of action of botulinum toxin?
There are 7 immunlogically disatinct types of botulinum toxins—A, B, C1, D, E, F, G.
a. A heavy chain and a light chain is bound by a disulfide bridge. Heavy chain binds to its specific neuronal *ecto* acceptor resulting in membrane translocation and endocytosis by intracellular synaptic vesicles. The light chain of A and E cleaves SNAP 25-which inhibits presynaptic membrane protein required for fusion of neurotransmitter containing vesicles. B, D, and F cleave VAMP (vesicle-associated membrane protein).
   C cleaves syntaxin.
   Analgesic effect on sensory system—partly due to block of acetyl choline—multiple antinociceptive mechanisms exist—making the BT usable in many painful disorders—musculoskeletal, neurologic, pelvic, perineal, osteoarticular, headache.
b. Effect on afferent limb BoNT A
c. Blocks neurotransmitter release at sympathetic and parasympathetic autonomic nervous systems.

Quiz 5

What is botulism?
Food poisoning is the result of eating food contaminated with *Clostridium botulinum* spores. Originally thought to be from sausages—the word botulism is derived from German for sausages.

Toxins A, B, and F are proteolytic and digest the meat with putrify meat with smell. Some types of B, C, D, E F are not proteolytic, do not digest meat and, therefore, have no smell.

Quiz 6

What are the types of botulism?

a. Food borne
b. Wound botulism
c. Infant botulism.

Quiz 7

What are the clinical features of botulism?

Clinical features of botulism include:

a. Ptosis
b. Diplopia
c. Dysphagia
d. Muscle fatigue, weakness in adults; Floppy baby syndrome in infants due to blocking at NMJ, flaccid paralysis. Honey could be the source.
e. Respiratory muscle fatigue, paralysis, respiratory failure
f. ANS—dry mouth, throat, postural hypotension, constipation.

Quiz 8

What are causes of death in botulism?

Causes of death: Paralysis of respiratory muscles—respiratory arrest, respiratory failure.

Quiz 9

What are the complications of botulism?

a. Prolonged fatigue
b. Prolonged muscle weakness
c. Breathlessness
d. Respiratory failure which may need ventilator.

What are the various roles botulism toxin can play?

a. Food poisoning
b. Bioterrorism
c. Treatment of cosmetic disorders—wrinkles
d. Treatment of painful conditions—muscle pain
e. Treatment of strabismus
f. Treatment of excessive of underarm sweating
g. Treatment of conditions characterized by abnormal muscle contractions—Torticollis, achalasia, spasmodic dysphonia, strabismus, oromandibular dystonia, cervical dystonia, strabismus.

101. Rashes on the Trunk

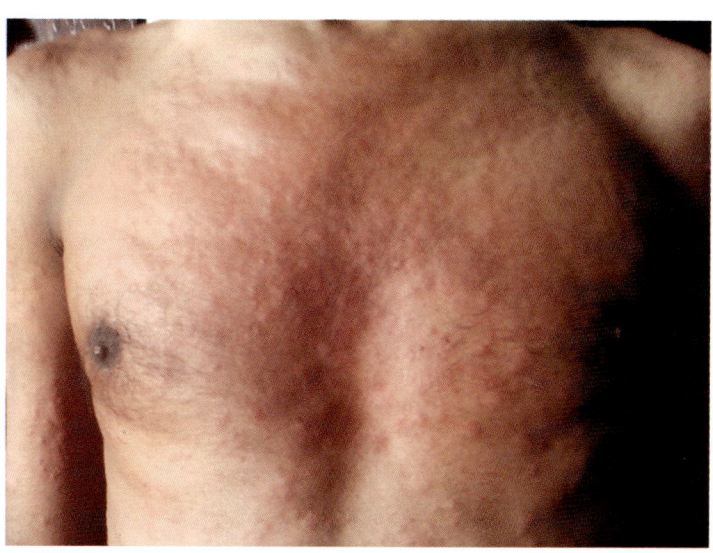

Quiz 1

What are the observations?

Widespread maculopapular rashes on the body with erythema.

Quiz 2

What are the differential diagnoses?

a. Viral examthemata—usually a wild with systemic features—fever, malaise, diarrhea
b. Chickenpox—"dewdrops on rose petal"—vesicles on erythematous papules; crops of lesions in different stages; contagious
c. Urticaria—raised, edematous lesions which wax and wane. History of drug/food/substance exposure
d. Taenia corporis—scaly progressive, annular lesions with central clearing
e. Roseola/Exanthem subitum/sixth disease—child < 3, macules and paules on trunk, neck, extrimities—spontaneous and sudden resolution
f. Miliaria rubra—erythematous papules on trunk, back, neck. Related to heat, fever.
g. Insect bites—urticarial papules and plaques
h. Erythema infectiosum/fifth disease—"slapped cheek" appeaence, sparing of periorbital area and the bridge of the nose; Erythema on trunk, extrimities, buttocks (In adults-arthralgias).
i. Drug eruption—allopurinol, β lactam antibiotics, sulfas, anticonvulsants, ACE inhibitors, NSAIDs, OHAs, thiazide diuretics—usually within 1–4 weeks of initiation of the drug.
j. Rarer causes—rickettseal pox (papule → vesicle → crust. Palm and soles); rubella (macules and papules on face, neck, trunk, extrimities
k. Secondary syphilis—generalized, non urticarial, involves palm and soles.

102. Elephantiasis Right Foot

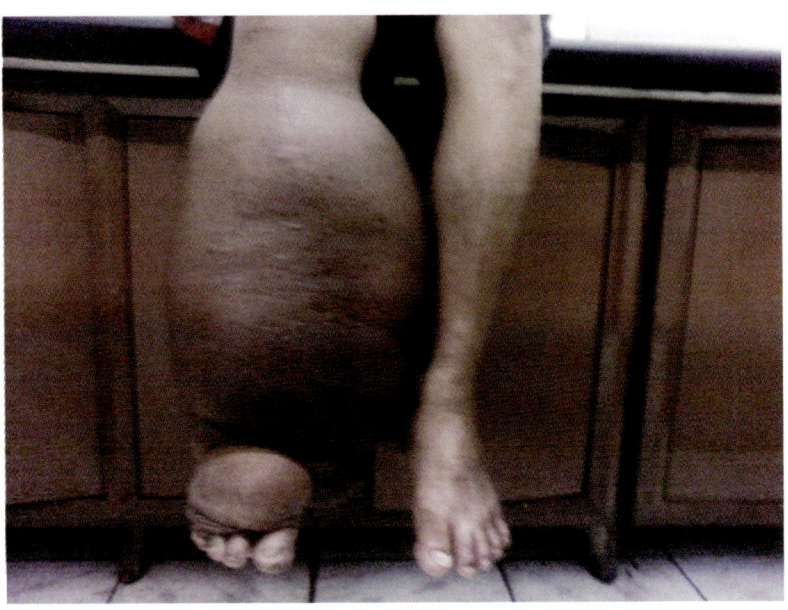

Quiz 1

What are the observations?

Hypertrophy and thickening of skin and subcutaneous tissue of foot (usually seen in extremities, hands, feet, scrotum, vulva, penis).

Quiz 2

What is the cause?

Filarial—*Wuchereria bancrofti*, *Brugia malayi*, *Brugia timori*. *Wolbechia bacteria* in the worm, host factors, opportunistic infections may have a role. Elephantiasis tropica/elephantiasis arabum.

Podoconiosis—non-filarial due to persistent contact with irritant soils—red clay with alkali metals containing sodium, potassium, associated with volcanic activity.

103. Bleeding from the Mouth

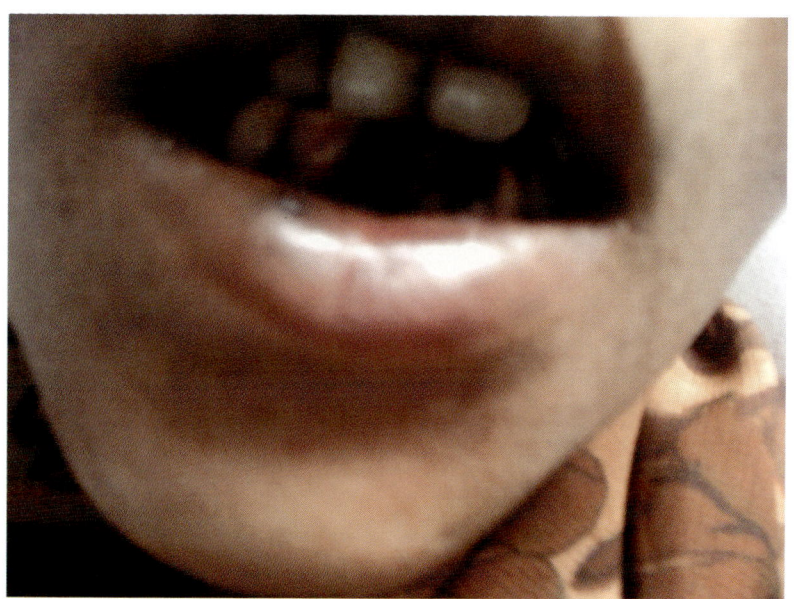

Quiz 1

What are the observations?
- Bleeding from the mouth
- Blood stained teeth.

Quiz 2

What are the differential diagnoses of bleeding in the mouth?
- Thrombocytopenia
- Leukemia—acute myelomonocytic leukemia with/without ulceration
- Primary biliary cirrhosis
- Acute organ failure—acute liver failure, acute kidney failure
- Coagulation disorders
- Anticoagulant overdose
- Bone marrow suppression
- Infections—Candida, herpes simplex, viral hemorrhagic fevers, dengue
- Vitamin deficiency—scurvey.

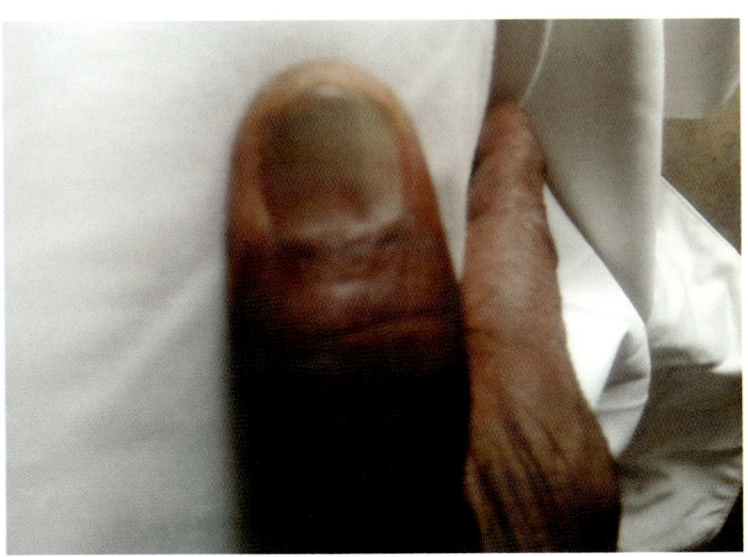

Quiz 1

What are the observations?

Discoloration of the distal half of the nail with a blackish color.

Possibility—trauma.

Quiz 2

What are the examples of nail discolorations/lines?

a. Terry's nails—proximal paleness extending well beyond half the nail overshadowing the lunula; distal band darker.

 Seen in stress related disorders—liver cirrhosis, CHF, old age, DM 2

b. Lindsay's nails—half and half nails—distal brown transverse band caused by pigment deposition in renal failure.

c. Beau's lines—transverse depressed ridges.

 Seen in severe infection, hypotension AMI, shock, hypocalcemia, malnutrition, cance chemotherapy.

d. Muehrcke's lines—transvers, non-depressed lines, usually 2 or more seen in hypoproteine- mia < 2.2 gm/dl (decreased synthesis/increased loss), cancer chemotherapy, nephrotic syndrome.

e. Mee's lines—transverse, non-depressed white lines, one per nail; disappears on pressure over the line;

 Seen in arsenic poisoning, thallium poisoning, other heavy metal poisoning.

f. Acral lentigenous melanoma—on palm, sole, mouth, within the nails. Involves periungua lesions.

g. Splinter hemorrhage—non-specific—seen in trauma, infective endocarditis, scleroderma.

h. Nail pitting—seen in psoriasis. Additional lesions include—oncycholysis, thickening, oil spot lesions—yellow patches on the nail.

i. Quitter's nails—distal pigmentation (due to tobacco staining) and proximal lack of it (as the patient has quit/switched over to low tar cigarette).

j. Paronychia—inflammation of the nail folds resulting in red, swollen, tender nails. Seen in professions involving frequent dipping of hands in water.

105. A Man using Tobacco Snuff

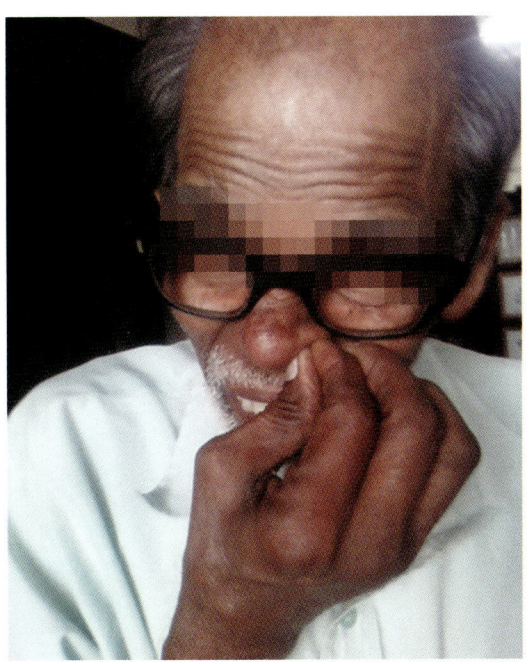

Quiz 1

What are your observations?

A man is seen using the tobacco snuff.

Quiz 2

What is snuff?

Snuff is a smokeless tobacco made using pulverized tobacco leaves.

Quiz 3

How is snuff used?

A pinch (observe the position of fingers) of tobacco is insufflated into each nostril. It delivers a swift hit of nicotine. The snuff may be flavoured.

Quiz 4

Is there a lung cancer risk?
No specific lung cancer risk but other cancer risk is more than non users of tobacco.

Quiz 5

There is also no exposure to carbon monoxide and nitrous oxide gases.
Also there is no risk of bronchitis, emphysema, lung cancer.

Quiz 6

Which medicines have been used as snuff?
a. Pituitary snuff—prepared from posterior pituitary lobes of porcine origin used in the past to treat nocturnal enuresis in children.
   Can result in allergic alveolitis (with precipitating antibodies) which can progress to pulmonary fibrosis (which may be irreversible). Miliary mottling may be seen which may be transient or progress to fibrosis.

106. Plexiform Neurofibroma

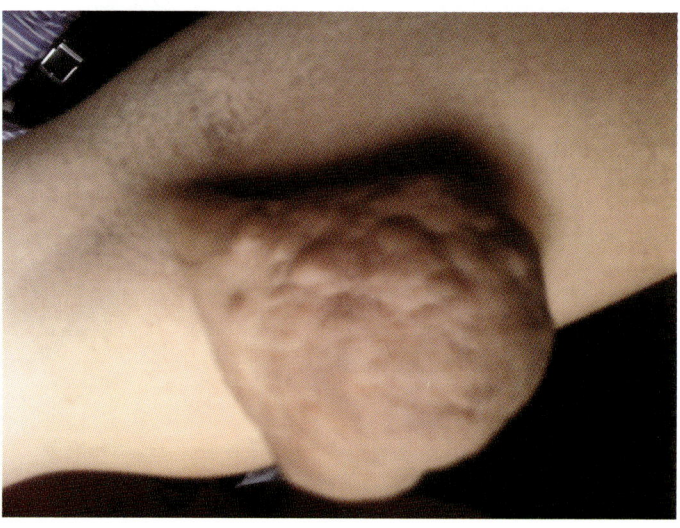

Quiz 1

What is your observation?
Pedunculated plexiform neurofibroma arising from forearm near the elbow.

Quiz 2

What are the locations for plexiform neurofibromas?
Face, eye socket, arm, chest, leg, back, abdomen.
Seen at any age even in children.

What are the complications?

Plexiform neurofibromas form a part of NF 1.

Complications of NF 1 include:

a. CNS/PNS—cognitive problems; epilepsy, stroke; hydrocephalus
b. Unsightly appearance (particularly if on face, if large) causing anxiety and emotional distress
c. Skeletal problems—hemivertebrae leading to scoliosis, osteoporosis
d. Visual problems—if arises from the optic nerve
e. Increase in neurofibromatosis—related to hormonal changes of puberty, pregnancy, menopause
f. CVS—hypertension (pheochromocytoma)
g. Devolopment of cancer <10%—plexiform neurofibromas
    Clues for possible malignant transformation increase in size, persistent pain, ulceration.
h. Increased risk of development of other cancers—breast, leukemia, brain, soft tissue cancer.

107. Excessive Bruisability or Bleeding Tendency

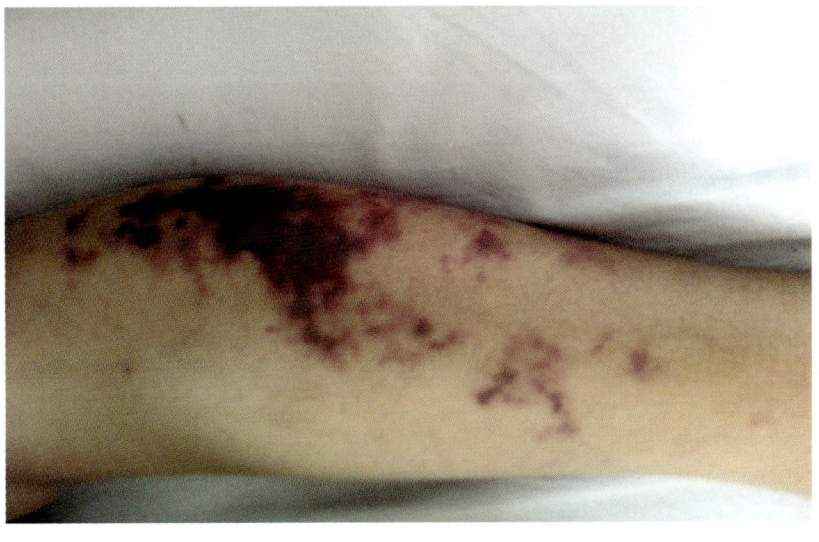

Quiz 1

What are the observations?

Ecchymosis around the knee joint associated with petichiae.

Quiz 2

What are the differential diagnoses for these?

a. Trauma—may be associated with petechiae. History of trauma may be there.
    Absence of history of trauma suggests a bleeding disorder.

b. By inhibiting clotting factors—heparin, warfarin

By producing autoimmune thrombocytopenia—penicillin, quinine, quinidine, DPH, carbamazepine, methyldopa.

By inhibiting platelet aggregation—aspirin, NSAIDs.

c. Vasculitis

Palpable and tender petechiae/purpura

Precipitated by drug hypersensitivity; by CTD (RA and SLE); by infections in hepatitis C.

Associated with systemic features—fever, arthritis.

d. Vitamin K deficiency—see to malabsorption, chronic liver disease.

e. Cholesterol emboli—a purpuric lividoreticularis, cyanosis in patients with advanced atherosclerosis seen in legs, feet. Onset often coincides with aortic catheterization.

f. Scurvey—vitamin C deficiency, characterized by painful perifollicular hemorrhages, ecchymoses, bleeding into muscles, bleeding from gums.

g. Warfarin necrosis—starts as painful erythema, progress to purpura, and then into subcutaneous fat necrosis.

h. HSP-Henoch scholein purpura—purpura > ecchymoses, abdominal pain, joint pain, hematuria, melena, systemic features like fever, headache, urticaria, edema, arthralgia.

i. Bacteremia—

Endocarditis—petechiae in extremities, skin, mucosa, splinter haemorrhages in the nailbed.

Meningococcemia-rapidly developing hemorrhagic lesions on trunk

Rockey mountain spotted fever—pink macules on wrist, palm, soles ankles, spreading centripetally.

j. Anticoagulant overdose.

k. Circulating anticoagulants—RA, SLE, AIDS, penicillin, postpartum state.

l. DIC—bleeding from multiple sites, acrocyanosis (due to microthrombi),

Seen in medical (snake bite, septicemia, heat stroke, transfusion reaction) conditions; surgical conditions (fracture femur, metastatic malignancies, massive trauma); obstretic conditions (amniotic fluid embolism).

m. Hemophilia—bleeding into skin, muscle, mucus membrane, into the joints following trauma, minor surgery.

Quiz 3

What are the disorders related to bleeding and coagulation seen in liver disease?

a. Reduced protein synthesis (including the coagulation factors) resulting in coagulation factor deficiency

b. Thrombocytopenia

c. Increased fibrinolysis

d. Vitamin K deficiency

Quiz 4

Which coagulation factor/s is/are NOT synthesized by the liver?

Factor VIIII only!

108. Elephantiasis of the Scrotum

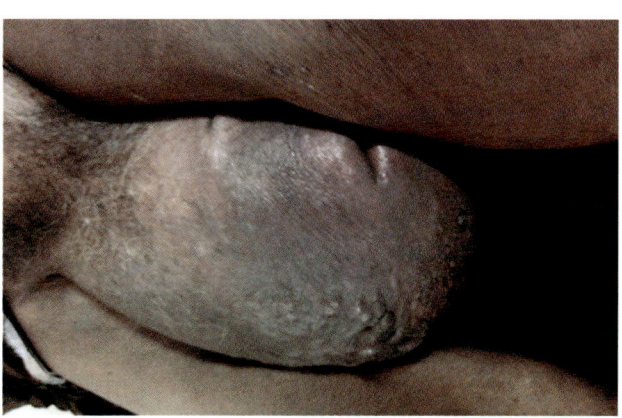

Quiz 1

What is the observation?

A large scrotum with hardly seen penis—elephantiasis of the scrotum.

Quiz 2

What is the most likely cause?

Filarial. There could be a small hydrocele; a large hydrocele; thickening of the scrotal skin and subcutaneous tissues.

Filarial elephantiasis is a manifestation of progression of lymphedema which may also involve limbs, breast, vulva, vagina, penis.

Quiz 3

What is "Lymph scrotum?"

Distended lymph containing vesicles on the skin of the scrotum seen in some patients of filarial elephantiasis. These patients may get recurrent attacks of acute dermato-lymphangio-adenitis (ADLA) involving skin and genitalia.

Quiz 4

What are the other genitourinary manifestations of filariasis?

a. Acute epididymo orchitis, funiculitis.
b. Hematuria
c. Chyluria
d. Chylocele.

Quiz 5

What are the features of advanced filarial lymphedema?

a. Increased in the size of limb/genitalia

b. Thickened skin

c. Increased skin folds

d. Hypertrichosis

e. Black pigmentation

f. Nodules, warty growth.

Quiz 6

Can it be non filarial?

Yes, due to contact with alkaline soil rich in sodium and potassium in Kenya, Egypt, Rwanda and due to presence of high concentration of mercury in the lake water in Ethiopia. This variant is known as Podoconiosis.

Quiz 7

What are the complications?

a. Secondary infection—resulting in pyocele—an emergency requiring immediate surgery.

b. Mechanical—impediment to walking and day to day activities, if very big.

c. Social embarrassment and shame leading to absence from school, work.

d. Hampered marriage prospects especially among young females.

109. Subconjunctival Hemorrhage

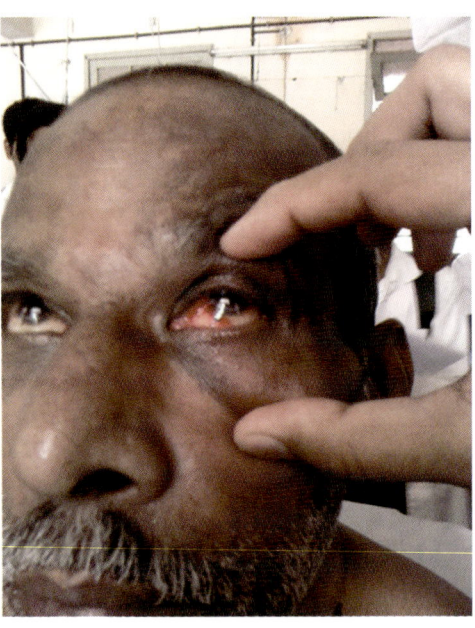

Quiz 1

What is the observation?

Subconjunctival hemorrhage.

Quiz 2

What is the mechanism?

Due to rupture of small blood vessels below the conjunctiva.

Quiz 3

What are the causes?

a. Infection—leptospirosis, whooping cough
b. Acute hemorrhagic conjunctivitis—pneumococal, enterovirus 70, coxsackie A virus
c. Trauma
d. Hypertension
e. Drugs—side effects—aspirin
f. Increased venous pressure—straining, coughing violently, choking, vomiting.

Quiz 4

What is the approach to a patient with sub-conjunctival hemorrhage?

a. Look for fever—infection—leptospira
b. Look for history of whooping cough, violent cough, forceful vomiting
c. Look for jaundice—leptospira, bleeding tendency
d. History of trauma
e. Check BP for hypertension
f. History of drugs—aspirin
g. Fundus examination for bleeding tendency/vessels.

110. Red Colored Nail due to Fungal Infection

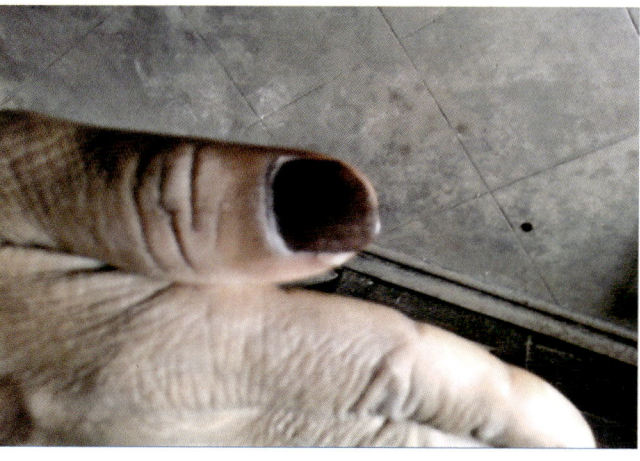

Quiz 1

What are the observations?

Red colored nail of the right thumb.

Quiz 2

What are the causes?

a. Nail polish
b. Trichophyton rubrum fungus infection—resulting in red colored nail without application of nail polish.

Quiz 3

Give causes for discoloration of nails

a. Pale nails—anemia—especially if associated with pallor of conjunctiva, palm, soft palate spoon nails/koilonychias in iron deficiency anemia.
b. Blue green nails—hallmark of pseudomonal infection.
c. White nails—opaque white nails with pink tips seen in cirrhosis and nephrotic syndrome.
d. Half and half nails
   A red brown distal band occupying 20 to 50% of the nail seen in cirrhosis, CCF, DM (Terry's nails).
   A brown distal pigmentation due to melanin deposition seen in renal failure (Lindsay nails).
e. Yellow nails
   Psoriasis—yellow oil droplet lesion on the nail
   Dermatophyte infection
   "Yellow nail syndrome"—Yellow nails without cuticles (associated with pleural effusion) seen in chronic chest infections, lymphedema.
f. Blue lunulae—seen in hepatolenticular degeneration (Wilson's disease), argyria (silver), antimalarial therapy
   Blue nails—cyanosis, polycythemia.
g. Red lunulae
   Cherry red lunulae—carbon monoxide poisoning; half moon-shaped in CCF.
   Red nails—trychophyton rubrum infection.
h. Black longitudinal streak—natural dark patients, melanomas, Peutz-Jeghers syndrome, junctional naevus.

111. Gingival Hyperplasia

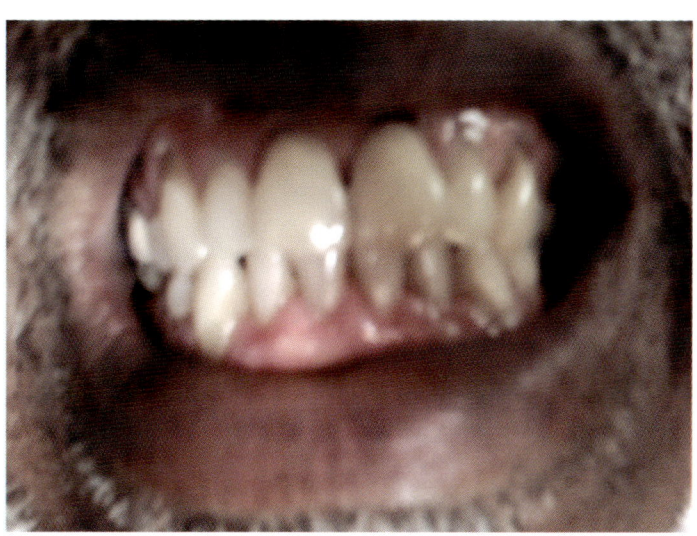

Quiz 1

What are the observations?

Gingival hyperplasia.

Quiz 2

What are the causes?

a. Drug induced—
   - Anticonvulsants—DPH, lamotrigine, valproate
   - Calcium channel blockes—nifedipine, amlodipine, verapamil
   - Immunosuppressant—cyclosporine
b. Systemic causes—pregnancy, scurvey, AML, Wegener's granulomatosis
c. Inflammatory enlargement due to dental related causes.

Quiz 3

What are the factors responsible for he gingival hyperplasia?

a. Oral hygiene, plaques (resulting in local accumulation of DPH, cyclosporine)
b. Susceptibility of subpopulations of keratinocytes and fibroblasts to DPH and cyclosporine.
c. Interaction between the said drugs and the susceptible fibroblasts and keratinocytes possibly resulting in a modulation of inflammatory process.

112. Peau d'Orange Appearance

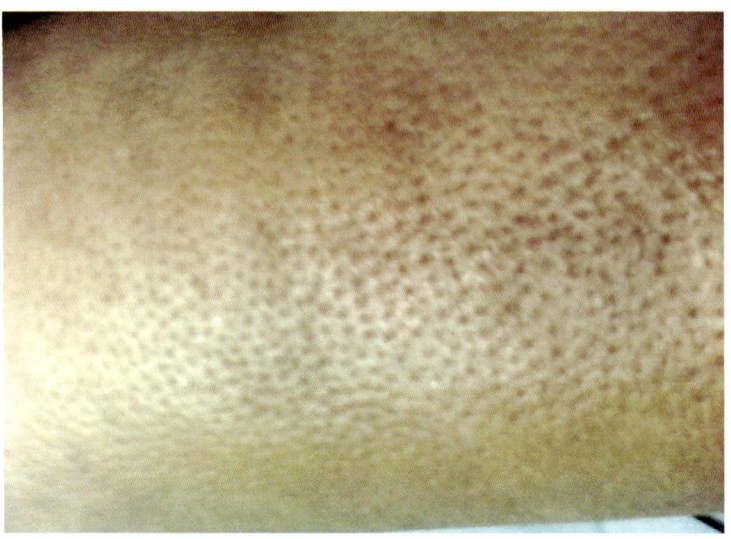

Quiz 1

What is your observation?

Skin (of the thigh) showing "peau d' orange" appearance.

Quiz 2

What is peau d' orange appearance?

Skin with a dimpled texture like that of an orange peel.

Quiz 3

What is the reason for it?

Due to a combination of cutaneous lymphatic obstruction—resulting in edema + stromal infiltration—together resulting in orange peel appearance.

Quiz 4

Which conditions produce it?

a. Ductal carcinoma of the breast

b. Lymphangitis carcinomatosa.

c. Beaks in Bruch's membrane in angioid streaks—a fundus appearene

Quiz 5

What are the causes of edema of the breast?

a. Obstruction to valveless subepithelial lymphatic plexus constituted by dermal papillary and subpapillary channels (described by Handley) by tumor invasion of the lymphatics/ by tumor emboli.

b. Other causes of lymphedema—obstruction to lymphatics, removal of LN and lymphatics (radical surgery), irradiation
c. Occlusion of the sublavian vein
d. Mastitis
e. CCF
f. Axillary lymph node disease—TB.

113. Increased Interdigital Space between Great Toe and 2nd Toe

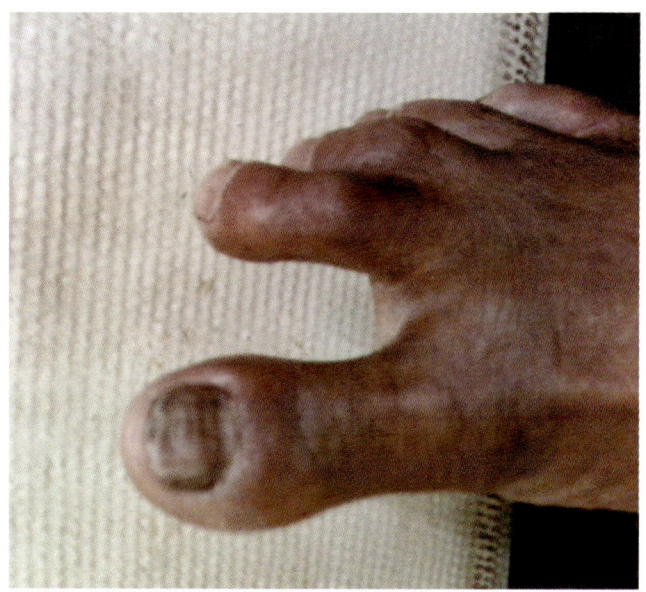

Quiz 1

What are the observations?
a. Increased space between the great and the 2nd toes.
b. Unhealthy nails.

Quiz 2

What are the conditions where this is seen?
a. As an isolated anomaly
b. Down's syndrome
c. Apert syndrome—acrocephalosyndactyly (malformations of face, skull, hands, feet)—first branchial (pharyngeal) arch syndrome. Similar skull may be found in Crouzon syndrome and Pfeiffer syndrome.
   Hand in apert syndrome—increase in the first webspace—short thumb with radial deviation + complex syndactyly of index, middle and ring fingers.
   "Spade palm"—side to side fusion of middle 3 fingers

"Mitten palm"—Fusion of fingertops forming concave palm
"Rosebud palm"—Tight fusion of all digits forming one conjoined nail
AD inheritance.
Defect on chromosome no 10—fibroblast growth factor receptor 2 gene.

Quiz 3

What is the nerve supply to the 1st interdigital space of foot?
Deep peroneal nerve (on the dorsal aspect); medial plantar nerve (on the plantar aspect).

Quiz 4

What are the causes of pain in the foot in that area?
Pain on the dorsal aspect of the foot
a. Avascular necrosis of 2nd metatarsal head—Freidberg's infarction
b. Morton's neuroma (interdigital neuroma).
   Pain on the plantar aspect of the foot
a. Metatarsalgia.

114. New Names for Old Diseases

Old name: CFS—chronic fatigue syndrome
New name: ME—myalgic encephalomyelitis

Quiz

What is it?
A complex disease involving a profound dysregulation of CNS and immune system, dysfunction of cellular energy metabolism and ion transport, and cardiovascular abnormalities.

115. Differential Diagnosis:
Hemorrhagic Lesions on the Sole of the Foot

1. Drug reactions—SJ syndrome
2. Hand, foot and mouth disease
3. Bleeding diathesis as a part of hematologic problem
4. Bleeding as a part of systemic disease
5. Anticoagulant overdose.

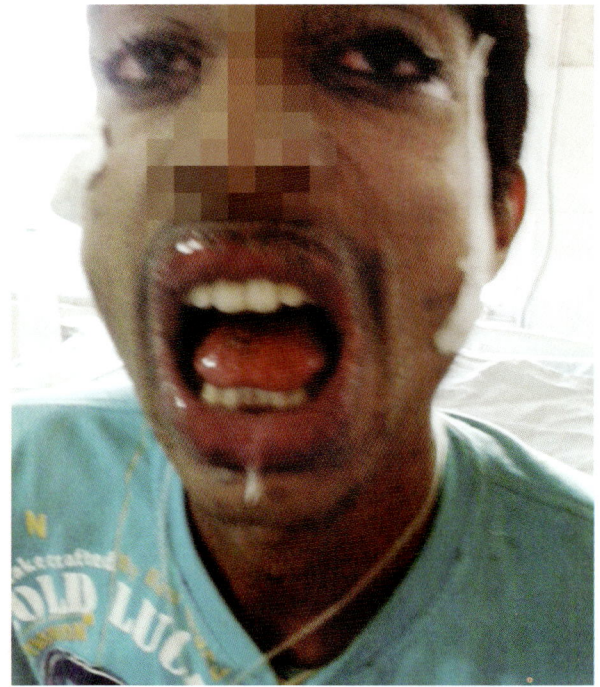

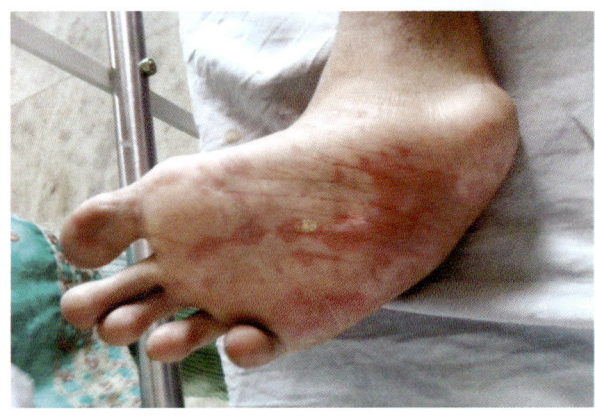

116. Gum Hyperplasia with Gum Bleeding

OBSERVATION

1. Gum hyperplasia
2. Gum bleeding
3. Adult patient.

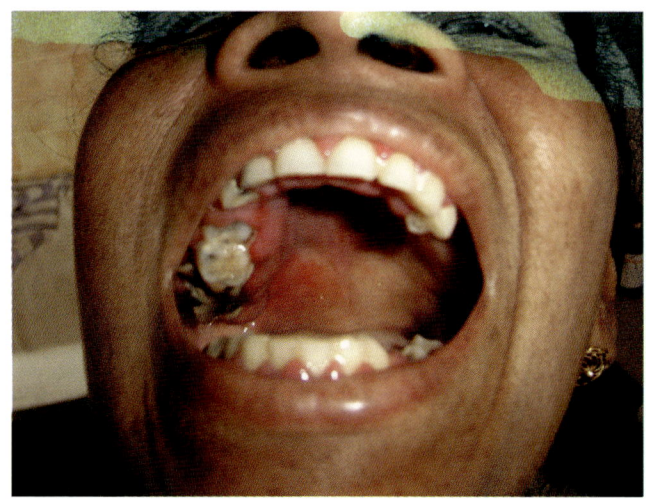

Possibilities

1. AML—acute monocytic leukemia FAB M5 > acute myelomonocytic M4, acute myelocytic M1, M2
2. Severe drug induced (phenytoin, cyclosporin, nifedipine) gum hyperplasia associated with underlying periodontal disease with increased vascularity
3. Scurvey—mainly gum bleeding

This patient was found to have AML-M5.

Syndromes Associated with AML

1. Down syndrome—trisomy 21
2. Kleinfelter's syndrome—XXY
3. Syndrome—trisomy 13
4. Fanconi anaemia
5. Ataxia telangiectasia
6. Kostmann syndrome.

Preleukemic Blood Disorders

1. Myelodysplastic syndrome (MDS)
2. Myeloproliferative disease (MPS).

OBSERVATION

1. Bilateral gynecomastia
2. Elderly patient.

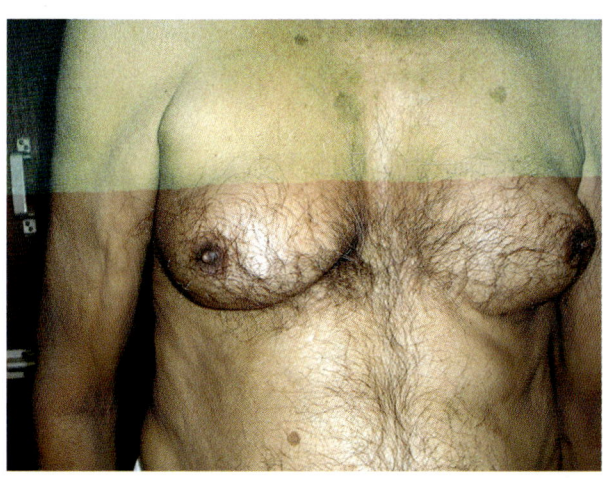

Causes of Gynecomastia

Unilateral/bilateral breast enlargement in males which is usually tender

1. Newborn—transient—Witch's milk
2. Adolescent—puberty—resolves in 2 years
3. Elderly—age-related testosterone deficiency
4. Drugs—ketoconazole, cimetidine
   - Gonadotrophin releasing hormone analogs
   - Human GH, HCG
   - Antiandrogens—bicalutamide, flutamide
   - Spiranolactone
   - 5 alpha reductase inhibitors—finasteride, dutasteride
   - Androgen deprivation therapy for prostate cancer
   - Hypogonadism—Klinefelter's syndrome
   - Endocrine—hyperthyroidism, hypopituitarism, hypogonadism
   - Organ failure related—liver failure with cirrhosis; CRF
   - Tumors—testicular (Leydig cell, Sertoli cell); adrenocortical (Cushing)
   - Lung—bronchogenic carcinoma

This patient had Klinefelter's syndrome

47 chromosomes XXY—an extra X chromosome—aneuploidy

Hypogonadism, reduced fertility, gynecomastia, osteoporosis, varicose veins, hernias

C/F seen more often in female patients: Autoimmune disorders, carcinoma breast, osteoporosis, venous thromboembolism.

Cases in Medicine

187

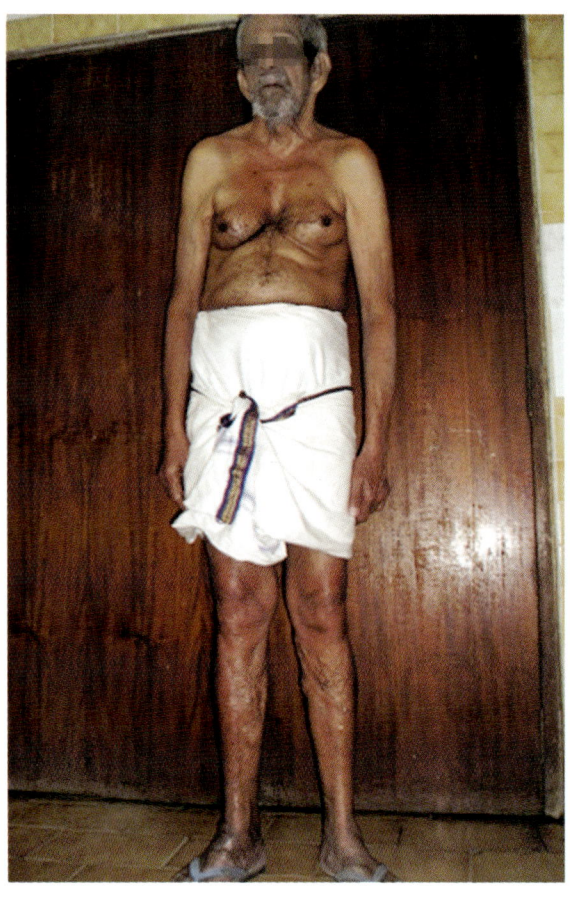

1. Klinefelter's syndrome—an example of pre-pubertal hypogonadism—hypergonadotrophic hypogonadism
2. Kallmann's syndrome—hypogonadotrophic hypogonadism—deficiency of testosterone (men) and estrogen and progesterone (women) + Anosmia
3. Hypogonadotrophic hypogonadism
   Primary HH—Kallmann's syndrome, charge, GnRH insensitivity
4. Secondary/acquired HH—brain tumor, pituitary tumor, pituitary apoplexy, head injury, drugs
5. Delayed puberty.

Varicose Veins Seen in a Patient of Klinefelter's Syndrome

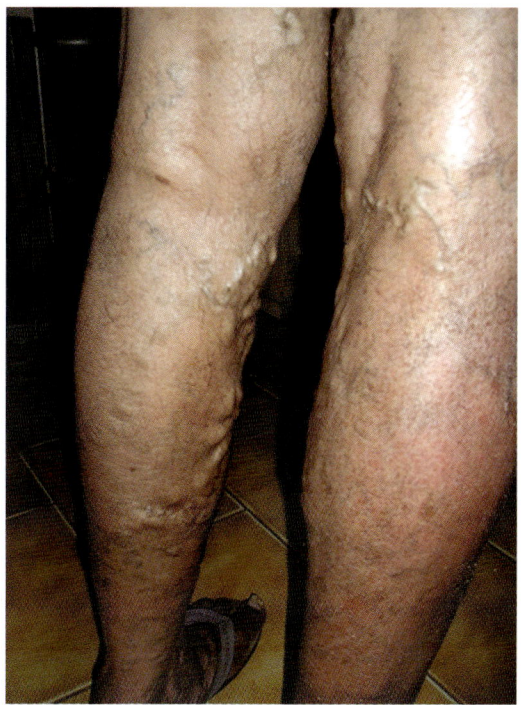

Tissue laxity giving rise to hernias and varicose veins.

Approach to Varicose Veins

Look for

1. Varicocele
2. Varicose ulcer
3. Tenderness—superficial thrombophlebitis
4. Deep vein thrombosis—development of new varicose veins.

Complications

1. Superficial thrombophlebitis
2. DVT
3. Hemorrhage
4. Venous ulceration.

Anatomical Facts

1. Great saphenous vein accompanies saphenous nerve.
2. Small saphenous vein accompanies sural nerve.

120. Carrying Angle

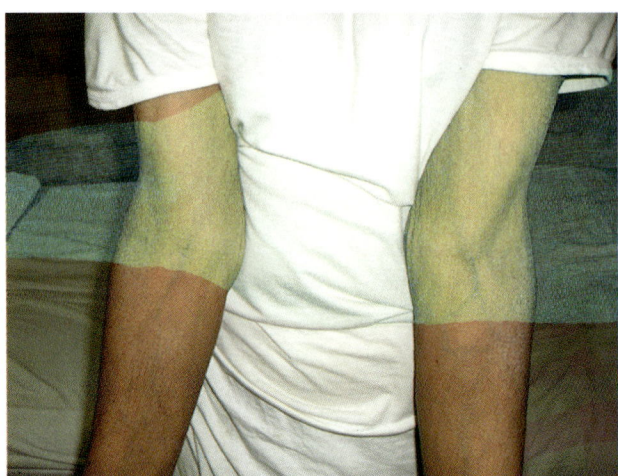

Angle formed between the elbow and sorearm when the arms are held besides the body with palm facing forward.

Normal carrying angle—5–15°.

Use of the carrying angle—helps forearms to clear hips while swinging during walking.

Increased carrying angle—cubitus valgus—certain fractures of elbow, Turner's syndrome, Noonan's syndrome.

Reduced carrying angle—"Gunstock deformity"—cubitus varus—supracondylar fracture of humerus.

Complication—subluxation of the ulnar nerve > ulnar neuropathy.

Quiz 1

What are the observations?

A swelling seen above the elbow—thikended ulnar nerve in leprosy.

Quiz 2

What are the causes for nerve thickening?

Differential diagnosis nerve thickening

1. Leprosy
2. Neurofibromatosis
3. Refsum's disease
4. Amyloidosis
5. Nerve tumors
6. Hereditary motor sensory neuropathy
7. Hypertrophic neuropathy—perineuronal/localized
8. Endocrine—acromegaly
9. Charcot-Marie-Tooth disease.

Cases in Medicine

Quiz 3

What is the method of palpation of the ulnar nerve?
Method of palpation
Using tips of index, middle and ring fingers
Roll the fingers backwards and forwards along the long axis of the thickened nerve
1. Ulnar nerve—palpated between the thumb and the middle finger in the upper arm behind the medial epicondyle.
2. Radial nerve—palpated with the thumb in the anatomical snuff box (even while shaking hands!).
3. Common peroneal nerve around the neck of fibula.

Quiz 4

Discuss in brief nerve thickening in leprosy and in other conditions.
Nerve thickening in leprosy
Hypertrophied thickened peripheral nerve with glove and stocking anesthesia with anesthetic patches (erythematous or hypopigmented) and autonomic features. AFB smear may be found.

Nerves known to be Thickened in Leprosy

1. Supraorbital
2. Cervical
3. Great auricular
4. Median
5. Ulnar
6. Radial
7. Radial cutaneous
8. Posterior tibial
9. Common peroneal.

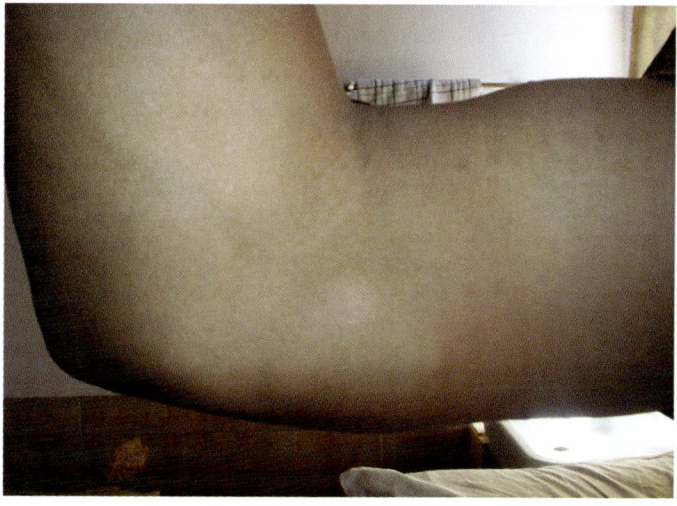

Thickening of the ulnar nerve in leprosy

Nerve Thickening in HSMN

In 30% patients—in demyelinated form (type 1) > axonal form (type 2).

Best nerve to palpate—great auricular nerve—head tilted away, neck muscles and skin tightened, fingers of the palpating hand drawn across the neck.

Nerve Thickening in other Conditions

Refsum's disease—nerve thickening + demyelinating polyneuropathy + ataxia + retinitis pigmentosa + hearing impairment. Due to phytanic acid deposition.

Primary Systemic Amyloidosis

Nerve infiltration with amyloid + palpable thickened nerves.

Sarcoidosis—nerve thickening unlikely—revise the diagnosis—rule out (RO) tuberculosis.

Localised Hypertrophic Polyneuropathy

Brachial plexus > femoral, ulnar

Brachial plexus thickening may also be seen in MADSAM—multifocal and demyelinating sensory and motor neuropathy. Biopsy shows "onion bulb" appearance.

Nerve Thickening in Nerve Tumors

von Recklinghausen's disease
- Thickening of peripheral nerves have been described.
- Bilateral greater auricular nerve thickening has been noticed.
- Swellings at entrapment sites, e.g. intervertebral foramen.
- Slowly progressive peripheral nerve lesions seen in type 2 neurofibromatosis.

Quiz 5

What are the alternate names of some peripheral nerves?
Alternate names of some peripheral nerves
1. Labourer's nerve—median nerve—responsible for coarse movements of the hand executed by the long flexors of forearm.
2. Musician's nerve—ulnar nerve—responsible for the fine movements executed by the small muscles of the hand.

Cases in Medicine

121. Arcus Senilis and Bilateral Cataracts

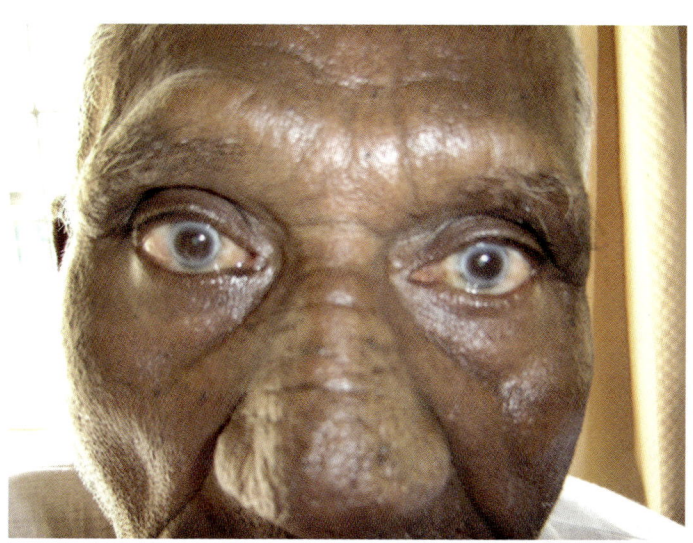

Differential Diagnosis: Cataracts

1. Old age—senile cataract
2. Congenital—Down's syndrome, myotonia dystrophica
3. Trauma—secondary to eye injury
4. Skin disease—atopic dermatitis
5. Drugs—steroid therapy
6. Eye diseases.

Differential Diagnosis: Arcus Senilis

1. Greyish opaque ring at the periphery of cornea within the corneoscleral junction. Due to deposition of phospholipid and cholesterol—could be complete or partial (arc).
2. Arcus juvenilis—same thing seen in younger people.
3. Kayser-Fleischer ring (KF ring)—grey corneal rings in dark eyes and brown rings in light colored eyes. Pathognomonic if Wilson's disease—ceruloplasmin deficiency resulting in excessive copper deposition in the viscera. Liver, eye, basal ganglia, myocardium, kidneys.

Located in the periphery of the cornea in the Descimet's membrane. Starts as a superior crescent. Then develops inferiorly and then later becomes circumferential. Best seen by slit lamp examination.

May disappear slowly with chelation therapy.

Treatment with zinc might help—by blocking excessive copper absorption.

Differential Diagnosis: Cataracts Related to Medical Conditions

1. Metabolic—diabetes
2. Genetic diseases—Down syndrome
3. Infection—Rubella syndrome
4. Drugs—steroids
5. Eye diseases—glaucoma
6. Mechanical—sunlight exposure
7. Smoking.

Types of Cataract

Sunflower cataract—Wilson's disease.

---

122. Mass in the Pharynx—Possibly Enlarged Tonsil

OBSERVATION

A huge (?tonsillar) mass.

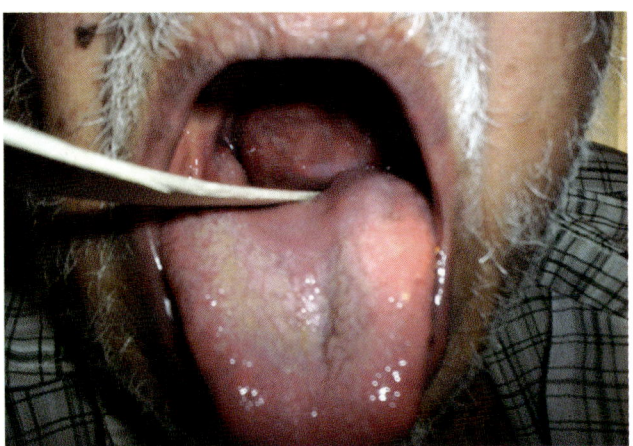

Differential Diagnosis: Huge Tonsils

1. Hypertrophied tonsils—due to recurrent pharyngitis—kissing tonsils
2. Tonsillar abscess—hot potato voice
3. Storage disorders
4. Lymphoma.

Waldeyer's Ring

Composition

Lymphatic ring formed by the annular arrangement of lymphoid tissues in the pharynx. From superior to inferior consists of:
- Two pharyngeal tonsils (adenoids when inflamed)
- Two tubal tonsils where each eusthachian tube opens into the nasopharynx

- Two palatine/faucial tonsils located in oropharynx
- One lingual tonsil (on the posterior tongue)
- Involved in non-Hodgkin's lymphoma.

Tangier Disease—Hypoalphalipoproteinemia

Mutations in gene 9q31 lead to tangier disease characterised by hypoalphalipoproteinemia + reduced HDL due to ABCA1 transporter (ATP binding casette transporter A1) deficiency (thus not helping transfer of cholesterol and phospholipids out of the cell) + hypertriglyceridemia + orange tonsils + premature atherosclerosis + corneal clouding + hepatomegaly + splenomegaly + neuropathy + thrombocytopenia.

AR inheritance.

123. Subcutaneous Nodule in the Neck

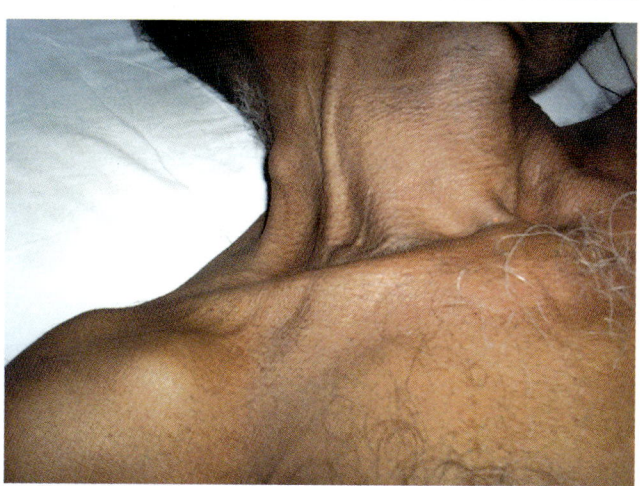

Differential Diagnosis

1. Lymph nodes
2. Lipoma.

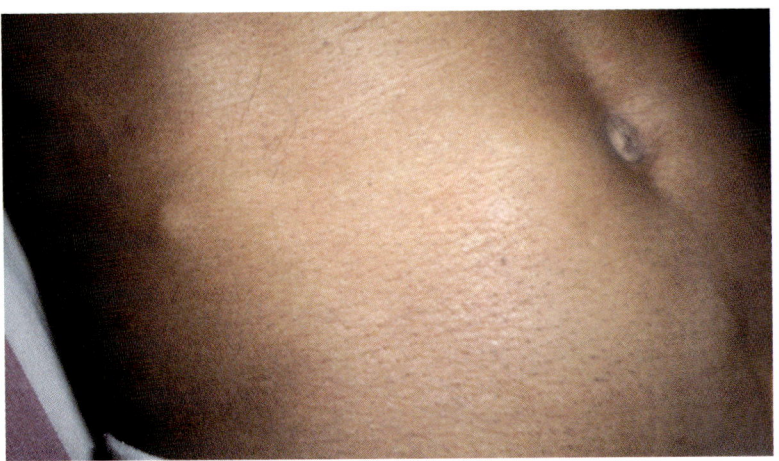

1. *Face*
   - Leprosy
   - Gouty tophi
   - Xanthomas.

2. *Neck*
   - LN
   - Jugulodigastric node—tonsillar LN
   - Delphian LN—paratracheal
   - Virchow's node
   - Neurofibromata
   - Rheumatic fever nodules.

3. *Limbs*
   - Neurofibromata
   - LN
   - Granulomas—infective
   - Palpable purpura.

4. *Hands*
   - Heberden's nodes
   - Bouchard's nodes
   - Rheumatoid nodules.

5. *Skin*
   - LN
   - Granulomas
   - Rheumatoid nodules

- Neurofibromas
- Primary skin conditions—lipomas
- Metastasis.

6. *Abdominal wall*
   - Sister Mary Joseph's nodule
   - Rheumatoid nodule.

125. Hemochromatosis—CRF (Patient of CRF on Hemodialysis)

OBSERVATION

1. Darkening skin
2. Increasing blood sugar (not known to be a diabetic).

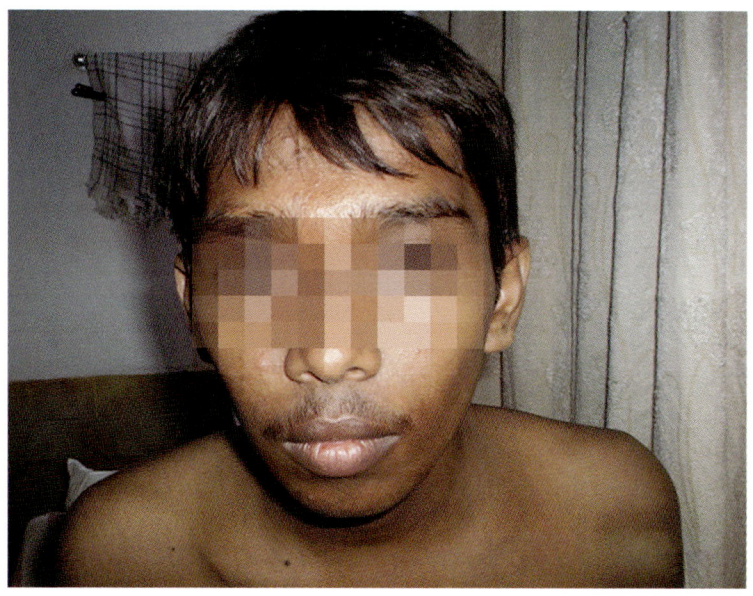

Diagnosis

Hemochromatosis due to repeated blood transfusions—pancreatic damage resulting in diabetes.

126. Unilateral Ptosis—Right Side

OBSERVATION

1. Unilateral ptosis
2. Slight facial asymmetry suggesting possibility of unilateral right sided facial palsy.

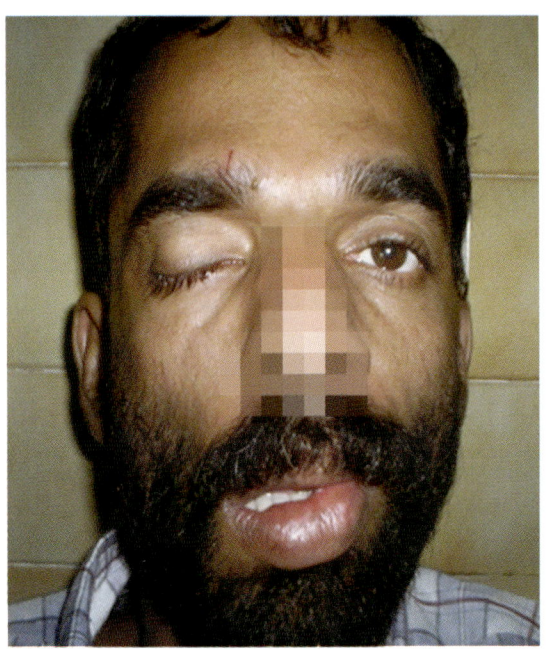

Inference and Discussion

Unilateral ptosis due to unilateral 3rd nerve involvement.

Course of the 3rd nerve.

Nuclear portion—at the midbrain.

Fascicular intraparenchymal portion (near red nucleus)—emerges from the cerebral peduncle

Fascicular intraparenchymal portion—meninges, PCA aneurysm (between PCA and internal carotid).

Fascicular cavernous portion—sella tursica between petroclinoid ligament below and interclinoid above.

Fascicular orbital portion—superior orbital fissure.

Midbrain Fascicular Syndromes

1. Weber's syndrome 3rd nerve + contralateral hemiplegia (lesion—base of midbrain).
2. Nothnagel syndrome 3rd nerve + contralateral cerebellum (tectum of midbrain).
3. Benedikt's syndrome 3rd nerve + contralateral hemiplegia, athetosis, tremors (lesion tegmentum of midbrain involving corticospinal tract and red nucleus).

Rules to be Remembered

1. Axons run ipsilateral

    Exceptions: Superior rectus—also innervated from contralateral 3rd nerve fibers—unilateral 3rd nerve lesion can also have contralateral ptosis milder than the ipsilateral ptosis.

    Levator palpebrae superiporis—bilateral innervations

2. Pupillary and accommodation reflex—Edinger-Westphal nucleus-ipsilateral

    Why PCA aneurysm involves pupils and diabetes and hypertension spare the pupil?

    Compression due to PCA aneurysm involves superficially placed papillary fibers whereas the ischemic lesions in diabetes and hypertension involve the core of the nerve thus sparing the papillary fibers.

Differential Diagnosis: Painful Ophthalmoplegia Syndromes

1. Diabetes
2. Tolosa-Hunt syndrome
3. PCA aneurysm
4. Migraine.

Differential Diagnosis: Unilateral Dilated Pupil

1. 3rd nerve palsy
2. Optic atrophy (loss of direct LR and AR + presence of consentual LR)
3. Holmes adies pupil (unilateral + loss of knee jerk + stubborn young females + slow reaction of the pupil to LR and mydriatics)
4. Sympathetic overactivity
5. Drugs—mydriatic eyedrops.

Cuases of Lesions in the Cavernous Sinus Resulting in 3rd Nerve Palsy

Tumors: Pituitary, craniopharyngioma, meningioma

Cavernous sinus thrombosis

Inflammatory: Tolosa-Hunt syndrome (non-caseating granuloma/non-granulomatous inflammation at the cavernous sinus or superior orbital fissure.

Microvascular disease causing ischemia to vasa nervosa

Mononeuritis multiplex.

Differential Diagnosis: Emergency Situations Causing 3rd Nerve Involvement

- Coning
- Myesthenia
- Aneurysms
- Migraine
- Giant cell arteritis.

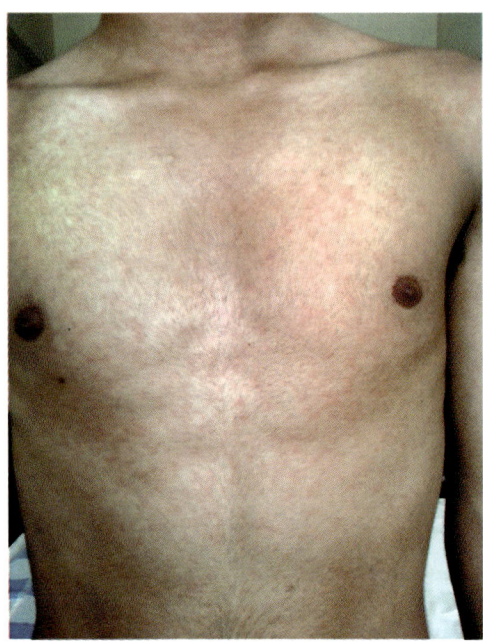

Causes

ITP

Drugs used in the Treatment of ITP

1. Steroids + splenectomy
2. Steroid sparing cytotoxic drugs
3. IVIG
4. Thrombopoiesis stimulating: Romiplostim—thrombopoiesis stimulating Fc peptide fusion protein (peptibody) SC inj.
   Thrombopoiesis stimulating oral eltrombopag drug with similar action.
5. Dapsone—second line drug.
6. Splenectomy sparing: Rituximab—chimeric monoclonal antibody—against B cell surface antigen CD 20—possibly an effective alternative to splenectomy.
7. Tamatinib—kinase inhibitor.

Mechanisms of Thrombocytopenia

a. Reduced production—marrow infiltrative disorders
b. Increased destruction—DIC, sepsis, infection, drugs including heparin
c. Sequesteration—hypersplenism
d. Dilution—massive transfusion, gestational thrombocytopenia—rare

Infection induced: Dengue, malaria, CMV, HCV, HIV 1

Meningococcal septicemia, DIC

Drug induced: Reduced production: Radiotherapy, chemotherapy, antifolates (DPH)

Increased destruction—heparin, rifampicin, sulfas, quinine, thiazide diuretics, sodium valproate, heavy metals.

Immune mediated: Autoimmune: ITP; Secondary to connective tissue disorders; lympho-proliferative disorders; drugs.

Alloimmune: Post-transfusion purpura PTP (1 week after platelet transfusion). Due to antibodies against P1(A1) antigen (HPA-1a) allele and P1 (a2) (HPA-1b) alleleor platelet receptor GP IIb/IIIa. IV gamma globulin helps.

Primary bone marrow disorders: Megaloblastic anemia, aplastic anemia, myelodysplastic syndrome, acute leukemia, myelofibrosis, metabolic disorders involving the marrow.

Hypersplenism: Congestive splenomegaly—thrombocytopenia as a part of pancytopenia. Portal hypertension with or without cirrhosis is the commonest cause.

C/F of thrombocytopenia:

Skin: Petechiae, purpura, echymoses.

Mucosa: Epistaxis, gum bleeding, GI bleeding, hematuria, menorrhagia.

Subconjuctival hemorrhage, retinal hemorrhage, intracranial hemorrhage

Rare: Hemarthrosis, muscle hematoma

Approach to purpura

1. History of known drugs
2. GE:
    Joint pains—connective tissue diseases
    Anemia—bone marrow suppression, leukemia
    Fever—dengue, HIV, leptospirosis, malaria
    Jaundice—leptospirosis, malaria
3. Systemic exam:
    Splenomegaly—ITP unlikely—consider lymphoma, leukemia, hypersplenism.

Differential Diagnosis: Thrombocytopenia + Thrombosis

1. HIT—heparin induced thrombocytopenia—recent exposure to heparin—thrombosis—arterial/venous.
2. TTP (pentad)—microangiopathy, thrombocytopenia, renal dysfunction, neurological symptoms, fever.
3. HUS (triad)—microangiopathy, renal failure, thrombocytopenia.
4. DIC—underlying condition producing DIC, bleeding manifestations, thrombotic mani-festations, coagulation abnormalities, elevated D dimer
5. APLA syndrome—thrombosis (venous/arterial), fetal wastage, associated ITP.

Causes of DIC

1. Medical—sepsis, shock, hypotension, cancer
2. Surgical—trauma, sepsis, extensive surgery
3. OBG—HELLP syndrome, pre-eclampsia
4. Miscellaneous

Bone Marrow Finding in ITP

Increases number of megakaryocytes.

Mechanism of Platelet Destruction in ITP

Peripheral autoimmune destruction of platelets.

Heparin-induced Thrombocytopenia (HIT)

Time interval (exposure to C/F): First exposure—5 to 10 days; reexposue (after receiving heparin within past 3–6 monthes:within 24 hours.
Mechanism: Antibody formation against the complex of heparin and PF4 (platelet factor 4)
C/F: Less severe bleeding (less severe thrombocytopenia).
Thrombosis: Venous/arterial > limb loss.
Diagnosis: Drop in platelet count > 50%
Demonstration of antiheparin antibodies
Treatment:
Stop heparin
Thrombosis prevention and treatment by using a quick acting alternative anticoagulant—Fondaparinux/lepirudin/dabigatran (newer oral anticoagulant).

Role of Peripheral Smear in the Diagnosis and Evaluation of Thrombocytopenia

1. Platelets small—production problem
2. Platelets large—destruction problem
3. RBCs:
   - Schistocytes in MAHA
   - Spherocytes—Evan's syndrome
   - Contain MP in malaria.

Role of Blood Biochemistry

1. Hemolysis—indirect hyperbilirubinemia, high LDH, low haptoglobin.
2. Liver dysfunction (acute—viral hepatitis or chronic—portal hypertension with or without cirrhosis).
3. Renal dysfunction—in patients with TTP/HUS/DIC/SLE.

Principles of Management

1. Identification and treatment of the underlying cause
2. Improving the platelet count
   - Reduced production—platelet transfusion
   - Increased destruction—to be prevented—IVIG/CST
3. Non-specific hemostatic agents
   - Antifibrinolytic—tranexamic acid
   - Recombinant activated factor VII.

Platelet Transfusions

a. Contra indicated—TTP, HIT—bleeding is rare, thrombosis is the major event.
b. Not indicated—ITP, hypersplenism—ineffective.
c. Indicated—primary marrow disorders, dilutional thrombocytopenia, DIC—helpful.

128. Bleeding Tendency

OBSERVATION

1. Purpura, ecchymoses
2. Bleeding from sites of venepuncture.

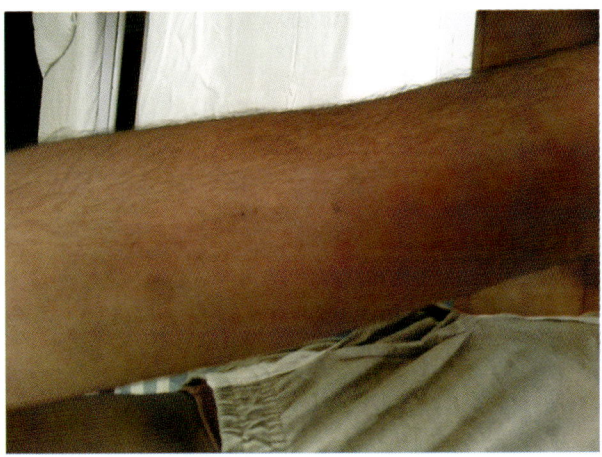

Causes

1. Organ failure—liver acute/chronic
2. Systemic diseases—connective tissue disorders, vasculitis
3. Bleeding disorders—thrombocytopenias,
4. Drugs—warfarin, streptokinase, heparin.

Antiplatelet Drugs and Anticoagulants and their Sites of Action

1. Aspirin—inhibits platelet aggregation by reducing thromboxane A2 production
2. Dipyridamole—inhibits platelet aggregation—inhibits cyclic nucleotide phosphodiesterase, thereby increasing cyclic AMP levels
3. Clopidogrel, ticlopidine—antiplatelet
4. GP IIb, IIIa inhibitors: Abciximab, eptifibatide, tirofiban
5. Warfarin—inhibits epoxide reductase. Vitamin K dependant coagulation factors are inhibited—factors II, VII, IX, X and proteins C and S
6. Heparin—potentiates the activity of antithrombin III
7. Low molecular weight heparin—enoxaparin
8. Direct thrombin inhibitors—lepirudin
9. Factor Xa inhibitor—fondaparinox
10. Streptokinase (protein produced by beta hemolytic streptococci)—converts plasminogen to plasmin which is involving in lysis of fibrin clots.
11. tPA—thrombolytic agent (IV)—activates plasminogen. Recombinant human enzyme—not inactivated rapidly by antibodies from previous streptococcal infections (unlike streptokinase).

Cases in Medicine

Features of Acute Liver Failure

1. Coagulopathy
2. Jaundice
3. Ascites
4. Encephalopathy.

129. Isolated XII Nerve Palsy

OBSERVATION

Tongue deviated to the left side.

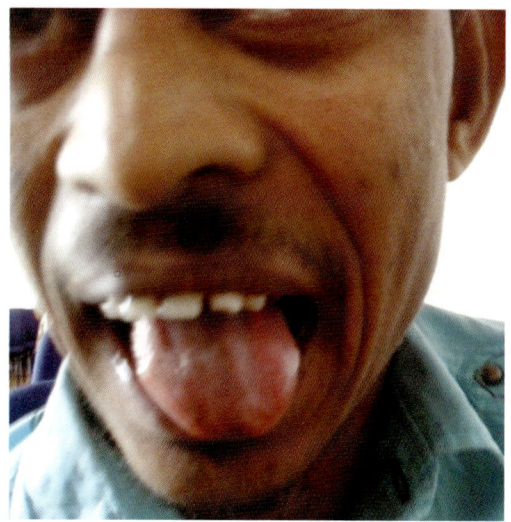

Inference

Paralysis of the XII nerve on the left side—tongue points to the affected side.
XII nerve supplies all muscles of the tongue except palatoglossus (supplied by IX nerve).

Mechanism

Involvement of the muscle—genioglossus—supplied by the XII nerve. Genioglossus tends to push the tongue to the opposite side—if paralysed on the left side, the tongue points to the left side.

Identifying the Lesion as LMN

1. Wrinkling of the mucous membrane
2. Wasting of tongue on that side
3. Fissuring of tongue.

Result of XII Nerve Paralysis

Dysarthria—peripheral.

130. Differential Diagnosis: Single Transverse Palmar Crease

Synonym: Simian crease

Usually proximal
1. Down syndrome
2. Turner's syndrome
3. Aarskog syndrome
4. Fetal alcohol syndrome
5. Can be associated with fused carpal bones.

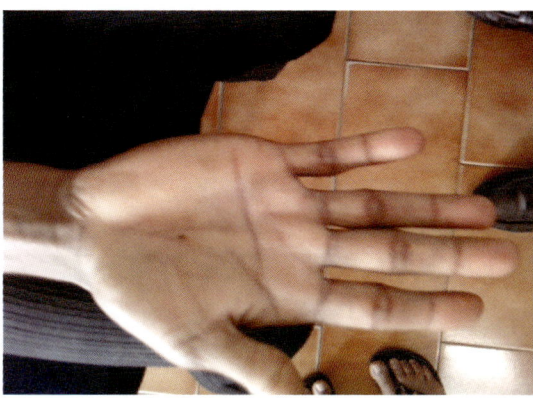 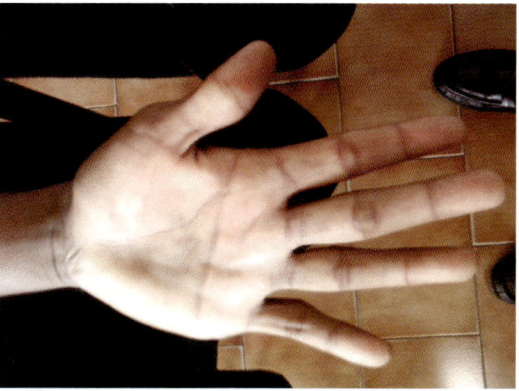

131. Target Lesions of Erythema Multiforme

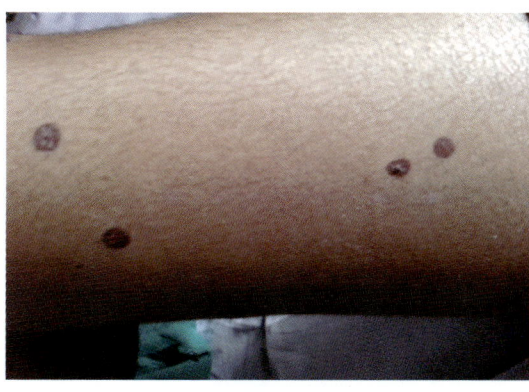 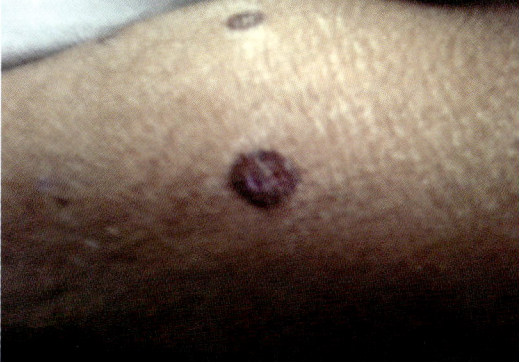

Classic Target Lesion

Seen in erythema multiforme (EM)—it has 3 zones:
- Central—dusky purpura(central bulla)
- Surrounding pale edematous zone
- Surrounding macular erythema.

Target lesions seen in SJS have only 2 zones:
- Central—dusky purpura (central bulla)
- Surrounding macular erythema.

Complications
1. Necrosis of skin, GI tract, respiratory tract
2. Mucosal scarring
3. Esophageal stricture
4. Corneal ulcer
5. Acute tubular necrosis, renal failure.

Stevens-Johnson syndrome is a immune complex mediated hypersensitivity disorder. Involves skin (purpuric macules, targetoid lesions, full thickness epidermal necrosis) + mucosa. precipitated by infections (viral, mycoplasma); drugs and chemicals. Mortality 5%.

Toxic epidermal necrolysis (TEN): Serious, sometimes fatal form of the disease.

SJS/ten overlap

SCAR: Severe cutaneous adverse reactions the entire spectrum

EM: Erythema multiforme—earlier considered cutaneous variant without mucosal involvement.

Now considered to be clinically and etiologically a separate disease entity. Target lesions are typical of erythema multiforme.

132. Ulcer on the Tongue

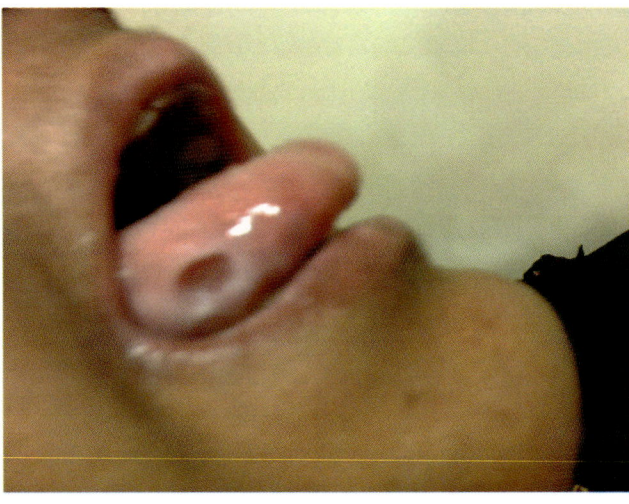

1. Sharp tooth—trauma
2. Sepsis
3. Syphilis
4. Aphthous ulcer

5. Tuberculosis
6. Scleroderma and other CTD
7. Squamous cell carcinoma.

Ulcers in Agranulocytosis

Ulceration without pus formation—seen in the throat.

133. Leonine Facies

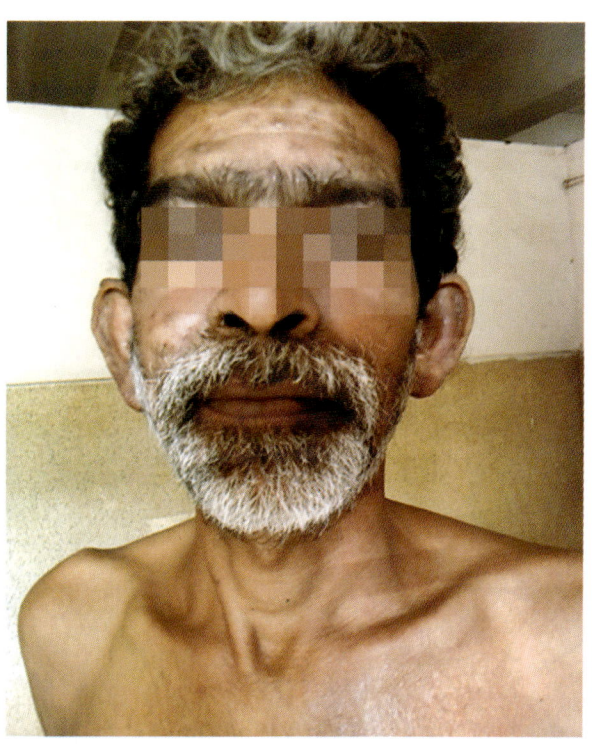

A face resembling lion's face.

Differential Diagnosis for Leonine Facies

1. Lepromatous leprosy
2. Paget's disease of the bone
3. Mycosis fungoides
4. Leishmaniasis
5. Amyloidosis
6. Mastocytosis
7. Hyperimmunoglobulin E syndrome
8. Pachydermoperiostosis.

Components of Leonine Facies in Leprosy

1. Thickened skin over face, ears, scalp
2. Thickened earlobes
3. Nodules on face
4. Madarosis—bilateral loss of the eyebrows on lateral 1/3.

Pachydermoperiostosis/Primary Hypertrophic Osteoarthropathy

Synonym: Touraine-Solente-Gole Syndrome

1. Pachydermo—thick skin over scalp and face with gyrations, thickened skin over extrimities
2. Periostosis—excessive bone formation
3. Finger clubbung
4. Mechanical ptosis—due to thick and coarse eyelids.

Inheritance

AD/AR.

134. Lepra Nodules on Forearm and Elbow

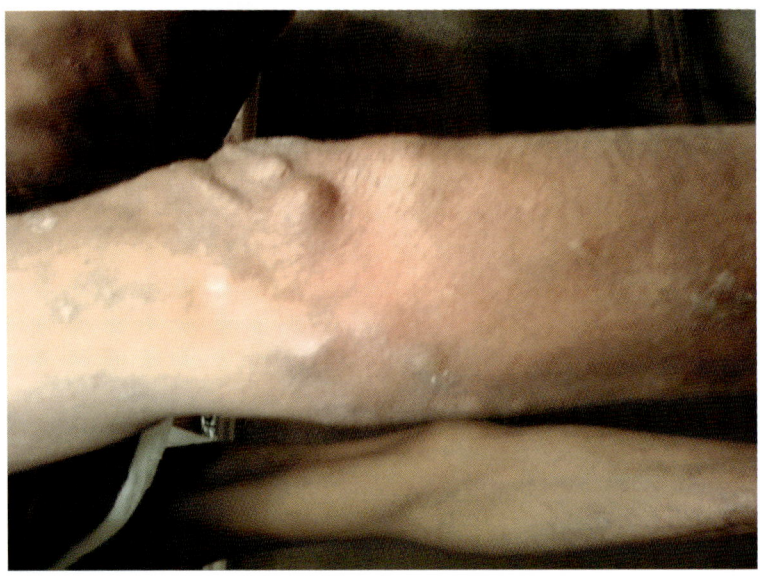

Nodules in Leprosy

1. Most advanced form of leprosy
2. Painless
3. Variable progress—may take months
4. Well circumscribed
5. Varying size and shape
6. Located on mucous membrane and skin

7. Commonest locations—face and earlobes
8. Can ulcerate—true lepromatous ulcers—discharge *M. leprae*
9. Histoid nodules of Wade—rare and painless—highly positive for *M. leprae*.

Features of Macular Lepromatous Leprosy

1. Location—face, buttocks, trunk, extensor aspect of extrimities
2. Patches—multiple—hypopigmented/erythematous
3. Texture—Waxy, smooth/erythematous
4. Margin—not well defined—merges into the surrounding area
5. Sensory deficit—none at the beginning
6. Sweating may be lost (later than in tuberculoid leprosy)
7. Increased sweating in other areas (compensatory)
8. No nerve thickening
9. AFB positive in scrapings from skin and nasal mucosa.

135. Lepra Nodules on Wrist and Hand

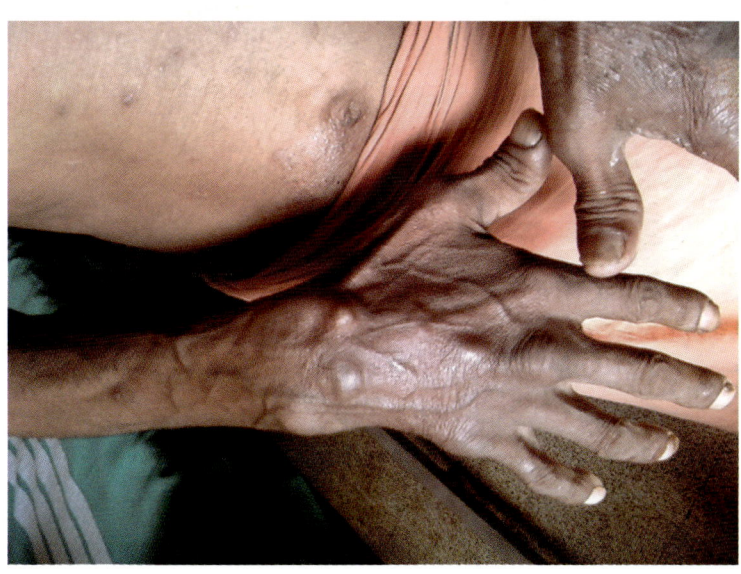

Clinical Features of Advanced Lepromatous Leprosy

1. Nerve involvement—"glove and stocking anesthesia"
   • Nerves involved—ulnar, median, radial, lateral popliteal, posterior tibial, facial
   • Nerves are tender and painful in ENL (erythema nodosum leprosum)
2. Nose—block, epistaxis, destruction of the nose bridge
3. Larynx—spead from epiglottis—hoarseness of voice
   Laryngeal edema—rare. May need tracheostomy

4. Eye—nodules on conjunctiva, sclera
  - Keratitis → blindness
  - Iridocyclitis (acute) in ENL
  - Iridocyclitis (chronic) → glaucoma
5. Testicular destruction—gynecomastia, gynecotelia (female type of nipples)
6. ENL—painful and tender nerves, painful and tender nodules, fresh "crop" of nodules, thalidomide may help.

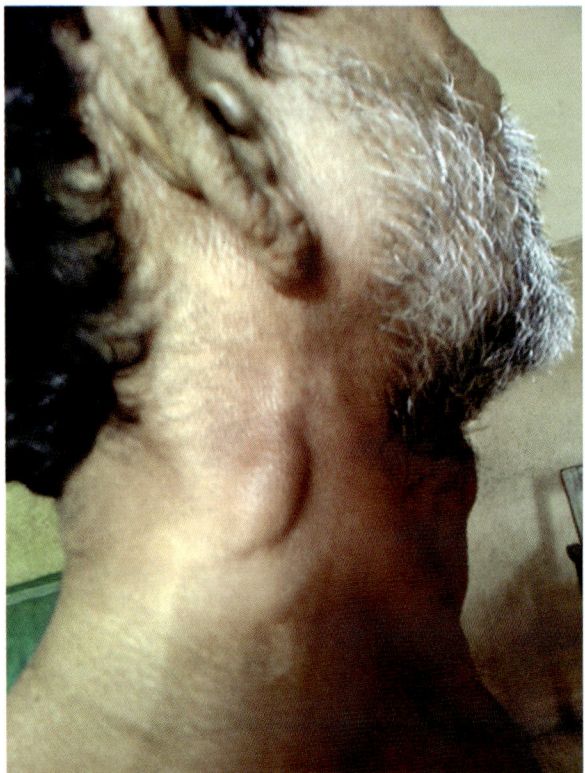

Quiz 1

What are your observations?

Thickened earlobe + thickened nerve on the neck.

Quiz 2

What are the causes of thickened nerves in the neck?

Differential diagnosis or causes of thickened nerves in the neck.

Congenital: Neurofibromatosis

Traumatic: Repeated trauma to exposed nerves—ulnar nerve at the elbow

Inflammatiry: Leprosy

Infiltrations: Sarcoid, amyloid

Incidental finding in a thin person.

Quiz 3

Which are the various nerves that could be thickened and palpable in the neck?

Nerves that could be thickened and palpable in the neck

1. Great occipital
2. Lesser occipital
3. Thrid occipital
4. Great auricular
5. Nerve to levator scapulae
6. Accessory nerve
7. Medial supraclavicular nerve
8. Nerve to levator scapulae
9. Anterior cutaneous nerve of neck
10. Anterior branch of facial nerve.

Location of the thickened great auricular nerve
- Comes out behind the posterior border of sternomastoid
- Crosses the sternomastoid.

Can be confused with dilated external jugular venous system

Usually seen in tuberculoid leprosy.

Quiz 4

What are the cardinal features of tuberculoid leprosy?

- Cardinal features of tuberculoid leprosy
- Nerve thickening—great auricular crossing the sternomastoid, ulnat at the elbow, lateral peroneal around the fibula
- Anesthesia.

Quiz 5

What are the 2 major types of LR (lepra reactions)?

1. Type 1 LR—"reversal reaction"—type IV hypersensitivity—seen in borderline leprosy in patients with cellular immune responses to *M. leprae* antigenic determinants.
   Features—acute inflammation in pre-existing lesions; appearance of new lesions; neuritis.
2. Type 2 LR—erythema nodosum leprosum (ENL)—most commn manifestation—immunologically mediated complication of LL. Most occur during first 2 years of MDT.
   Presents with red, tender and painful skin and subcutaneous lesions + fever + systemic inflammation—involving nerves, eyes, joints, testes, LN. Most occur during first year of MDT.

Quiz 6

What are the consequences of the LRs?

Permanent nerve damage, deformity, disability—in 10% paucibacillary and 40% multibacillary lesions in type 1 LR.

"Silent neuropathy" may be taking place in all patients and 30% damage to nerves must occur before sensory involvement becomes detectable.

What are the biomarkers of LRs?
IL-6—in both types of LR
TNF alpha—to monitor progress and response to steroids
Neopterin—a macrophage activation marker.

136. Clubbing

Synonym: Hippocratic fingers.

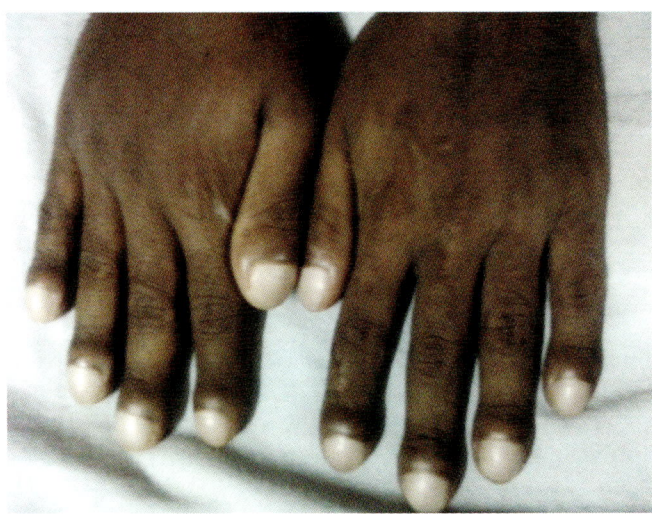

Main Features of Clubbing

1. Loss of nailbed angle
2. Increased nail curvature
3. Fluctuation at the nailbed
4. Drumstick like swelling of the terminal phalanx.

Stages of Clubbing

1. Swelling of subcutaneous tissues over the base of the nail
2. Increased curvature of the nail
3. Swelling of the pulp of the fingers in all dimentions
4. HPOA—pain and swellings of hands, wrist, feet, knees, ankles.

Signs in Clubbing

1. Lovibond's sign—obliteration of the angle between the base of the nail and the skin
2. Schamroth's sign—a lozenge-shape seen when both the thumb nails are held in apposition

Starting location of clubbing: Thumb and index finger.

Causes of Clubbing

1. Congenital, idiopathic.
2. RS—lung abscess, Ca bronchus, bronchiectasis, COPD emphysema, pneumoconiosis, TB sequelae, mesothelioma, ILD.
3. CVS—CCHD, infective endocarditis.
4. GIT—cirrhosis (primary biliary), hepatoma, ulcerative colitis.

Tender Clubbing

1. Carcinoma bronchus
2. Suppurative lung disease.

Unilateral Clubbing

1. Localised vascular anomalies—subclavian artery aneurysm, AV malformation, aortic aneurysm
2. Pancoast tumor (same side)
3. Hemiplegia
4. Trauma.

Unidigital Clubbing

1. Median nerve injury
2. Trauma.

Differential Clubbing

PDA with PH (LL > UL).

Reversible Clubbing

1. Suppurative lung diseases—lung abscess, empyema.
2. Other curable causes of clubbing.

Rapid Clubbing/Acute Clubbing

1. Lung abscess
2. Carcinoma bronchus.

Drumstick Clubbing

1. CCHD—Fallot's tetralogy
2. Bronchiectasis.

Parrot Beak Clubbing

Carcinoma bronchus.

Pseudoclubbing

1. Thyroid acropachy
   - Painful
   - No nailfold edema

- X-ray shows soap bubble appeaeence of new bone formation
- Thumb, index finger > other fingers
2. Pachydermoperiostosis
3. Scleroderma
4. Acromegalic bony enlargement
5. Acrosteolysis—pseudoclubbing seen in people working with vinylchloride

Commonest pneumoconiosis associated with clubbing—asbestosis.

Tuberculosis and Clubbing

1. Uncomplicated tuberculosis usually not associated with clubbing
2. Clubbing in tuberculosis is rare and late—indicates a complication or sequelae

HPOA—Marie-Bamberger Syndrome

1. Lung abscess
2. Carcinoma bronchus
3. Pleural mesothelioma.

Rare Causes of Clubbing

1. CVS—LA myxoma
2. RS—pulmonary AV malformation
3. Mediastinal—lymphoma, thymoma, carcinoma esophagus
4. Extrathoracic—thyroid carcinoma, purgative abuse, pachydermoperiostosis.

Syndromes Associated with Clubbing

1. Marie-Bamberger syndrome
2. Kartagener's syndrome.

137. Gynecomastia and Spider Nevus

Synonym: Nevus araneus, spider angioma.

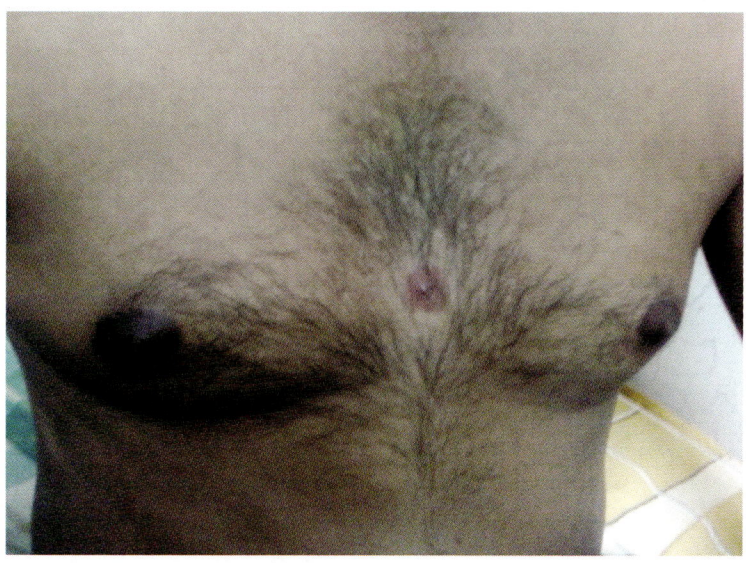

What are they?

1. Vascular lesions—seen in some conditions and occasionally in normal people
2. Solitary/multiple.

Parts

1. Central red arteriole/punctum—body of the spider—pulsations may occasionally be felt over the punctum
2. Radial pattern of thin-walled capillaries—legs of the spider
3. Diascopy (pressure with a glass slide) → temporary blanching and obliteration of the lesion with rapid return on release
4. Location—exposed areas—face, neck, upper trunk, above the nipple line, arms. In children—back of the hands and fingers

Mechanism: Dilatation of pre-existing vessels.

Conditions Where Seen

1. Cirrhosis of the liver—associated with gynecomastia, palmar erythema, testicular atrophy, leukonychia, muscle atrophy, ascites, jaundice. Number of lesions may indicate extent of fibrosis. [Niederau C, Liv. Int. 2008; 28(5); 659–666.]
2. Pregnancy
3. Thyrotoxicosis.

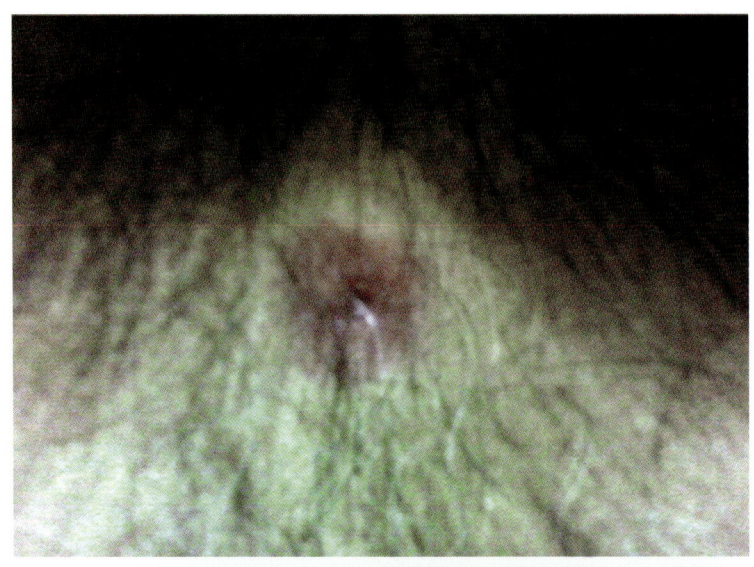

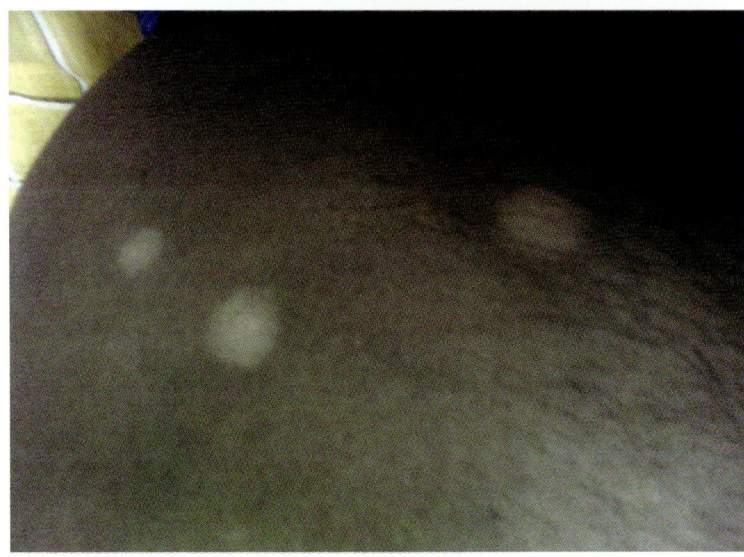

139. Onychomadesis

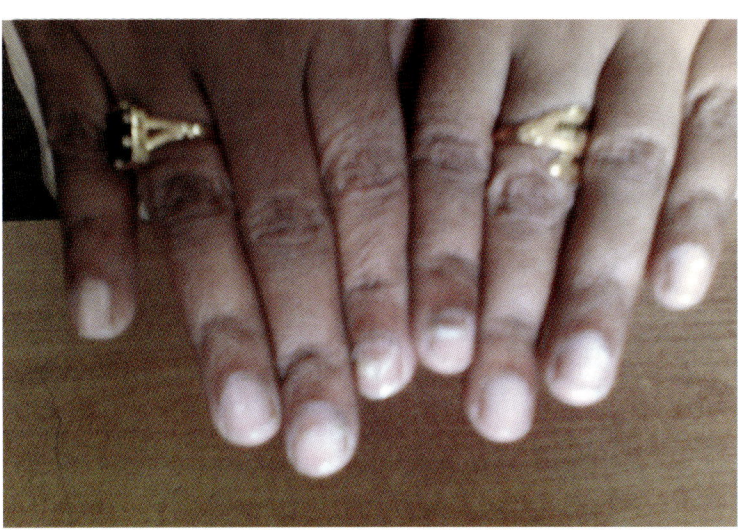

Quiz 1

What are the observations?

Unhealthy looking nails with varying degrees of white color in them—onychomadesis.

Quiz 2

What is it?

Periodic shedding of the complete nails usually beginning at the proximal end associated with a systemic disease.

Quiz 3

What is the mechanism?

Mechanism of onychomadesis:

Temperory arrest of the function of the nail matrix.

Quiz 4

What are the conditions associated with onychomadesis?

Infections—hand, foot and mouth disease, fungal (Candida) infections. This adult patient had a history of hand, foot and mouth disease.

- Cutaneous T cell lymphoma
- Pemphigus vulgaris
- Kawasaki disease
- Peritoneal dialysis
- Drugs—antineoplastic, retinoids, azithromycin.

Quiz 5

Give some examples of diseases affecting the nails?
a. Shell nail syndrome (resembles clubbing but the nailbed is NOT bulbous but atrophic)—seen in bronchiectasis.
b. Congenital onychodysplasia of nail of index fingers—seen at birth—dysplasic nails in index finger (uni/bilateral).
c. Onychorrhexis—brittle nails—repeated exposure to soap water, nail polish; hypothyroidism. Improvement observed with biotin.
d. Racquet nails—broad short square nail situated on a short distal phalanx—AD.
e. Hapalonychia—thin, soft, easily bendable nails—seen in malnutrition, myxedema, RA, leprosy.
f. Onycholysis—spontaneous separation of the nailbed—may start as "oil spot". May be associated with green discoloration (pyocyanin) in Pseudomonas infection.
g. Hangnail—overextension of the cuticle.
h. Omega nail/pincer nail/trumpet nail—lateral edges overlap each other—AD.
i. Retronychia—nail plate grows into the proximal nailfold.

Quiz 6

Give examples of nail involvement in systemic disease
a. Koilonychia—in iron deficiency anemia
b. Psoriasis—Beau's lines—transverse depressions, crumbling nail plate, leukonychia, pitting, oil spots, green discoloration in the area of onycholysis
c. Nail patella syndrome—yellow nail syndrome—yellow nail + pleural effusion + bronchiectasis
d. Green nails—onycholysis with Pseudomonas infection
e. Alopecia areata—spotted lunulae
f. Anonychia—ectodermal defects, sequel to SJ syndrome, Cooks syndrome—nail hypoplasia of digits 1, 2, 3; nail absence of digits 4,5; DOOR syndrome—deafness, onycho-osteodystrophy, mental retardation; glossopalatine syndrome—abnormal mouth, tongue attached to the TM joint.

140. The Third Mogul Sign

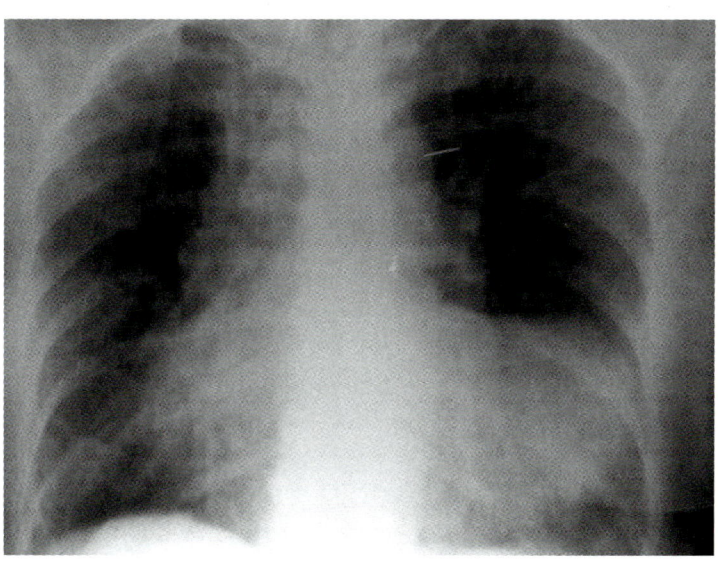

Quiz 1

What are the observations?

A bulge seen on the cardiac outline on the left side on the lower part of the cardiac silhouette.

Quiz 2

What are moguls?

Moguls are ice heaps encountered most often unexpectedly during skiing down the slopes of the snow covered Swiss Alps. Similar unexpected bulges on the cardiac silhouette mainly on the left side gives it the name.

Quiz 3

What is a third Mogul sign?

First and second bulges come from expected routinely encountered structures aorta and the pulmonary artery. The third bulge comes from unexpected source which could be variable-LV aneurysm arising out of weakness of the LV wall following acute MI; from an enlarged left atrium and hence is more popular and well known. Hence the third Mogul sign is best known.

Quiz 4

What are the various structures that could result in a positive third Mogul sign?

a. Enlarged LA appendage
b. LV aneurysm
c. Pericardial cysts

Cases in Medicine

d. Thymic enlargement

e. Lymphadenopathy

f. Coronary artery fistula and aneurysms.

Quiz 5

What causes coronary artery aneurysms in childhood?

Kawasaki's disease—children <5 years—mucocutaneous lymph node syndrome, fever, cervical lymphadenopathy, desquamative rashes on the palm, multisystem vasculitis—coronaries preferentially involved with aneurysms and thrombosis, myocarditis, pericarditis, valvulitis, AV node conduction anomalies.

Quiz 6

What is the treatment of Kawasaki's disease?

IV immunoglobulins, aspirin.

Corticosteroids may cause aneurysm rupture.

Quiz 7

What is the most likely cause for the 3rd Mogul sign in this case?

LV aneurysm.

141. A Large Goiter

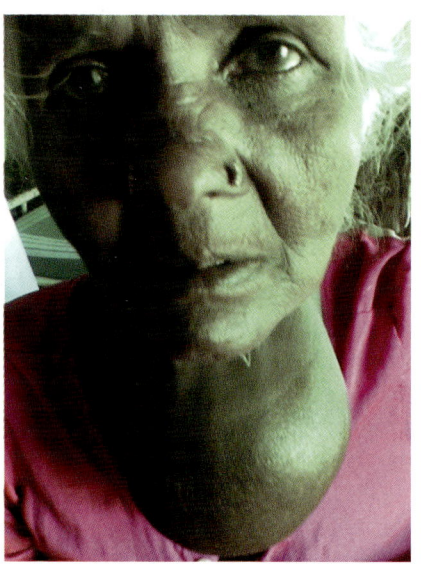

Quiz 1

What are the observations?

A really large goiter—a swelling in front of the neck possibly arising from the thyroid gland.

Quiz 2

How do you say that the swelling is arising from the thyroid gland?
If the swelling moves with deglutition (swallowing) it usually suggests origin from the thyroid gland—a goiter.

Quiz 3

How do you determine whether the goiter has a mediastinum (retrosternal) extension?
Tests to know whether there is a retrosternal extension:
a. Inspection—look for the visibility of the lower border of the thyroid gland while the patient swallows
b. Palpation—try to feel the lower end of the thyroid gland when the patient is trying to swallow
c. Percussion—percussion just below the suprasternal notch is dull and this dullness continues with the dullness elicited over the goiter.

Quiz 4

What are the other things that you look for when you examine goiter?
1. Displacement of the trachea
2. Palpability of the carotid arteries (absence of pulsations indicates possible malignant infiltration into the carotid sheath—Berry's sign)
3. Presence of hard masses—lateral lobes/lymph nodes (metastatic)
4. Features of thyrotoxicosis—fine tremors, eye signs
5. CVS examination—atrial fibrillation, evidences of cardiac failure.

Quiz 5

What are the evidences of a goiter being toxic?
a. Goiter—diffuse, soft/firm in Graves' disease.
b. Eye signs
c. Ophthalmopathy
d. Dermopathy
e. Bruit over the thyroid
f. Fine tremors
g. Atrial fibrillation
h. Cardiac failure
i. Thyroid acropachy.

Quiz 6

What are the features of Graves' disease?
1. Diffuse goiter—symmetric.
2. Bruit—due to increased intrathyroidal blood flow.
3. Ophthalmopathy—may precede, accompany or follow Graves' disease—exophthalmos due to the retro-orbital infiltration with lymphocytes, fat and in later stages, fibrosis; increasing the retro-ocular pressure and impeding the function of extraocular muscles. Ophthalmopathy can result in ophthalmoplegia, diplopia, cheimosis, papilledema, corneal ulcer.

4. Dermopathy—shin (pretibial myxedema) > toes, forehead, neck, areas of trauma—painless thickening of skin with hyperpigmented nodules/plaques.
5. Thyroid acropachy—clubbing with subperiosteal new bone formation (with soap bubble appearance).
6. Radioiodine uptake—high (as against a low uptake in painless thyroiditis).

Quiz 7

What are the types of toxic nodular goiter?
a. Diffuse toxic goiter—ophthalmopathy, dermopathy; RAIU elevated; elevated T3, T4—N/ elevated; suppression test—abnormal
b. Toxic nodular goiter
   • Uninodular
   • Type I multinodular
   • Type II multinodular—non-homogenous
c. Thyroid carcinoma.

Quiz 8

What are the features of struma ovarii?
Abdominal mass with or without ascites.

Quiz 9

What are the named signs of thyrotoxicosis?
a. *Connected to the goiter*
   1. Guttman's sign—bruit over the goiter in the neck
   2. Pemberton's sign—engorgement of face and dilated veins on neck, arms, chest on elevation of both arms over the head due to pressure of the retrosternal goiter on the great vessels
   3. Berry's sign—absence of carotid pulsation in the neck often due to malignant infiltration of the carotid sheath by the thyroid cancer
   4. Maire sign—fine tremors in the extrimities.

b. *Ocular signs:*
   1. Von Graefe's sign—upper eyelid lags behind while the eyeball slowly moves down. Suddenly a rim of sclera is seen above the eyeball due to the momentary lagging behind of the upper eyelid
   2. Dalrymple's sign—widened palpebral fissure due to exophthalmos
   3. Jellinek's sign—brownish pigmentation of the eyelid (upper > lower)
   4. Boston's sign—jerking of the lagging lid on elevation of the eyeball
   5. Graves' sign—failure of the eyelids to close fully during sleep
   6. Backer's sign—increased pulsations of the retinal arteries
   7. Cowen's sign—jerky consensual papillary reaction
   8. Enroth's sign—edema of eyelids (upper near the supraorbital margin > lower)
   9. Griffith's sign—lagging of the lower eyelid on the eyeball looking up
   10. Knife's sign—unequal papillary dilatation

11. Rosenbach's sign—fine tremors of the upper eyelids on gentle closure of the eyelids.
12. Stellwag's sign—infrequent and incomplete blinking of the eyelids.
13. Wilder's sign—slight twitch of the eyeball on moving from adduction to abduction or *vice versa*.

Quiz 10

What is subclinical hyperthyroidism?

Suppressed TSH associated with normal free T3 and T4.

Importance—can be associated with
1. Progression to nodular thyroid enlargement with hyperthyroidism
2. Increased risk of atrial fibrillation (X3 in elderly) and influence on the LV ejection fraction particularly in response to exercise
3. Decreased bone mineral density in postmenopausal women.

Quiz 11

How do you interpret T3, T4 and TSH reports in varying combinations?

a. Elevated free T3/T4 + low TSH
   • Primary hyperthyroidism—Graves', multinodular goiter, toxic nodule
   • Transient thyroiditis—postpartum
   • Rare—thyroxin ingestion, struma ovarii, amiodarone therapy
   • Rare + pregnancy test + ve—hyperemesis, hydatidiform mole.

b. Normal free T3/T4 + low TSH
   • Subclinical hyperthyroidism, thyroxin ingestion
   • Rare—CST therapy, dopamine/dobutamine infusion.

c. Low free T3/T4 + low/normal TSH
   • Recent treatment of hyperthyroidism (TSH remains suppressed)
   • Pituitary deficiency (secondary hyperthyroidism)
   • Congenital TSH/TRH deficiency.

d. Low free T3/T4 + elevated TSH
   • Primary hypothyroidism of any cause
   • Autoimmune, postradiation, post-thyroidectomy,
   • Drugs—amiodarone, lithium, interferons, IL2
   • Iodone deficiency/iodine excess, goitrogens, amyloid goiter, Reidel's thyroiditis
   • Congenital absence of the thyroid tissue associated with TSH receptor, PAX8 and TTF2 mutations
   • Iodine transport defect, thyroglobulin synthesis defect, resistance to TSH.

e. Normal T4/T3 + elevated TSH
   • Subclinical autoimmune hypothyroidism
   • Drugs—amiodarone, sertraline, cholestyramine
   • TSH receptor defects/resistance; Pendred's syndrome (SN deafness, goiter).

f. Elevated T4/T3 + normal/elevated TSH
   • TPO antibodies interfering with thyroid hormones

- Amiodarone
- Thyroid hormone resistance
- Intermittant T3/T4 overdose.

Quiz 12

What are the situations where TSH alone might be misleading?
Common—recent treatment of thyrotoxicosis, pituitary disease, non-thyroidal illness.
Rare—TSH secreting pituitary tumor, thyroid hormone resistance.

Quiz 13

What are the common errors in the interpretation of the results of thyroid function tests?
1. Low T3/T4 + low TSH = profound hypothyroidism (can be mistaken for persistent hyperthyroism)
2. High T3/T4 + low TSH = self resolving thyroiditis (can be mistaken for established thyrotoxicosis)
3. Low/normal T3/T4 + low/normal TSH = non-thyroidal illness (can be mistaken for hypothyroid)
4. T3/T4 not tested + TSH normal = possibly hypothyroid (can be mistaken for euthyroid)
5. Normal T3/T4 + high TSH = possible interfering antibody/heterophile antibody.

Quiz 14

What are the indications for thyroid ultrasound?
1. To confirm the presence of thyroid nodule when the clinical examination is equivocal
2. To measure accurately the size, structure and vascularity
3. To distinguish between the benign and malignant masses (by U/S)
4. To distinguish between the thyroid nodule and the other neck masses—LN, thyroglossal cyst, cystic hygroma.
5. To evaluate diffuse changes in thyroid parenchyma
6. To identify residual/recurrent thyroid and identify mets in the cervical LN
7. To screen patients at high risk for thyroid cancer—familial thyroid ca, MEN2, neck irradiation in childhood.
8. For guiding diagnostic (FNAC, biopsy) and therapeutic interventional procedures.

Quiz 15

Briefly discuss development of thyroid and its anomalies
Median eminence on the floor of the primitive pharynx (foramen caecum—4th week of gestation) → primitive primordium desends through anterior portion of the neck to below thyroid cartilage (7th wk IUL) → thyroid retains attachment to the pharynx (by an epithelial stalk (thyroglossal duct (obliterated by 8–10th week IUL) → thyroid section starts at 11th week of IUL.

Anomalies
1. Additonal thyroid tissue along the thyroglossal duct—pyramidal lobe attached to the distal end of thyroglossal duct and left side of the isthmus (50% of population)
2. Thyroglossal cyst—persistent thyroglossal duct—a midline swelling at the level of hyoid bone/thyroid cartilage
3. Ectopic thyroid sites—midline—sublingual, suprahyoid, infrahyoid
4. Congenital agenesis/hypoplasia—lobe/isthmus—absent isthmus with lobes on either side of the trachea.

Quiz 16

Mention some classical U/S appearences in thyroid diseases

1. "Spoke and wheel like appearance"—benign adenoma—central and peripheral vascularity on color Doppler
2. "Spongiform appearance"—multiple internal cystic spaces
3. "Ring down artifact"—cystic nodule
4. "Thyroid inferno"—Graves' disease due to generalized hypervascularity
5. Perithyroidal satellite lymph nodes—delphian lymph nodes cephalad to isthmus—in Hashimotos thyroiditis (non-tender)
6. Pretracheal level VI chain LN in de Quervain's thyroiditis (tender—initially hyperthyroid, later euthyroid, then hypothyroid)
7. Ill-defined margins with fibrosis + displaced/deformed trachea—Reidel's thyroiditis.

Quiz 17

Mention some relevant facts about thyroid hormones

1. Thyroid gland produces T3 and T4 from iodinated tyrosine
2. 80% of the hormone produced is T4-thyroxine)—80 micrograms/day
3. T3 is produced from T4 in the peripheral tissues
4. Thyroid hormones affect all tissues and metabolic pathways.

Quiz 18

What are the clinical consequences of iodine deficiency?

Abnormal thyroid function, endemic goiter, endemic cretinism, perinatal death, infant mortality, infertility.

Quiz 19

How do the various thyroid malignancies classically behave?

1. Papillary—lymphatic spread
2. Follicular—vascular spread
3. Anaplastic—very aggressive with local invasion; poor prognosis
4. Huerthle cell—behavior cannot be predicted by histopathology
5. Medullary—associated with MEN II
6. Lymphoma—associated with Hashimoto's thyroiditis.

Quiz 20

What are the symptoms and signs of nodular goiter?

1. Lump in the neck—develops slowly
2. Thyrotoxicosis of insidious onset
3. Dysphagia
4. Cough
5. Sudden enlargement of goiter
6. Sudden neck pain
7. Stridor
8. Hoarseness of voice-suggesting carcinoma.

142. Syndactyly

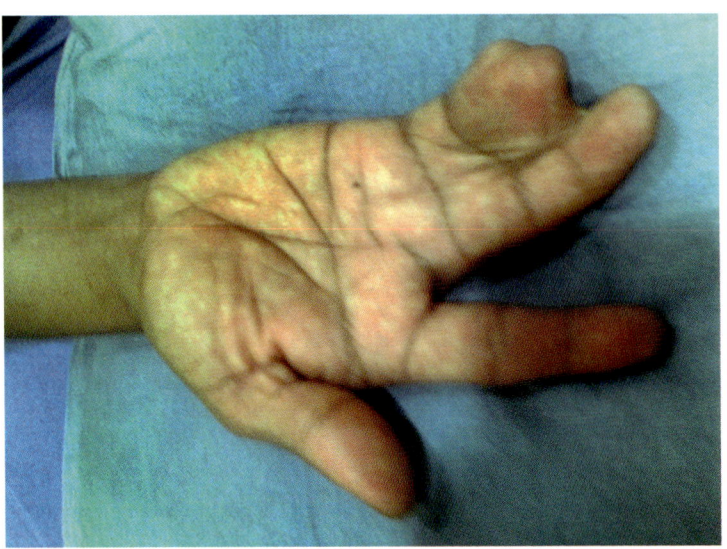

Quiz 1

What are the observations?
Webbing of ring, little and the lateral part of the middle finger—syndactyly.

Quiz 2

What is syndactyly?
Webbing of fingers and/or toes—fusion of ring and the little finger in this patient, along with skin continuity between the middle and the ring fingers.

Quiz 3

How common is it?
Syndactyly is the most common congenital anomaly of the limbs—seen once in 2000–3000 live births.

Quiz 4

What type of syndactyly is seen between the middle and the ring fingers?
The fusion between the middle and ring fingers indicate simple syndactyly—involving only the soft tissues.

Quiz 5

What type of syndactyly is seen between the ring and the little fingers?
The fusion between the ring and the little fingers indicates complex syndactyly—possibly involving the bones.

Quiz 6

What are the syndromes associated with syndactyly?

Syndromes associated with syndactyly include:

1. Alport's syndrome—usually associated with complex syndactyly
   - Components of Alport syndrome:
   - Short thumb with radial deviation
   - Complex syndactyly of index, middle and ring finger
   - Simple syndactyly of fourth webspace
   - Genetics
   - AD inheritance
   - C to G mutation on FGFR2 gene on chromosome 10.
2. Amniotic band syndrome—the skin is joined in the most part of the digits. However, there is a gap with normal skin in the proximal portion.
3. Fraser syndrome—cryptophthalmos, cutaneous syndactyly, abnormal genitalia, nose and ear malformation, laryngeal atresia, cleft palate, renal agenensis, mental retardation.
4. Smith-Lemli-Opitz syndrome—syndactyly toes II-III, microcephaly, hypoplastic kidneys, male pseudohermaphroditism, severe mental retardation.
5. Tsukahara syndrome—syndactyly, microcephaly, pachygyria, renal dysplasia, abnormal genitalia.
6. QT prolongation syndrome.

143. Syndactyly Associated with Transverse Palmar Crease

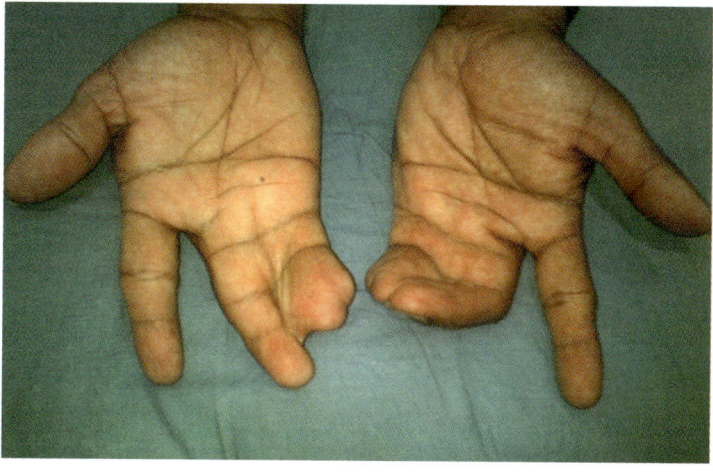

Quiz 1

What are the observations?

- Syndactyly.
- One of the tranverse creases is long and extends to the ulnar border of the palm.

What are the types of long palmar creases?
a. Normal—all creases proxinmal and distal are present and are normal.
b. Simian crease—seen in Down syndrome. Proximal palmar crease is long and extends to the ulnar border. Distal transverse crease is absent.
c. Sydney line—proximal crease extends to the ulnar border of the palm. Distal crease is present.

144. X-ray Features of a Large Long-Standing Goiter

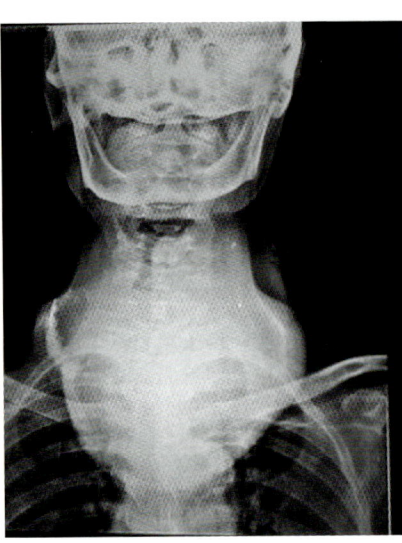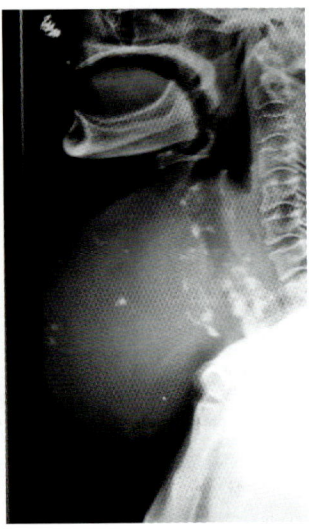

Quiz 1

What are the observations?

Observations in the PA view
1. Calcification—linear calcification in the periphery and speckled calcification in the substance of the goiter
2. Trachea—displaced and curved—"Scabbard trachea"—resembling the protective sheath of the sword.
3. Soft tissue shadow in the neck—well seen in both PA and lateral views
4. Soft tissue shadow extends into the superior mediastinum partially overlapping the aortic shadow—indicating the retrosternal extension
5. Also note the age-related calcification in the aortic knuckle.

Observations in the lateral view
1. A large soft tissue swelling projecting anteriorly and descending well down on to the chest wall
2. Evidence of calcification at multiple different sites.

Quiz 2

What is the difference between retrosternal extension and a retrosternal goiter?

When a cervical goiter also extends partially into the mediastinum, it is called retrosternal extension.

When most of the goiter (>51%) is in the mediastinum, it is called retrosternal goiter. Most of the retrosternal goiters (79%) are cervicomediastinal. 21% are completely intrathoracic.

Quiz 3

What are the presentations of a retrosternal goiter?

a. A neck mass (75%)

b. Asthma like presentation with breathlessness (70%)

c. Hoarseness of voice (40%)

d. Dysphagia (30%)

e. Stridor (20%)

f. SVC syndrome (6%) → thrombosis

g. Cerebral hypoperfusion (due to arterial compression, thyrocervical steal)

h. Involvement of nerves—phrenic, recurrent laryngeal nerve, Horner's syndrome

i. Pleural effusion, chylothorax

j. Pericardial effusion.

Quiz 4

What are the serious complications of a retrosternal goiter?

1. Pressure symptoms including airways obstruction.
2. Stimulation of the carotid sinus during surgery resulting in severe bradycardia and even death.
3. Damage to the recurrent laryngeal nerve during clearance of the thyroid cancer.

Quiz 5

What is the importance of involvement of the carotid sheath/artery?

• Suggests a malignant process.

• Berry's sign—inability to feel the carotid pulsation in the neck due to malignant infiltration of the carotid sheath.

Quiz 6

What are the effects of thyroid mets?

• Local infiltration of the neighboring structures

• Hormone producing mets—thyroxine produced from the mets to lungs and the bones from follicular carcinoma.

Quiz 7

What is the association of MEN 2 and the thyroid cancer?

Patients with MEN 2 are at a higher risk for the development of early medullary cancer of the thyroid gland. Early thyroidectomy is indicated, if they carry a mutation of the proto-oncogene.

Quiz 8

What is lingual thyroid and what is its embryology?

Embryologically thyroid devolops from the 3rd and the 4th branchial arches and descends from the foramen caecum to the neck. Devolopmental arrest can lead to formation of a lingual thyroid.

The diagnosis is done with a thallium/technetium scan.

Biopsy may be dangerous as it can cause excessive bleeding and there is a risk of aspiration.

Quiz 9

What is hyperthyroidism? What are the causes?

Hyperthyroidism is overfunction of the thyroid gland associated with a clinical state of thyrotoxicosis.

Causes

1. Graves' disease
2. Toxic nodular goiter
3. Destructive thyroiditis
4. Iodine excess—Jod-Basedow effect
5. Amiodarone
6. TSHoma.

Quiz 10

What are the features of Graves' disease?

Autoimmune thyroiditis with a triad

1. Autoimmune thyroiditis
2. Eye disease (die to involvement of retro-orbital space)
3. Pretibial myxedema (involvement of skin); thyroid acropachy (fingers involved).

Quiz 11

What kind of goiter is seen in Graves' disease?

Diffuse goiter with a bruit.

Quiz 12

Mention some salient features of hyperthyroidism

1. Graves' disease and nodular goiter are common causes
2. Graves' disease associated with ophthalmopathy, dermopathy, acropachy, other autoimmune features
3. Atrial fibrillation and fever indicate severe disease
4. Thyroid storm may be due to iatrogenic reasons
5. Usually TSH is very low or undetectable in thyrotoxicosis
6. Treatment options include antithyroid drugs, radioiodine, thyroidectomy.

Quiz 13

What are the features of various types of thyroiditis?

1. Hashimoto's thyroiditis lymphocytic
2. Graves' thyroiditis

3. Postpartum—painful lymphocytic thyroiditis + triphasic thyroid function
4. De Quervain's—painless inflammatory giant cell thyroiditis + high ESR
5. Riedel—hard goiter + fibrosing thyroiditis + midline fibrosis.

Quiz 14

What is triphasic thyroid function in postpartum thyroiditis?

- 1st phase—elevated S. Free T4–<6 months of delivery—euthyroid/mildly thyrotoxic
- 2nd phase—4–12 months after delivery—hypothyroidism
- 3rd phase—recovers normal thyroid function.

Quiz 15

What are the salient features of hypothyroidism?

1. Hashimoto's thyroiditis is the main cause
2. Insidious onset with multiorgan involvement
3. Characteristically associated with delayed relaxation of tendon jerks
4. Elevated S. TSH
5. Dose change done not before 6 months
6. In patients with heart disease—start low and go slow.

Quiz 16

Give salient features of thyroid disease in pregnancy

1. Postpartum thyroiditis can last for about 1 year
2. Extra thyroxine may be needed if there is pre-existing hypothyroidism
3. Autoimmune thyroid disease improves during pregnancy
4. Due to transplacental transmission of TSH, maternal thyrotoxicosis may be associated with fetal thyrotoxicosis.

Quiz 17

Which thyroid related substances are transferred transplacentally?

Iodine, antithyroid drugs, propranolol, TRH, thyroid stimulating antibodies are transferred transplacentally.
T3, T4, and TSH do not cross the placenta.

145. Pancreatic Calcification

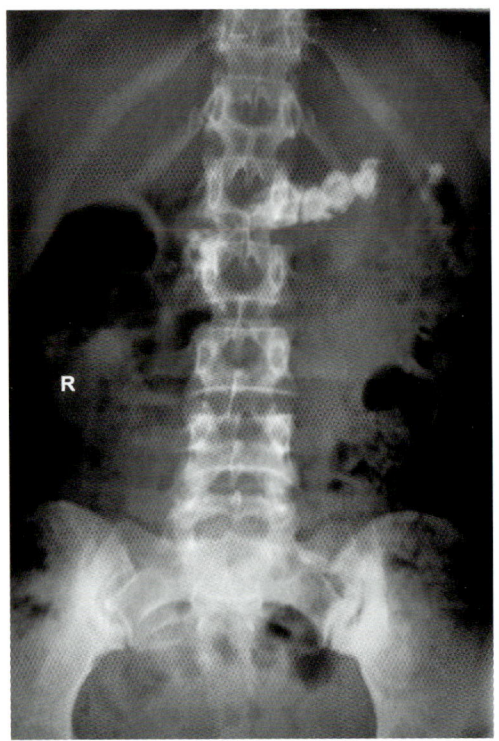

Quiz 1

What are the observations?
Horizontal calcifications mainly at the level of L1 (and some also at the level of L2).

Quiz 2

What is the commonest cause of pancreatic calcification?
Chronic alcoholic calcific pancreatitis.

Quiz 3

What are the causes of pancreatic calcification?
1. Chronic alcoholic pancreatitis
2. Hereditary pancreatitis
3. Hyperparathyroidism
4. Kwashiorkor—chronic protein malnutrition
5. Cystic fibrosis
6. Pseudocyst of the pancreas
7. Tumors.

Quiz 4

What are the characteristic features of various conditions causing pancreatic calcification?

Characteristic features of pancreatic calcification:

1. Chronic alcoholic pancreatitis intraductal calculi (numerous irregular concretions of varying size)—mainly limited to the head/tail; may extend throughout the pancreas as seen in this patient.
2. Hereditary pancreatitis—AD; calculi tend to be larger and rounder calculi found in younger, non-alcoholic patients.
3. Hyperparathyroidism associated with renal calcification—nephrocalcinosis and nephrolithiasis. Simultaneous coexistence of pancreatic and renal calcification should suggest the possibility of hyperparathyroidism.
4. Chronic protein malnutrition (kwashiorkor)—associated with excessive alcohol consumption/malnutrition.
5. Cystic fibrosis—AR inheritance; calcification seen in the areas of fibrosis. Calcification seen in very young (sometimes as young as 4 years) + associated diabetes mellitus—"painless pancreatitis".
6. Serous cystadenomas—"Sunburst calcifications" central calcification with calcification in the septa radiating outwards.
7. Pseudocyst of the pancreas—parenchymal calcification of the pancreas + calcification of the rim of the pseudocyst.
8. Metastasis—metastatic renal cell carcinoma, metastatic colonic carcinoma.
9. Idiopathic, senescent pancreatic calcification.

Quiz 5

What are the mimics of pancreatic calcification?

a. Splenic artery calcification
b. Calcified gallstones in the distal CBD
c. Retained contrast in the duodenal diverticula.

Quiz 6

Mention some interesting phenomena observed in pancreatic calcification.

Some phenomena observed in pancreatic calcification include:

1. Disappearing calcification—malignancy, chronic pancreatitis (rare observation)
2. Displacement of calcification—pseudocyst of the pancreas
3. Painless pancreatitis associated with calcification—cystic fibrosis.

Quiz 7

What is the role of gallstones in the precipitation of acute pancreatitis?

Role of gall stones is well known. Microlithiasis and biliary sludge also have a role

Microlithiases are small stones of <3 mm diameter

Biliary sludge is defined as a suspension of crystals (cholesterol monohydrate), mucin, glycoproteins, cellular debris, proteinaceous material within bile. Sludge may be visualized by abdominal US or EUS. Microscopic examination is needed to identify the crystals.

Quiz 8

What are the conditions associated with recurrent "idiopathic pancreatitis"?

a. Autoimmune pancreatitis—elevated total IgG, IgG4. ANA positive.
b. Diagnosable with ERCP (70% in one study)—microlithiasis, sludge (27.5%), sphincter of Oddi dysfunction type II (35%), pancreas divisum (7.5%).
c. EUS—endoscopic US—biliary sludge (in patients with gall bladder *in situ*), microlithiasis may reduce the need for ERCP. EUS + duodenal bile sampling will reduce the need for ERCP.
d. Also exclude—concealed alcohol use, hereditary pancreatitis, drug induced, infections, recent abdominal trauma, systemic diseases.
e. Metabolic causes—hypercalcemia, hypertriglyceridemia.
f. CT abdomen—gallstones, pancreatic neoplasm, chronic pancreatitis.
Rapid bolus contrast technique—to diagnose pancreatic necrosis, small neoplasms.

Quiz 9

What is the role of genetic testing?

Particularly when the family history is positive in recurrent idiopathic pancreatitis
a. Genetic testing for cationic trypsinogen gene (TRSS1)
b. Cystic fibrosis transmembrane conductance regulator gene (CFTR)
c. Mutations in trypsin inhibitor gene (SPINK1)
However, the exact role in the genetic testing of these genes is not clear and is controversial.

Quiz 10

What tests may prove useful for recurrent acute pancreatitis in future?

MR cholangiopancreatography may be a useful noninvasive strategy to identify bile duct stones and to evaluate for pancreatic divisum.

146. Unilateral Red Eye

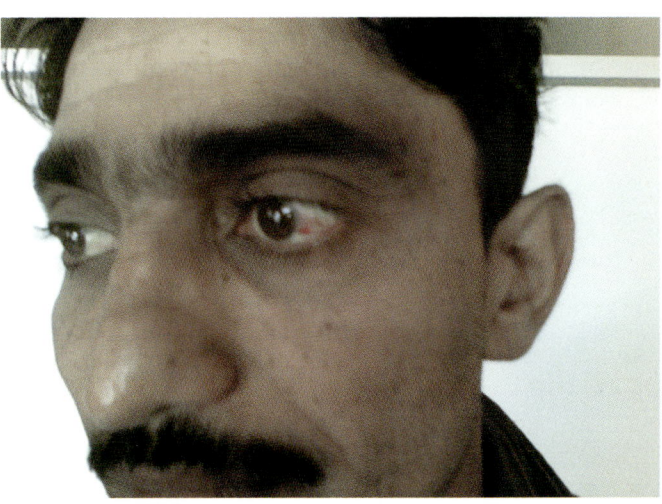

Quiz 1

What are the observations?
Unilateral subconjunctival hemorrhage.

Quiz 2

What is the synonym?
Hyposphagma. It is bleeding under the conjunctiva.

Quiz 3

What are the common causes?
a. Trauma—including operations like Lasik in the eye
b. Aspirin
c. Whooping cough
d. Leptospirosis
e. Acute hemorrhagic conjunctivitis—enterovirus 70/coxsackie A
f. Increased venous pressure—straining, vomiting, coughing
g. Scurvey.

Quiz 4

In a patient of high fever, conjunctival suffusion, subconjunctival hemorrhage, what else do you look for?
Jaundice, myalgia, high fever, hematuria, pulmonary hemorrhage.

Cases in Medicine

147. Unilateral Consolidation with Paratracheal Lymph Nodes Enlarged

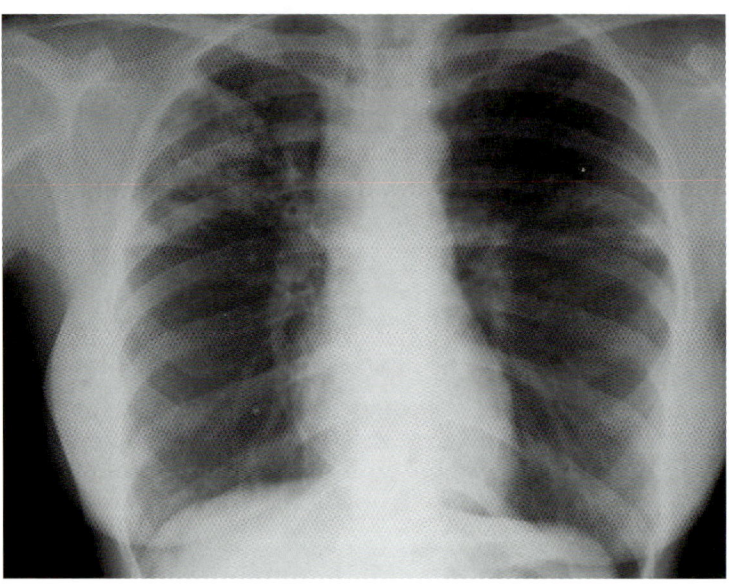

Quiz 1

What are the observations?

a. Parenchymal—right upper lobe infiltration with an "air bronchogram sign". A tendency for cavitation is also seen.
b. LN—right paratracheal lymphadenopathy
c. Pleural—there is a hint at the interlobar effusion—a thickened horizontal fissure partially seen on the right side.

Quiz 2

How do you analyse these observations?

1. In the right upper zone and a part of the midzone, air bronchogram sign is seen—that is to say, the air in the alveoli is replaced by inflammatory fluid (therefore, giving a white shadow on the CXR instead of the black one); while the bronchi still containing air cast a black shadow. Together they cast a black shadow (of air in the bronchi) overlapping a white shadow (of inflammatory fluid in the alveoli)—known as the air bronchogram. The presence of air bronchogram indicates the likelihood of the disease process being a consolidation.

2. Usually, pneumonia is not associated with enlargement of regional LN on the CXR. If however, the coexistence of enlarged lymph nodes is indeed visible, one has to seriously consider the possibility of tuberculosis/malignancy.

3. There is also a partially thickened interlobar fissure seen—suggesting a possibility of interlobar effusion.
4. A careful observation of this CXR shows the simultaneous presence of bronchogram sign (indicating consolidation), enlargement of right paratracheal lymph nodes, and an interlobar effusion in the horizontal fissure.

Quiz 3

What possibilities do you consider?

The possibilities considered include:

a. Tuberculosis—upper lobe parenchymal involvement, paratracheal LN involvement and interlobar effusions are fairly common and typical occurrences in TB.
b. Malignancy—possibility of an obstructive pneumonia has to be considered but this squamous cell malignancy usually involves hilar lymph nodes. Enlarged paratracheal LN do not cause obstructive pneumonia.
c. Paratracheal lymph nodes can also be involved in lymphomas—where the involvement is bilateral and consolidation infrequent. Multiple types of pleural effusion can also be seen in this condition.

Quiz 4

What is Garland triad?

Simultaneous coexistence of involvement of right paratracheal, right hilar and the left hilar lymph node masses constitute garland triad. It is also known as 1–2–3 sign or Pawnbroker's sign.

Lambda sign also gives the same information—involvement of bilateral hilar and the paratracheal LN.

These are classically seen in sarcoidosis.

Quiz 5

What are the syndromes described in sarcoidosis?

a. Heerfordt syndrome—fever, parotid enlargement, facial palsy, ocular involvedment. A variant of sarcoidosis.
b. Löfgren syndrome—fever, malaise, erythema nodosum, hilar adenopathy, arthritis, uveitis, parotitis.

148. Prominent Vessel on the Left Temple

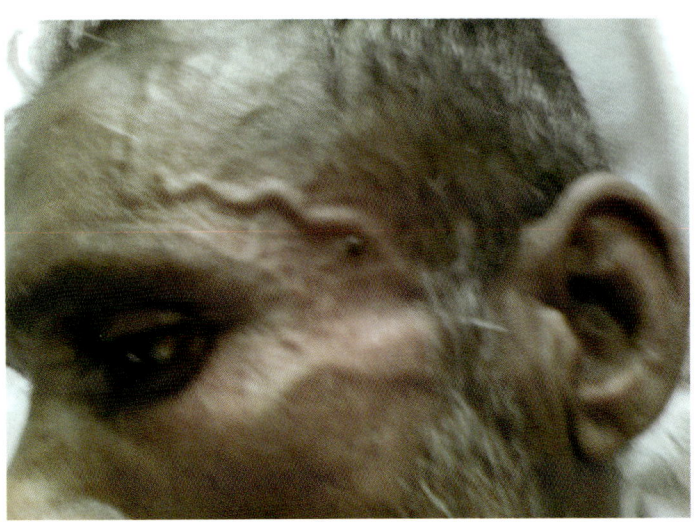

Quiz 1

What are the observations?

Enlarged, tortuous, prominent vessel on the left temporal region—most likely temporal artery.

Quiz 2

What are the possibilities?

a. May be a normal variation

b. If it is tender and feels like a thickened cord, look for other signs of connective tissue disease—history of headache, blindness/amaurosis fugax, jaw claudication, elevated ESR—consider possibility of giant cell arteritis.

Quiz 3

What are the examples of intermittent claudication?

1. Legs—peripheral vascular disease, Leriche's syndrome (intermittent claudication also involving legs, thighs, + impotence)
2. Legs—neurologic due to spinal canal stenosis
3. Upper limbs—TAO, peripheral vascular disease
4. Jaw—giant cell arteritis
5. Abdominal angina—mesenteric ischemia
6. Angina pectoris—stable angina also is an example.

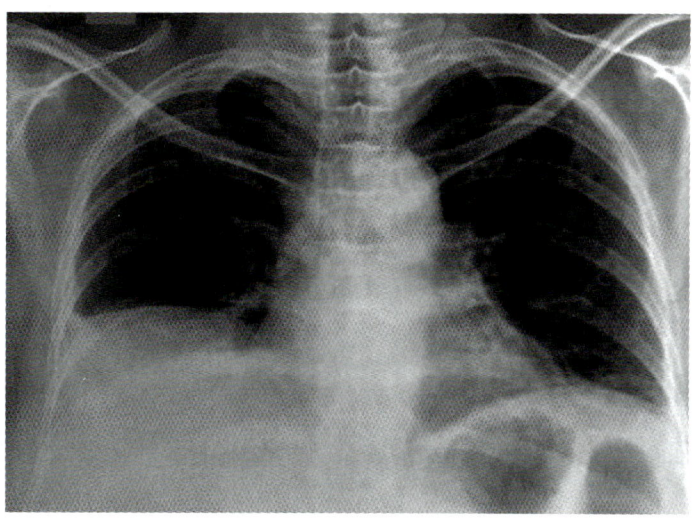

Quiz 1

What are the observations?

1. Elevated right hemidiaphragm
2. Loss of normal contour of the elevated diaphragmatic leaf
3. Lateral displacement of the peak of the diaphragm on right side
4. A small lamellar effusion—seen obliterating the right cardiophrenic angle.

Quiz 2

What are the infereneces?

Upward enlargement of the liver + sub-diaphragmatic effusion + a small pleural effusion.

Quiz 3

What is the most likely diagnosis?

Most likely cause—amoebic liver abscess.

Quiz 4

What other additional lesion can coexist hidden with these findings?

Right basal atelectasis.

Quiz 5

What are the complications of amoebic liver abscess?

a. Complications due to rupture of the amoebic liver abscess into:
   1. Pleura—empyema
   2. Pericardium—pericardial effusion, tamponade

Cases in Medicine

239

3. Peritoneal cavity—peritonitis
4. Outside the abdominal wall—direct or by incision—amoebiasis cutis
5. Into the intestine—natural evacuation
   b. Complications due to dissemination of the amoebic live abscess to:
      1. Lung-Lung abscess
      2. Brain-Brain abscess.

Quiz 6

What are the pulmonary manifestations of amoebiasis?

1. Pneumonia
2. Pleural effusion
3. Empyema—due to rupture of amoebic liver abscess into the pleural cavity—anchovy sauce pus.

Quiz 7

What are the clinical features of amoebic liver abscess?

a. Patient may give a history of right upper quadrant pain (due to the liver abscess) and right shoulder pain (referred pain due to the involvement of the diaphragmatic pleura laterally innervated by the phrenic nerve)
b. Fever—high, swinging temperature often exceeding 104°F
c. Toxic patient—ill, tachycardia, tachypnoea, hypotension
d. Jaundice may be seen if the abscess presses on the porta hepatis
e. Tender hepatomegaly
f. Intercostal tenderness
g. Upward enlargement of the liver
h. Relative immobility (reduced mobility) of the liver on deep inspiration
i. Reduced breath sounds on the lower portion of the right chest—due to upward enlargement of the tender liver and also due to pleural effusion.

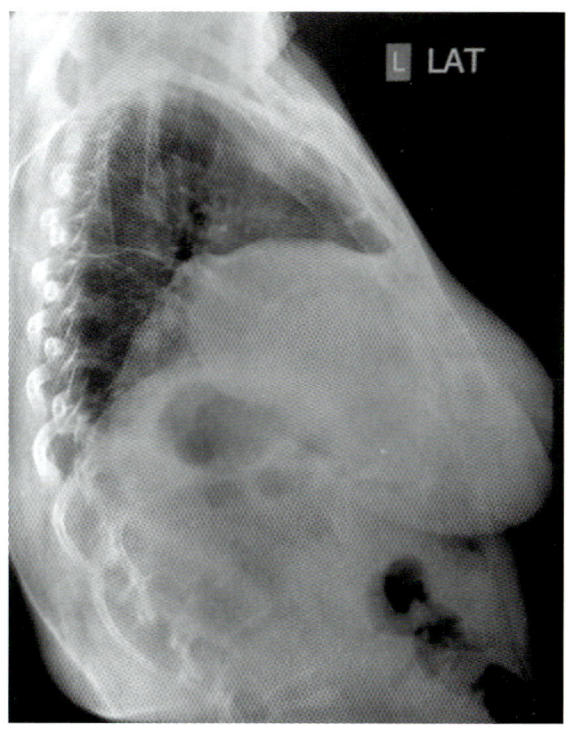

L LAT

Quiz

What are the observations?

1. Elevation of the right hemidiaphragm clearly seen
2. Anterior pleural recess obliterated suggestive of a small pleural effusion
3. Small collections of fluid also seen in the interlobar fissure.

151. Calcifications Related to the Cardiac Shadows

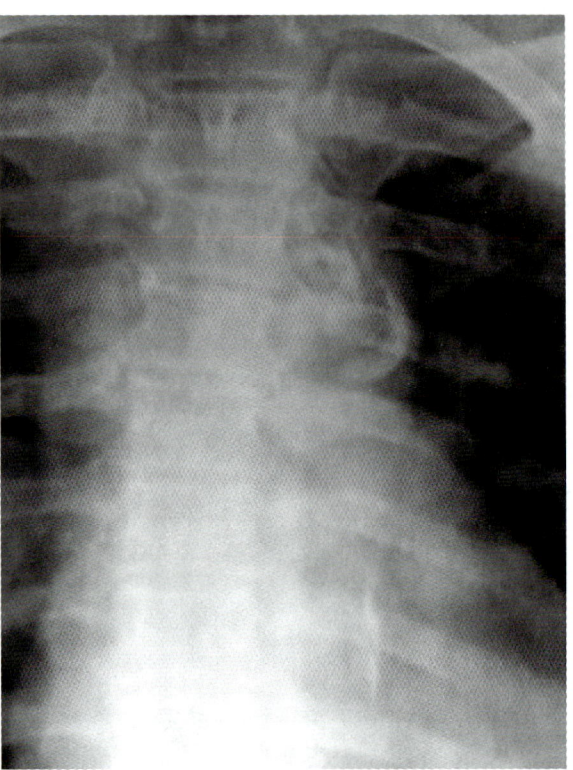

Quiz

What are the observations?

Two calcifications clearly seen

1. One related to the aortic knuckle—semilunar calcification
2. One linear calcification seen lower down on the left side—could be a calcified coronary artery.

Molecular basis of coronary artery calcification

Calcification is diffuse (not solely confined to intima)—due to GLa containing proteins with high affinity to hydroxyapatite.

Osteopontin (cell attachment protein), osteonetin (a protein associated with calcium) and osteocalcin (gamma carboxylated protein that regulates mineralization) also have a role.

Bone morphogenic factor 2a a potent factor for osteoblastic differentiation is noted in atherosclerotic plaque and it responds to transforming growth factor beta.

Teleologically calcification might have a role in myocardial protection.

Coronary remodelling is associated with progression of atherosclerosis.

Chest X-ray is an inexpensive tool in detecting coronary artery calcification but its sensitivity remains low.

152. Mediastinal Mass

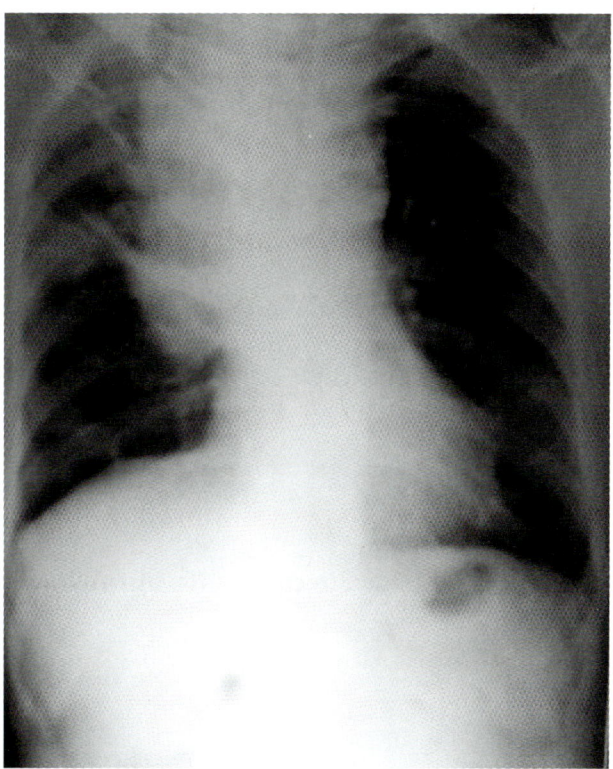

Quiz 1

What are the observations?

1. Mediastinal enlargement with multiple enlarged lymph node masses mainly on the right side—predominantly disease condition involving the lymph node component of the mediastinum.
2. A closer scrutiny as described below also reveals pleural component of the disease.
3. Elevated right hemidiaphragm probably due to the involvement of the phrenic nerve.

Quiz 2

What are the details of the observations?

1. Mediastinal enlargement—right upper zone, mid zone and a part of the lower zone
2. Mediastinal enlargement is mostly on the right side—in the region of known lymph nodes and the margin is scalloping—all these make lymph node enlargement the most likely cause of the enlarged mediastinum.

   Right paratracheal, tracheobronchial, hilar lymph node masses are seen. Possibly the subcarinal nodes are also involved.

3. Prominent horizontal fissure with displacememt upwards (in the distal portion) indicating possible obstruction to the lymphatic drainage and venous drainage.
4. Note the slight fullness seen on the left side above the aortic knuckle indicating the presence of lymph nodes on the left side also.
5. Also notice—obliteration of the cardiophrenic and the costophrenic angles (in the PA view) and the anterior and the posterior pleural recesses (in the lateral view) suggesting the presence of a pleural effusion. Also, the diaphragm has lost its contour and this is more obvious on the lateral view—suggesting the co-existence of a subpulmonic effusion on the right side.

Quiz 3

What is the most likely clinical presentation of this patient?
The syndrome of SVC obstruction—edema of the face and the upper limbs
- Non-pulsatile engorgement of the internal jugular vein–as the enlarged LN not only obstruct the free flow of blood into the heart (thereby causing the engorgement) but also prevent the transmission of the pulsations from the right atrium to the internal jugular vein (resulting in a non-pulsatile JVP)
- Cheimosis of the conjunctiva
- Cyanosis of the face, lips and oral mucosa
- Increasing cyanosis and cheimosis on pronged bending down
- Giddiness
- Dilated veins in the chest wall with the direction of the blood flow above downwards.

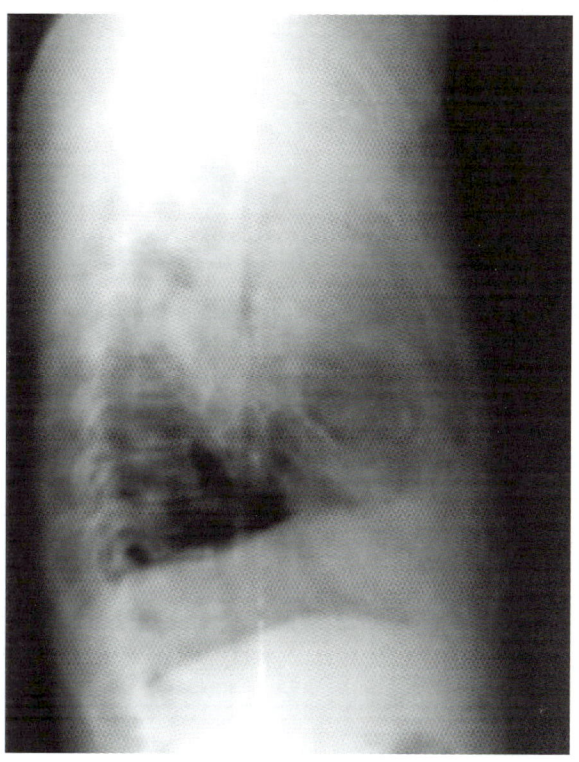

Quiz

What are the observations?

1. A large, dense mediastinal opacity involving the superior and the inferior (mainly the middle) mediastinum
2. An elevated right hemidiaphragm
3. Blunting of the anterior and the posterior pleural recesses indicating pleural effusion
4. Thickened interlobar fissure indicating interlobar effusion.

Cases in Medicine

154. Sequelae of Tuberculosis Associated with COPD

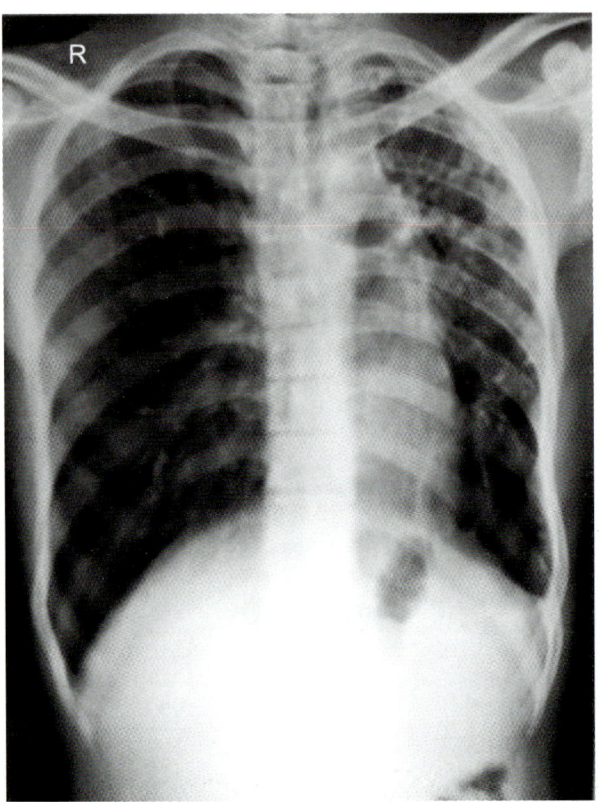

Quiz 1

What are the observations?

1. Emphysema as indicated mainly by the presence of horizontal ribs, hyperlucency with reduced pulmonary vasculature and flattened diaphragm.
2. Other evidences of parenchymal involvement—reduction in the size of the left hemithorax, mediastinal and tracheal shift to the left, involvement and calcification mainly on the left side
3. Blunting of the costophrenic angle mainly on the left side.
4. Compensatory emphysema on the right side
5. Some spots of calcification on the right side

Quiz 2

Are the findings recent or old?

Old.

First relates to emphysema.

Second, third and fourth indicate old scarring disease involving the parenchyma—possibly tuberculosis. The observations are basically the sequelae of tuberculosis.

a. Sequelae of tuberculosis:
1. Reduction in the size of the left hemithorax—indicating volume loss on the left side.
2. Trachea—shifted to the left side.
3. Obliteration of the left cardiophrenic angle with calcification—indicating fibrosed/calcified pleura secondary to old pleural effusion/empyema.
4. Diffuse, patchy calcification in the parenchyma and pleura more on the left side involving upper, mid and lower zones.
5. Diffuse, scattered specks of calcification are also seen on the right side occupying upper, mid and lower zones.
6. Calcification in the region of the hilar lymph nodes especially on the left side—suggesting a calcified primary complex—Renke's complex.
7. Heart is displaced to the left partly due to left sided volume loss due to fibrothorax and partly due to compensatory emphysema on the right side.

b. Features of COPD—better appreciated on the right side
• Hyperlucency
• Horizontally placed ribs
• Flattened diaphragm
• Diaphragm placed lower
• Relatively small heart
• Displacement of the heart to the left side—partly due to fibrothorax on the left side and partly due to compensatory emphysema on the right side.

155. Same Patient—Right Lateral View

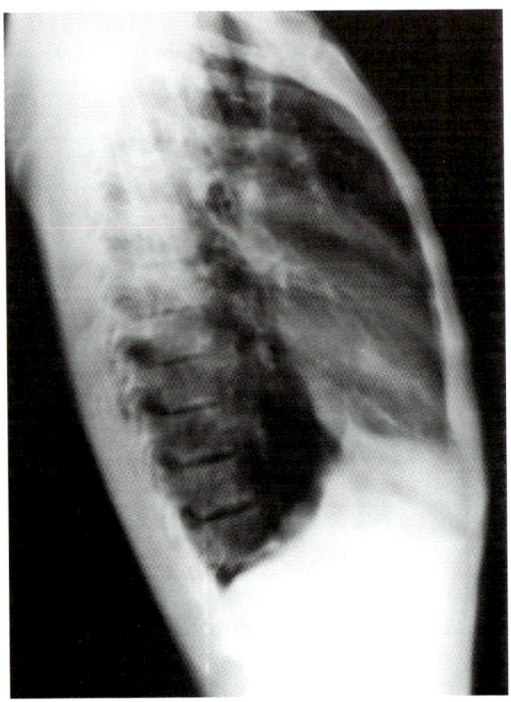

Quiz 1

What are the observations?

1. Scattred calcifications in the parenchyma and the pleura
2. Blunting of the anterior pleural recess
3. Increase hyperlucency in retrosternal and retrocardiac spaces.

Quiz 2

What are the inferences?

The findings are mainly due to sequelae of tuberculosis and some are suggestive of COPD. However, compensatory emphysema cannot be completely ruled out.

a. Features of sequelae of tuberculosis
   1. Scattered calcification in lung parenchyma and pleura.
   2. Calcification in the pleura, anterior and posterior pleural receses and adjacent portions of the pleura.
   3. Calcification of the hilar lymph node.
b. Features of COPD
   1. Hyperlucency particularly in the retrosternal and the retrocardiac spaces.
   2. Narrow, tubular heart.

156. Surgical Emphysema and Mediastinal Emphysema

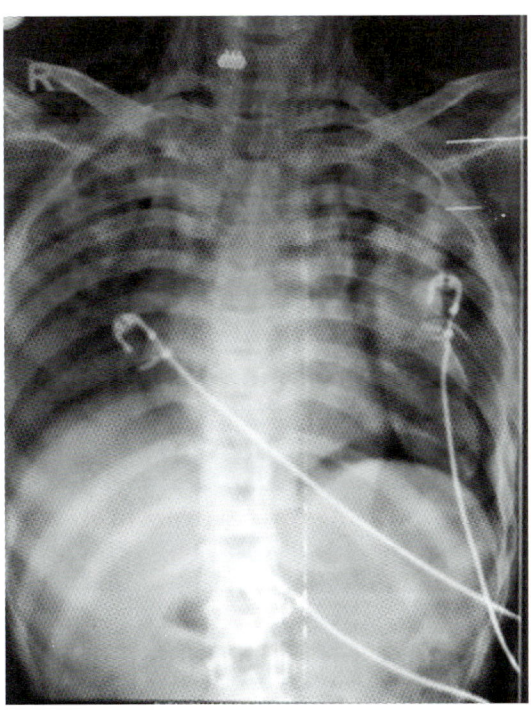

Quiz 1

What are the observations?

a. Features of surgical emphysema
  - Free air along the muscle plains seen adjacent to the neck and the upper chest wall.
  - Free air along the muscle plains of the chest wall.
b. Features of mediastinal emphysema
  Free air outlining the cardiac border.

Quiz 2

What is the approach to reading of such X-rays?

1. Look for a pneumothorax
2. Look for an intercostal tube
3. Look for # rib(s).
4. Look for accompanying hemothorax.

Quiz 3

What are the features of surgical emphysema?
Crepitus on palpation to the location of the surgical emphysema.

Quiz 4

What is the extent of spread if it starts in the chest? What are the common causes?

Common causes include:

a. Trauma (RTA)-# rib resulting in pneumothorax
b. IC tube insertion for pleural effusion/empyema
c. Rupture of emphysematous bulla
d. Severe asthma
e. Positive pressure ventilation.

Extent of spread

a. Starts at the alveoli (e.g. severe asthma) → spreads proximally along the bronchial sleeves to the hilum → ascends up the mediastinum → deep fascia of the neck → descends along the arms—upper arm, forearm, hand; descends along the chest wall → to the anterior abdominal wall → limited by the inguinal ligament.
   From the neck it can ascend along the face → deforming the face.
b. Travels along the muscle plains.
c. Can co-exist with mediastinal emphysema.

Quiz 5

What are the mechanisms of causation of mediastinal emphysema?

a. Air entering from alveoli → asthma, emphysema → travels along the vascular sheath to the hilum.
b. Spontaneous pneumomediastinum—from rupture of esophagus stoma—usually in the lower 8 cm of esophagus (no connective tissue support on the left side; musculature here is inherently weak → due to increased intraluminal pressure secondary to—exercise, vomiting associated with failure of the cricopharyngeal sphincter to relax, increased intracranial pressure.
c. Rupture of trachea/bronchus usually during trauma—increased pressure in the trachea/bronchus over a closed glottis acts as a shearing force.
d. Air entering the mediastinum from the deep facial planes of the neck—during thyroidectomy and tonsillectomy.
e. Air entering mediastinum from the retroperitoneal space—air from the retroperitoneum enters the mediastinum along the aorta/esophagus usually following the perforation of the intestines/stomach.
f. Mixed etiology—spontaneous and trauma to the chest wall.

Quiz 6

What is "malignant pneumomediastinum"?

Pneumomediastinum producing increased mediastinal pressure and resulting in shock associated with dyspnoea, cyanosis, engorged non-Pulsatile neck veins, rapid thread pulse, hypotension. Untreated, it can proceed to pulmonary edema and circulatory failure.

How do you identify the mediastinal emphysema?

Clinical sign—to and fro crunching sound heard along with the heart beats. Best heard at the cardiac apex (Hamman's sign).

Radiological—CXR PA—air in the mediastinum seen as a sharp, distinct line running parallel to the left and sometimes to the right border of the heart.

CXR lateral view may show substernal air collection.

Quiz 7

What are the clinical features of mediastinal emphysema?

1. History sharp constricting retrosternal pain in the chest (due to dissection of the mediastinal tissues with air) with radiation to both shoulders and down both the arms, aggrevated by exertion and swallowing.
2. Signs include:
   - Surgical emphysema occasionally esulting in disfigurement of face and neck due to subcutaneous air collection—crepitus on palpation.
   - Apex beat may not be palpable.
   - Cardiac dullness may be reduced.
   - Auscultation over the surgical emphysema reveals superficial cracking sounds.
   - Auscultation over the mediastinal emphysema reveals Hamman's sign—A crunching sound best heard in the left parasternal region in the left 3rd to 6th IC spaces, heard in synchrony with the cardiac cycle (systole), best heard in the sitting up or the left lateral decubitus position. It is heard despite the presence of surgical emphysema so much so the presence of a positive Hamman's sign associated with surgical emphysema/ pneumothorax is highly suggestive of an accompanying mediastinal emphysema.
   - Auscultation over the cardia reveals distant heart sounds.
3. Features of an accompanying pneumothorax.

Quiz 8

What are the situations where a false positive Hamman's sign can be elicited?

Left-sided pneumothorax, dilated left esophagus, bullous emphysema of the lingular segments, diaphragmatic hernia with the high left diaphragm, gastric dilatation.

Quiz 9

What are the differential diagnoses for pneumomediastinum?

Esophageal rupture

In esophageal rupture shock occurs faster.

- X-ray chest PA view taken early might show a localized mediastinal emphysema in the lower part of the mediastinum.
- A lateral view of the neck view may show pushing forward of the larynx and the esophagus due to collection of air in the retrovisceral space.

157. Tetany, Carpal Spasm and Trousseau's Sign

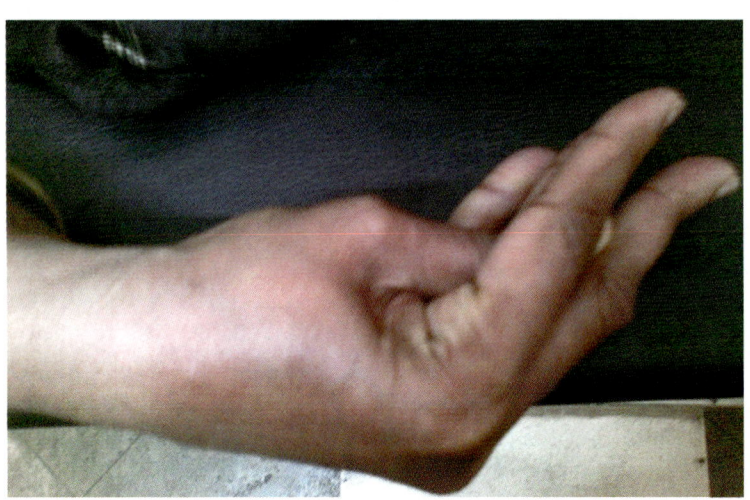

Quiz 1

What are the observations?

Carpal spasm—pedal spasm—a similar observation, if seen in the lower limbs.

Quiz 2

What are the common accompanying signs?

Accompanied by paresthesia.

Quiz 3

What is the significance of this observation?

May be spontaneously observed in tetany.

   If elicited by compresing the upper arm with a tourniquet/inflated BP cuff above the systolic for 3 minutes (only if not seen spontaneously) indicates latent tetany.

   Chvostek's sign—other sign of latent tetany elicited by percussing the facial nerve near the angle of the mandible-resulting in twitching of the angle of the mouth on the same side.

Quiz 4

What are the sequence of events if the serum calcium progressively reduces?

Sequence of events of progressive reduction in serum calcium

1. Neuromuscular irritability → paresthesias of hands, feet, perioral region (low serum calcium calcium reduces the excitation threshold of the nerves). → Chvostek's sign, Trousseau's sign.
2. Blepharospasm—bronchospasm, laryngospasm, tetany.

3. CNS—seizures, increased ICT

Chronic hypocalcemia → extrapyramidal features, parkinsonism +/− calcification of basal ganglia and dentate nucleus (presence of calcification—the features may not reverse with correction of the hypocalcemia).

4. CVS prologed QT syndrome, arrhythmias, CCF.

5. Eye features—lens deposits and cataracts.

Quiz 5

What are the causes of hypocalcemia?

Causes of hypocalcemia

1. Hypoparathyroidism—parathyroid removal during complete thyroidectomy
2. Polyglandular autoimmune syndrome I—hypoparathyroidism + hypoadrenalism + chronic mucocutaneous candidiasis.
3. Damage to the parathyroids—disease, vascular insufficiency, radiation
4. Hypomagnesemia—inhibition of secretion and end organ resistance to the action of PTH.
5. Activating mutations of receptors to sense higher than existing levels of calcium and hence resulting in persistent abnormal low PTH levels despite low serum calcium levels (hypercalciuria aggrevated by Vit D analog treatment.
6. Pseudohypoparathyroidism (Fuller Albright)—resistence to PTH confined to the kidneys → short stature, round face, short metacarpals (knuckle knuckle dimple dimple syndrome), obesity, basal ganglia calcification. Various types of vitamin resistant rickets have been described.
7. Chronic renal insufficiency—due to hyperphosphatemia and reduced activation of Vit D in the kidneys.
8. Hyperphosphatemia—due to tumor lysis, malignant hyperthermia, rhabdomyolysis acute pancreatitis—chelation of calcium by FFA
9. Osteoblastic metastasis (prostate and breast)—as calcium is used up for the bone formation
10. Toxic shock and sepsis
11. Biphosphonate administration
12. "Hungry bone syndrome"—after parathyroid tumor resection, cure of hyperthyroidism.

Cases in Medicine

158. Bilateral Hilar Adenopathy

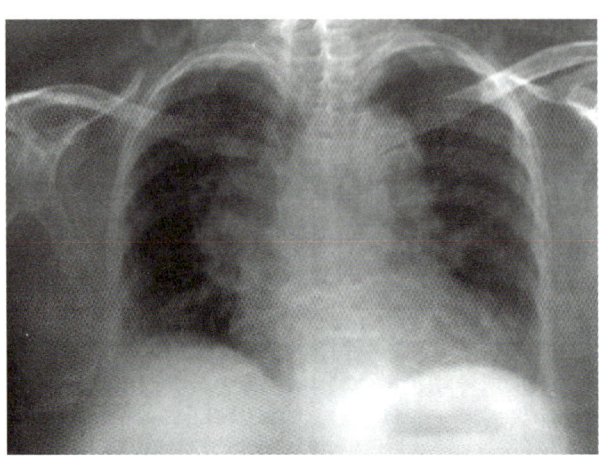

Quiz 1

What are the observations?
1. Bilateral hilar prominences
2. Scalloping outline better seen on the right side—suggests a lymph node mass
3. Bilateral hilar adenopathy (BHA)
4. Reticulonodular shadows seen at the bases better seen on the right base.

Quiz 2

What is the approach to read an X-ray with BHA?
Approach to a CXR with BHA (bilateral hilar adenopathy)
1. Look for other lymph nodes—paratracheal, tracheobronchial, subcarinal mediastinal, etc.
2. Look for reticulonodular shadows at the bases.

Quiz 3

What are the causes of BHA?
Cauases of BHA
1. Granulomatous dieases—sarcoidosis
2. Granulomatous infections—tuberculosis
3. Infections—HIV, mycoplasma, fungal infections
4. Malignancies—lymphoma—non-Hodgkin's > Hodgkin's
5. Pneumoconiosis—silicosis
6. Immunologic—Churg-Strauss syndrome, adult Still's disease.

Quiz 4

What are the chest X-ray features of sarcoidosis?
Chest X-ray patterns include:
0—normal chest X-ray

I—BHA
II—BHA + lung infiltration
III—lung infiltration without BHL (only parenchymal disease)
IV—lung fibrosis, scarring, retraction of both the lungs at the hila, + no BHA (end stage lung disease).

Quiz 5

What is Garland sign?

Garland sign/1-2-3 sign/Pawnbroker's sign

Simultaneous presence of right paratracheal LN group and the BHA.

Suggests sarcoidosis.

159. Bilateral Gynecomastia and Spider Nevi

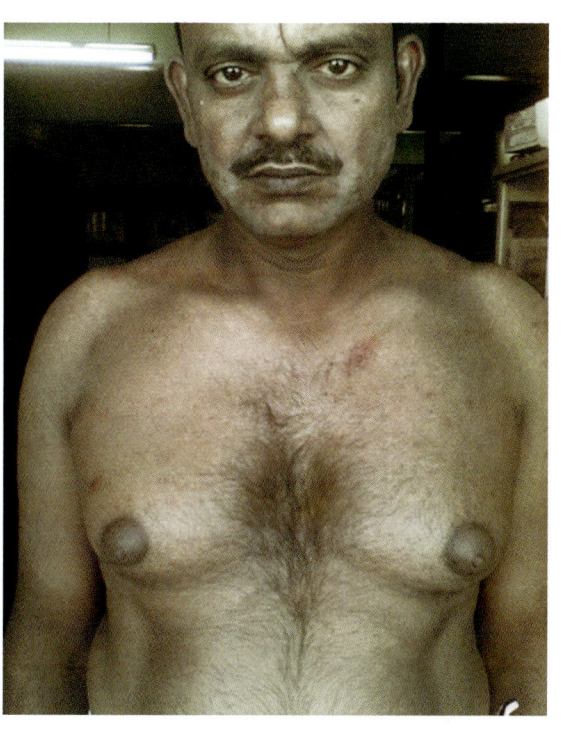

Quiz 1

What are the observations?

1. Bilateral gynecomastia
2. Multiple spider nevi—biggest seen below the left side of the neck, at least 3 are seen on the left side of the chest and at least 1 on the right side of the chest.
3. Co-existence of the two should suggest liver disease—cirrhosis of the liver.

Quiz 2

What are spider nevi?

Synonyms:
1. Arterial spider
2. Spider telangiectasia
3. Spider angioma.

Location:
- Vascular territory of the SVC above a line joining the nipples.
- Commonly at the necklace area, face, forearm, dorsum of the hand.

Quiz 3

What are the components of spider nevi?

A small arteriole

Small vessels radiating from the central arteriole—resembling the silk threads in the American dollar—" Paper money skin".

Quiz 4

What are white spots?

White spots are—spots seen on arms and buttocks on coling the skin—they represent the beginnings of the spider nevi.

Quiz 5

Which are the conditions where spider nevi are seen?

a. Liver disorders—cirrhosis—old ones increase in numbers/new ones appear
b. Pregnancy—2nd to 5th months. Disappear within 2 monthes after delivery.

Quiz 6

What are the differential diagnoses for spider nevi?

1. Hereditary hemorrhagic telangiectasis—seen in cirrhosis, primary biliary cirrhosis, Raynaud's phenomenon, CREST syndrome
2. Campbell de Morgan's spots—bright red spots increasing with age
3. Venous star—seen with elevated pressure—seen on a main tributary of the vein with increased pressure. Seen on foot, legs, back, lower border of ribs. Not obliterated by pressure.

160. Vitiligo

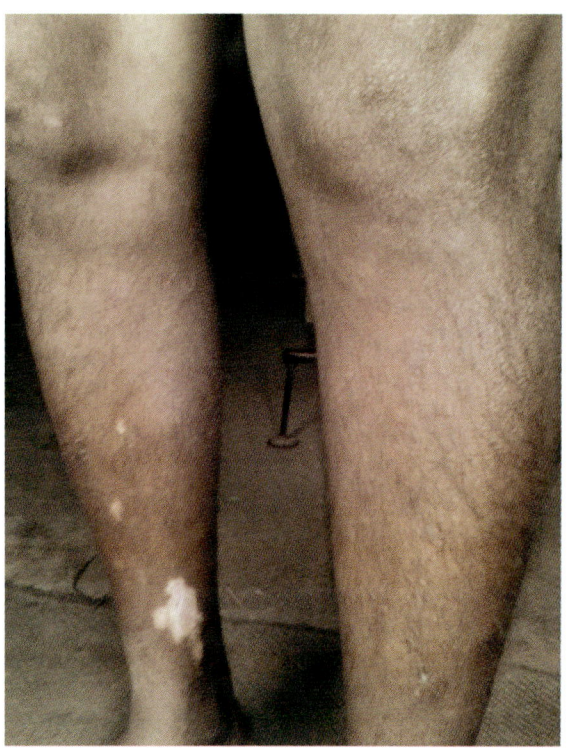

Quiz 1

What are your observations?

Patches of vitiligo—one big on the right foot and many tiny one on both feet.

Quiz 2

What are the causes of vitiligo?

Autoimmune—solo manifestation or a part of autoimmune syndrome

For example, pernicious anemia (megaloblastic anemia) due to autoimmune atrophic gastritis +
vitiligo +
1. Oxidative stress
2. Exposure to some chemicals
3. Sunburn.

Quiz 3

What are the syndromes associated with vitiligo?
1. Addison's disease.
2. Polyendocrine deficiency syndrome—hypogonadism, vitiligo, hypothyroidism, DM.

3. Stiff person syndrome—may be associated with DM, thyroiditis, vitiligo, pernicious anemia. Can be mistaken for Parkinson's disease, fibromyalgia, anxiety, multiple sclerosis.
4. Parry-Romberg syndrome—progressive facial hemiatrophy, vitiligo, seizures, trigeminal neuralgia.
5. Autoimmune disorders—autoimmune thyroiditis, autoimmune gastritis, alopecia areata.

Quiz 4

What are the differential diagnoses for vitiligo?
1. Waardenburg syndrome—AD, piebaldism, hypomelanotic macules, bilateral deafness, heterochromia iridis, broad bridge of the nose, white forelock.
2. Tuberous sclerosis—hypopigmented macules with a confetti-like pattern, ash leaf macules, low intelligence, epilepsy, pituitary—adrenal dysfunction.
3. Diffuse scleroderma with hypopigmented macules.
4. Melanoma assoiated vitiliginous depigmentation.
   Vitiligo begins centrally (chin, trunk, neck) and spreads distally (hands, feet).
   Vitiliginous depigmentation starts distally and spreads proximally (trunk).

161. An Excellent X-ray for Developing Skills of Observation

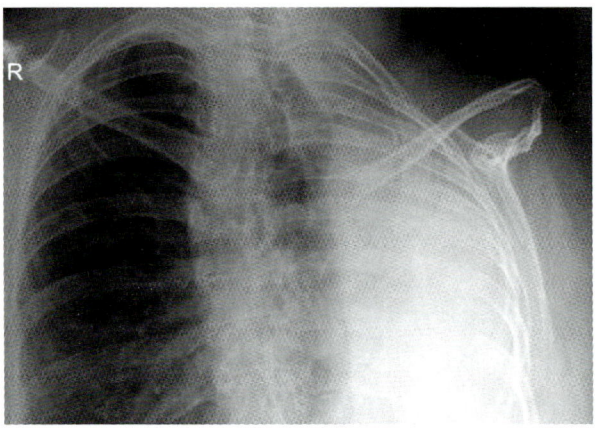

Quiz 1

What are your observations?
The observations include:
1. Asymmetry of the bones—bones on the left side are smaller and underdeveloped.
2. 1st, 2nd, 3rd, 4th ribs are not only smaller but also not properly positioned—apparent crowding.
3. Left clavicle is hypoplastic and so is the left scapula.
4. Placement of the medial end of the clavicle is abnormal and unnatural—much lower than expected.
5. Scoliosis with hemivertebra.
6. Trachea shifted to the right side.

7. White opacity on the entire left side—in fact, no lung is visible! Part of the blackness is due to the shifted trachea; part of it is due to herniation of the right lung into the left hemithorax.
8. Now observe carefully—there is no humerus seen on the left side—in fact the entire left upper limb is missing!

Quiz 2

What is the diagnosis?
Amelia with agenesis of the left lung.
This patient also had agenesis of the left kidney on abdominal ultrasound examination.

Quiz 3

What is amelia?
A birth defect with lack of one or more limbs. All 4 limbs are absent in tetra amelia.

Quiz 4

What is the mechanism of development of amelia?
Interfernce with the limb development process between 24th and 36th day of embryonic life.

Quiz 5

What are the conditions seen in association with amelia?
Cleft lip/palate, body wall defects, neural tube defects, agenesis of lung, kidney, diaphragmatic leaf on that side.

162. Diffuse Bilateral Parenchymal Shadows

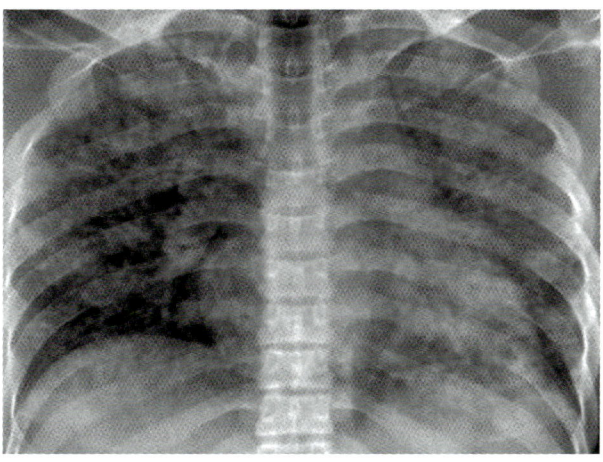

Quiz 1

What are your observations?
1. Air bronchogram—seen on both sides—appearance better appreciated on the left side.
2. The shadows are rather dense.

Quiz 2

What is your diagnosis?

Pulmonary alveolar hemorrhage.

Quiz 3

What are the possible clincal presentations.

Hemoptysis

Possible associations include:

1. Connective tissue disorders—Wegener's granulomatosis, SLE, Goodpasture syndrome
2. Leptospirosis
3. Anticoagulant overdose
4. Superwarfarin poisoning
5. Coagulation failure—acute fulminant hepatitis
6. Pulmonary hemosiderosis
7. ATRA syndrome—all transretinoic acid syndrome—patients with acute promyelocytic leukemia on treatment with ATRA. CXR shows increased CT ratio, ground glass opacities, peribronchial cuffing, septal lines, pleural effusion
8. Post-bone marrow transplantation.

Quiz 4

What is the classification of diffuse pulmonary hemorrhage?

a. Pauci-immune disease involving pulmonary capillaries
   Pulmonary capillaritis + ANCA positive—CTD, APLA, HSP, acute transplant rejection
   No pulmonary capillaries—SLE, Goodpasture, idiopathic pulmonary hemosiderosis, penicillamine, VOD
b. Syndromes caused by immune deposits + positive immunofluorescence
c. Large miscellaneous group including—drug reactions, infections, idiopathic diseases.

Quiz 5

What are the examples of vasculitis involving medium caliber vessels?

- Polyarteritis nodosa
- Kawasaki disease.

Quiz 6

What are the examples of small vessel vasculitis

a. IF (immunofluorescence) negative + ANCA positive
   1. Microscopic polyangiitis—vasculitis + no asthma + no granuloma
   2. Wegener's granulomatosis—vasculitis + no asthma + granulomas +
   3. Churg-Strauss syndrome—vasculits + eosinophilia + asthma + granulomas.
b. IF positive + immune complexes in the vessels
   1. Cryoglobulinemic vasculitis—cryoglobulins in the blood or vessel walls
   2. Henoch-Schönlein purpura-IgA deposits in the vessel walls
   3. Lupus/rheumatoid vasculitis—SLE
   4. Other vasculitis due to immune complexes—other sources of immune complexes.

How do histology and immunology help in the diagnosis?
a. Antiglomerular BM antibodies with Linear IF pattern → Goodpasture syndrome
b. Anti GBM antibodies with granular immunofluorescent pattern → SLE, HSP, IgA nephrpathy.
c. ANCA + with negative IF (or Pauci-immune) → Wegener's MPA, Churg-Strauss
d. Unknown with no IF/pauci-immune → idiopathic pulmonary hemorrhage.

Quiz 8

What are the antibody findings in pauci-immune disease?
a. c-ANCA—cytoplasmic ANCA—proteinase 3 ANCA-Wegener's (75% 0 > MPA (40%). Churg- Strauss.
b. p-ANCA—perinuclear ANCA—myeloperoxidase ANCA Churg-Strauss (30%) > MPA (10%). Wegener's (5%).

163. Acute Pulmonary Edema—Predominantly Interstitial Edema

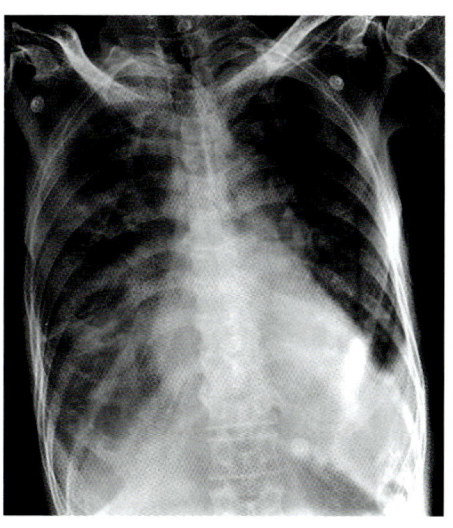

Quiz 1

What are the observations?
a. Cardiomegaly
b. Multiple linear interstitial shadows seen in all 3 zones more in mid and lower zones
c. Increase in visible vessels particularly in the upper zones mainly on the right side
d. Short, horizontal lines seen at the lower zone some abutting the pleura—Kerley B lines representing superficial lymphatics in the interlobar septa
e. Relatively long, fine linear shadows radiating from the hilum, situated deep within the lung parenchyma—deep lymphatics in the deep interlobar septa.

Quiz 2

What are Kerley lines?

They are septal lines seen on CXR due to thickened septa which are not usually visible. There are 4 types of Kerley lines: A, B, C, and D.

Quiz 3

What are Kerley A lines?

They are long, fine, linear shadows radiating from hila representing thickened deep lymphatics of the thickened interlobar septa.

Quiz 4

What are Kerley B lines?

They are horizontally oriented short, peripheral lines seen in lower zones extending to and perpendicular to and abutting the pleura at the costophrenic angle. They represent superficial lymphatics in the interlobar septa.

Quiz 5

What are Kerley C lines?

They arefine "lace like"/"spider web like"polygonal opacities seen in the peripheral/subpleural location usually due to pulmonary fibrosis. They represent visible subpleural lymphatic plexus.

Quiz 6

What are Kerley D lines?

They are due to criss crossing of Kerley A and B lines.

Quiz 7

At which stage of the pulmonary edema are Kerley A and B lines become visible?

When the PCWP increases to 17–22 mmHg, signs of interstitial edema appear and Kerley A and B lines become visible.

When the PCWP approaches 25 mmHg, alveolar edema appears.

Quiz 8

Which are the conditions where the Kerley lines/septal lines are seen?

a. Acute pulmonary edema/pulmonary venous hypertension
b. Pneumoconiosis
c. Pulmonary fibrosis
d. Interstitial pneumonitis
e. Deposition of hemosiderin in the septa
f. Lymphangiitis carcinomatosa
g. Lymphangiomyomatosis.

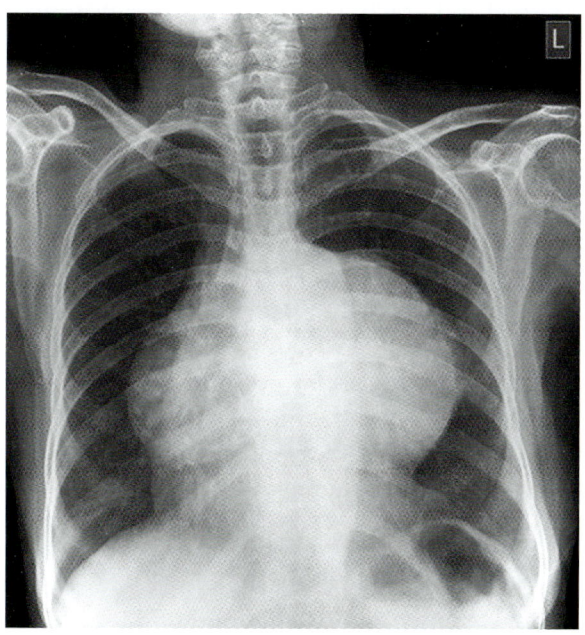

Quiz 1

What are your observations?

The observations include:

1. Cardiac silhouette looks grossly abnormal—looks like gross cardiomegaly at a superficial glance.
2. Careful observation shows that these are the dilatations of the ascending and the descending aorta—right atrium is visualized but ventricle is hardly seen.
3. Rim and the outline of the dilatations show calcification
   Linear calcification (mainly on the left side) and speckled calcification (mainly on the right side).
4. The overall appearences suggest aneurysm of the ascending and the descending aorta with calcified wall and calcified thrombus.

Quiz 2

What are the genetic disorders associated with thoracic aortic aneurysm?

a. Marfan's syndrome—aortic root dilatation—due to cystic medial degeneration (in Marfan's syndrome, Ehlers-Danlos syndrome) due to mutation in one of the genes for fibrillin 1 (a major component of microfibrils of elastin due to which the amount of elastin the aortic wall decreases.
b. Familial thoracic aortic aneurysm syndrome also consists of cystic medial degeneration. There is also a sporadic variety not associated with CTD/family history.

Cases in Medicine

c. Loeys-Dietz syndrome—bifid uvula, hypertelorism, craniostenosis, Marfan like features, arterial aneurysms/dissections
d. Genetic mutations associated with TAA and dissection
   TGFBR1
   TGFBR2 (transforming growth factor beta receptor type II)—thin skin, tortuous/aneurismal arteries' congenital contractural arachnodactyly/Beal's syndrome
   FBN1 (fibrillin 1—Marfan's syndrome—skeletal, ectopia lentis, dural ectasia
   ACTA2 (actin alpha 2) smooth muscle, aorta—associated with livedo reticularis, iris flocculi, bicuspid aortic valve, PDA
   MYH11 (smooth muscle specific beta myosin heavy chain)—associated with PDA
   COL3A1—thin skin; rupture of GI, arteries, gravid uterus
e. Turner's syndrome—bicuspid aortic valve, coarctation of the aorta, ascending aortic dilatation primary amenorrhea, karyotype 45XO, webbed neck, low hairline, broad chest. Increased risk of aortic dissection.
   Increased risk of aortic dissection, if bicuspid aortic valve, hypertension, pregnancy, coarctation of the aorta.
f. APKD—Berry aneurysms > aortic dissection resulting in subarachnoid hemorrhage
g. Noonan's syndrome
h. Ehlers-Danlos syndrome associated with cystic medial degeneration.
i. Bicuspid aortic valve—irrespective of the hemodynamic severity is always associated with aortic dilatation (earlier thought to be" post stenotic"). May be associated with cystic medial degeneration.

Quiz 3

Which are the inflammatory disorders associated with thoracic aortic aneurysm and dissection?

Aorta arteritis:

a. Takayasu arteritis—
   - Age <40—young women
   - TAA can be seen in the early (inflammatory) stage or late (sclerotic) stage.
   - Intermittent claudication
   - Reduced pulsations/bruit in subclavian artery, brachial artery
   - BP variation >10 mmHg between 2 arms.
b. Giant cell arteritis
   - Age >50. Usually involves temporal/cranial arteries. Also involves aorta.
   - Aneurysms may be TAA/AAA.
   - Headache + temporal artery tenderness + reduced pulsations
   - ESR >50
   - Biopsy—necrotising vasculitis.
c. Behcet disease
   - Ulcers—oral + genital ulcers
   - Uveitis, retinal vasculitis
   - Skin—erythema nodosum, pathergy.

d. Ankylosing spondylitis
  - Age <40 + backache + morning stiffness
  - There is inflammation of the fibrocartilage and is directed to the tissues rich in fibrillin 1 resulting in ascending aortic aneurysms.

Quiz 4

What are the other causes of TAA?

a. Atheroscerosis—involves descending aorta beyond the origin of the left subclavian artery.
b. Dissecting aneurysm—after dissection the outer wall of the false lumen is weakened further because its inner half (the intimal flap) has been dissected away, thereby giving rise to aneurysm.
c. Trauma—non-penetrating deceleration injuries. Can kill; can get diagnosed and treated; can get missed and develop into pseudoaneurysms. TAA is usually saccular.
d. Syphilis—latent period from spirochetal infection to complication is 10 to 30 years.
  - Route taken by the spirochetes and the sequence of events.
  - Secondary syphilis → spirochetes enter tunica media → obliterative end arteritis of vasa vasorum (proximal ascending thoracic aorta) → destruction of collagen and elastin fibres → aortic dilatation, fibrosis, calcification.
  - Longitudinal wrinkling → "tree barking" (radiologic pattern).
  - Aortic wall weakening → fusiform/saccular aneurysms.
  - Sites involved ascending A > arch > root.
  - Ascending aorta—can be associated with secondary aortic regurgitation.
  - Root involvement associated with ostial coronary artery stenosis.

Quiz 5

How do you treat a patient with Marfan's syndrome?

1. Good control, if hypertension—<140/90
   β blockers, ARBs (Losartan), ACE inhibitors used
2. Treat associated coronary artery disease
3. Treat dyslipidemia.

Quiz 6

Give examples of vascular calcifications

a. Calcific atherosclerosis
   Location and mechanism of calcification—intimal, ossification
   Associated diseases—atherosclerosis, osteoporosis, dyslipidemia, hypertension, inflammation.
b. Monkeberg's medial calcific sclerosis
   Location—tunica media
   Associated diseases—DM2, ESRD, hypophosphatemia, amputation.
c. Elastocalcinosis
   Location—internal elastic lamina
   Associated diseases—pseudoxanthoma elasticum, Marfan.
d. Calcific uremic arteriopathy
   Location and mechanism—microvessels, amorphous
   Associated diseases—ESRD, Warfarin.

e. Calcific aortic valvular stenosis
   Location—aortic face of leaflets
   Hyperlipidemia, congenital bicuspid valve, rheumatic HD.
f. Portal vein alcification
   Location—portal vein thrombus, venous wall
   Associated diseases—portal hypertension, liver disease.

Quiz 7

How does calcification help in the diagnosis of aortic dissection?
Increased (>1 cm) from aortic intimal calcification to the outer edge of the aortic shadow
Mediastinal widening on a single CXR
Both more so if they are new findings as compared to the old CXR.

Quiz 8

What are the other features?
Progressive widening of aortic shadow on PA/AP view.

Quiz 9

What are the syndromes caused by thoracic aortic aneurysms?
a. Chest pain—anterior/posterior
b. Esophageal compression → dysphagia
c. Recurrent laryngeal nerve compression → hoarseness of voice
d. SVC compression → SVC syndrome
e. Pulmonary artery/tracheal compression → cough/dyspnea/both
f. Aneurysmal erosion into pulmonary parenchyma/rupture into the bronchus → hemoptysis
g. Rupture into the pleural space → shock
h. Ostial lesions in syphilitic aortitis → angina.

Quiz 10

List the syndromes caused by abdominal aortic aneurysms
a. Pain—midabdominal/lumbar/pelvic
b. Rupture into peritoneal cavity → shock
c. Duodenal compression → intestinal obstruction
d. IVC compression → peripheral edema
e. Aneurysmal rupture into the duodenum → GI bleed
f. Aneurysmal rupture into the vena cava → high output cardiac failure
g. Thrombosis of aneurysm/embolization of the thrombus to legs → arterial insufficiency of the legs.

165. Luftsichel Sign

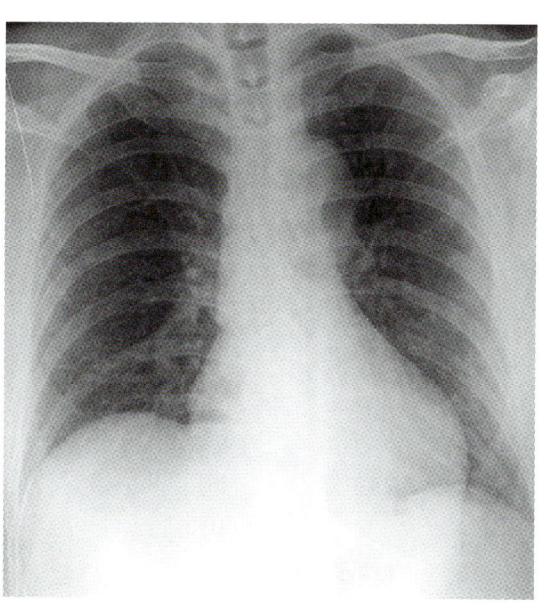

Quiz 1

What are the observations?
1. Multiple patchy lesions seen on the left side in upper and mid zones.
2. A strip of black lucency seen covering the aortic knuckle—represents the expanded apical segment of the lower lobe protruding and covering the aortic knuckle which is normally covered by upper lobe (the bronchopulmonary segments which have selectively collapsed due to disease process involving the upper lobe—most likely TB)—' the lucency covering the aortic knuckle resembles a sickle made of AIR—hence the name—Luftsichel sign or air sickle sign.

Quiz 2

What is the origin of the term Luftsichel sign?
Luft—air
Sichel—sickle
Classically there is a crescent of air between the aorta and the medial border of the collapsed lobe/segment of the left lung.
Aortic knuckle is clearly seen.

Quiz 3

What is the finding in the lateral view?
Left upper lobe always collapses anteriorly with a clear posterior margin.

Quiz 4

What is the other sign on the PA view which it may sometimes be associated with?
Juxtaphrenic peak sign—left hemidiaphragm becomes tented/peaked.

Quiz 5

What are the other signs of left upper lobe collapse that may be seen?
Sandwiching of the superior pulmonary vein between the aorta medially and the medial border of the collapsed upper lobe laterally.
Collapsed segment is tethered by the bronchus, left pulmonary artery and the superior pulmonary vein.

Direct signs of collapse
1. Displacement of the fissures
2. Loss of aeration
3. Crowding of vessels.

Indirect signs
1. Tracheal shift
2. Mediastinal shift
3. Rib crowding
4. Compensatory overinflation of the remaining lung
5. Hilar displacement.

Quiz 6

What are the differential diagnoses of the Luftsichel sign?
a. Right lung herniation—left lung collapse results in shift of the aorta to the left and mediastinal shift to right lung herniates behind the sternum to fill the space and produces a parasternal hyperlucency. In Luftsichel sign there is para-aortic lucency.
b. Mediastinal pneumothorax—accompanied by pneumothorax/surgical emphysema. No other signs of collapse.

Quiz 7

What investigation is essential for a patient of Luftsichel sign and why?
Bronchoscopy—to rule out endobronchial pathology.

166. Coarctation of the Aorta—Rib Notching

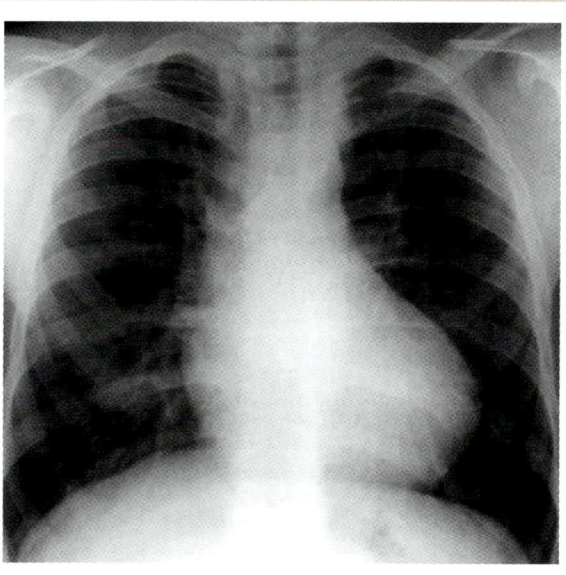

Quiz 1

What are the observations?

1. Borderline cardiomegaly.
2. Pulmonary hyperemia.
3. Absence of aortic knuckle/aortic notch shadow.
4. Sign of 3—
   Seen on the left side
   - Upper part of 3—slightly dilated aorta just above the coarctation
   - Narrow middle portion representing the coarctation
   - Lower portion of 3—slightly dilated aorta just below the coarctation—indicating the post-stenotic dilation of the coarctated aorta.
5. Rib notching—seen on the inferior margins of 5th, 6th, 7th, and 8th ribs due to repeated pulsations from the dilated and tortuous intercostal arteries acting as collaterals in coarctation of the aorta—Dock's sign.
   Rib notching usually becomes evident after the age of 8 years.
6. Superior intercostals vein may be seen as a projecting nipple from the aortic knob/knuckle—not seen in this CXR.

Quiz 2

What is the clinical sign related to Dock's sign?

Dock's sign (rib notching at the inferior margins from 3rd to 9th ribs) indicates the presence of intercostal collaterals. Clinically these patients can have visible and palpable arteries on the back and a Suzman's sign positive—a continuous murmur presents on a visible/palpable collateral seen on the back.

Quiz 3

What are the causes of rib notching?

1. Coarctation of the aorta (due to enlarged pulsating intercostal arteries)
2. Interrupted aorta—enlarged pulmonary artery
3. Subclavian artery obstruction
4. TOF
5. Pulmonary atresia
6. Tricuspid atresia
7. SVC obstruction—enlarged pulmonary vein
8. Neurofibroma—entangled intercostals nerve.

Quiz 4

Why rib notching is not seen below the age of 8 years?

It is caused by pressure erosion of the adjacent ribs by enlarged tortuous collaterals. So rib notching is rare in young children even in the presence of severe coarctation.
It is seen in the inferior aspects of the middle thirds of the posterior ribs—3rd to 8th ribs.

Quiz 5

Why are the first two ribs spared of notching in the coarctation of the aorta?

The first two ribs are spared as the first and the second intercostals arteries arise from the costocervical trunk of the subclavian artery.

Quiz 6

What are the collaterals involved in the coarctation of the aorta?

a. Main collateral route—internal mammary artery with retrograde flow below the coarctation with intercostals arteries 3 to 9
b. Internal epigastric arteries, scapular arteries, various mediastinal arteries.

Quiz 7

What are the causes of unilateral rib notching?

1. Ipsilateral Blalock-Taussig shunt—1st and 2nd ribs
2. Presubclavian coarctation.

Quiz 8

What are the causes of pseudo-rib notching?

1. Congenital—non-sclerotic margins of the adjacent bone
2. Hyperparathyroidism.

Quiz 9

What are the causes of superior rib notching?

1. Osteogenesis imperfecta
2. CTD—RA, Marfan's, SLE
3. Local pressure
4. Hyperparathyroidism (abnormal osteoclastic activity).

Quiz 10

What are the causes of superior and inferior rib notching?
Hyperparathyroidism.

Quiz 11

How does the rib notching of coarctation differ from that of neurofibromatosis?
a. In neurofibromatosis type 1, the inferior rib notching can be anywhere
b. It can be associated with soft tissue shadows.

Quiz 12

What are the clinical clues to the presence and the location of coarctation?
1. Hypertension + delayed and weakened femoral pulses compared to carotid and arm pulses
2. Differential cyanosis—suggests postductal coarctation with reversal of shunt—PDA
3. Hypertension (secondary)
4. LVH—secondary to hypertension
5. Suprasternal pulsations
6. Parasternal systolic murmur; interscapular systolic murmur—due to coarctation itself
7. Continuous murmurs on the intercostals collaterals
8. Aortic ejection click—bicuspid aortic valve
9. BP higher in upper limbs and low in lower limbs
10. Intermittent claudication/weakness of the lower limbs
11. BP higher in right upper limb—subclavian artery is also narrowed.

Quiz 13

What are the congenital anomalies associated with coarctation of the aorta?
a. Bicuspid aortic valve
b. MVP
c. VSD
d. Aneurysm of the sinus of Valsalva
e. Aneurysms of the circle of Willis (Berry aneurysms).

Quiz 14

What are the complications associated with the coarctation of the aorta?
1. CCF
2. Dissection of the proximal aorta
3. AS/AR
4. Bicuspid aortic valve → infective endocarditis
5. Hypertension → CVA
6. Berry aneurysms → subarachnoid hemorrhage
7. Aneurysm of the sinus of Valsalve → rupture.

Quiz 15

What are the syndromes associated with coarctation?
Turner's syndrome.

Mention some syndromes associated with congenital cardiac lesions

1. TAR syndrome—VSD
2. Syndactyly/polydactyly—VSD
3. Trisomy 13–15 VSD
4. Trisomy 17–18 VSD, PDA
5. Down syndrome ASD (endocardial cushion defect type)
6. Arachnodactyly ASD
7. Ellis-Van Creveld syndrome—ASD, single atrium
8. Holt-Oram syndrome—ASD familial
9. Rubella syndrome—PDA, PS
10. Turner's syndrome—coarctation of the aorta, AS, PS
11. William's syndrome—supravalvular AS, peripheral pulmonary artery stenosis
12. Hurler syndrome—MR/AR
13. Marfan's syndrome—incomplete coarctation, ASD, MVP, tulip bulb aorta, annuloaortic ectasia, fusiform aneurysm of the ascending aorta, PA aneurysm.

167. Barium Swallow in Coarctation of the Aorta

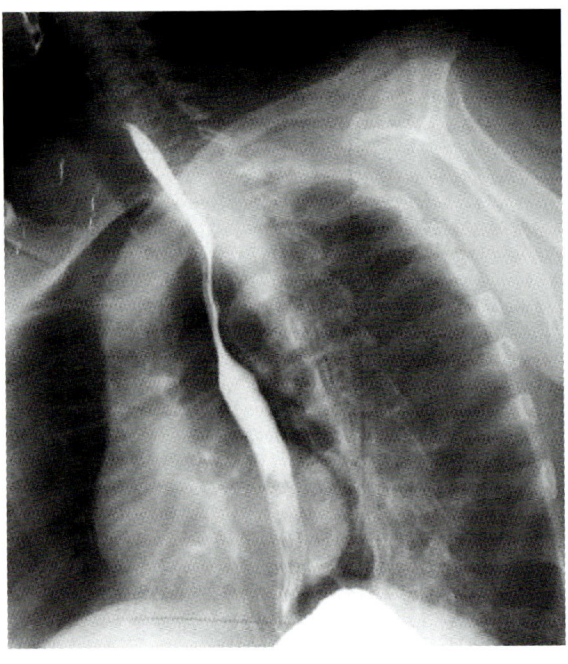

Quiz 1

What are the observations?

Barium filled esophagus with a reverse 3 sign.

Quiz 2

What is a reverse 3 sign"?

Reverse 3 sign
- A radiologic sign where the upper portion of the reverse 3 is formed by the indentation of the esophagus by the slightly dilated aorta
- Middle portion represents the coarctation of the aorta
- Lower portion is formed by the indentation of the oesophagus by the post stenotically dilated segment of the coarctated aorta
- This sign is specific for coarctation of the aorta.

Quiz 3

Where else do you find a reverse 3 sign/inverted 3 sign/sign of Epsilon?

In carcinoma of the pancreas the ampullary region of the duodenum may show this sign due to the projecting of the tumor above and below the ampulla.

Quiz 4

What is a reverse 5 sign?

Seen in hypoplastic left heart syndrome where the right heart border is only made up of two structures—SVC only in the upper part entering dilated RV at a striking angulation resembling reverse 5 (ascending aortic shadow is absent).

Quiz 5

What is coarctation?

- Localized narrowing of the aortic arch due to fibrous ring encircling the wall/shelf projecting into the lumen
- Juxtaductal narrowing may be preductal/postductal. Aorta distal to the narrowing is dilated and aneurysmal
- In infantile coarctation, the narrowing is diffuse, tubular and severe and presentation is with CCF
- In adult coarctation the narrowing is ring like, less severe and is detetected during evaluation for the hypertension.

Quiz 6

What is reverse coarctation?

Also called Takayasu's arteritis/pulseless disease the BP is low in upper limbs (mouths of the aortic branches are narrowed) and higher in the upper limbs.

Quiz 7

What are the salient features of Takayasu's disease?

- Described by a Japanese ophthalmologist
- Also called pulseless disease
- Affects aorta, brachiocephalic and pulmonary arteries
- Subclavian is the most commonly affected artery
- Asian women. Women 10 > 1 (men)
- Collaterlas rare as the ostia of the intercostals are narrowed—so inercostals cannot effectively participate in collateral circulation—rib notching rare.

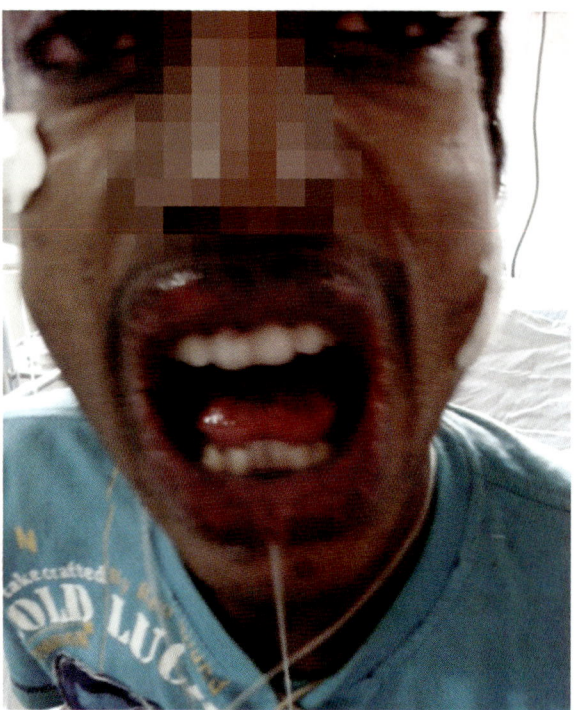

Quiz 1

What are the observations
1. Hyperemia of the conjunctiva—bilateral
2. Hyperemia of the lips, tongue and mouth.

Quiz 2

What do these observations suggest?
Involvement of the skin + mucosa after exposure to drugs/chemicals—suggests severe drug reaction—possibly Stevens-Johnson syndrome.

Quiz 3

What is the mechanism?
Hypersensitivity induced cell death causing separation of epidermis from the dermis—characterised by necrosis surrounded by inflammation.
SJ syndrome is the milder variant and toxic epidermal necrolysis is the more severe variant.
SJ syndrome has been reported after viral infections, bacterial infections and drugs.
Can be mistaken for erythema multiforme which is usually a type III hypersensitivity reaction to herpesvirus infection.

169. Wow! What is it?

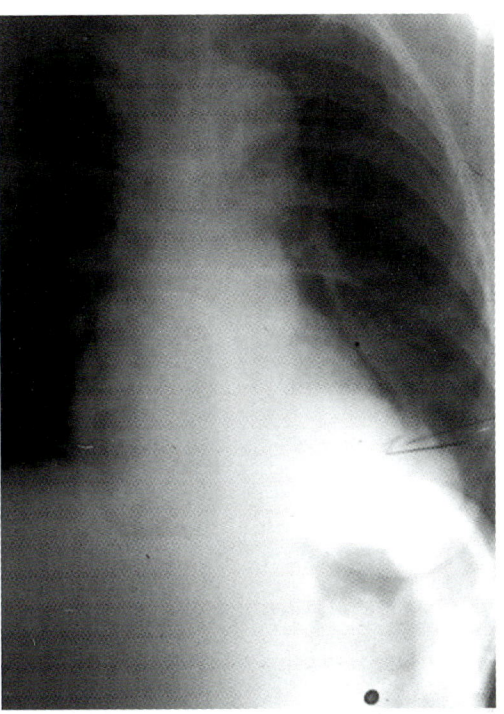

Quiz 1

What are the observations?

1. An obliquely placed oval mass is seen overlapping the lower portion of the cardiac silhouette and the left diaphragmatic leaf.
2. Silhouette sign is positive indicating that the said mass in anterior to the heart.

Quiz 2

What are the possibilities?

1. Mass—secondaries
2. Primary.

Quiz 3

What happened?

Discussion as per the cause being inconclusive, a biopsy, possibly excision biopsy was thought of.

Abdominal ultrasound done as a part of the work up revealed absence of both the kidneys in the abdomen—indicating that this "mass" is an ectopic kidney—in fact the only functioning kidney!

I owe this CXR to our urologist, Dr. GG Laxman Prabhu who narrated the episode in his own inimitable style!

Cases in Medicine

Quiz 4

What is the moral of the story?
However, certain the finding looks, one should carefully analyse and exclude other possibilities. Imagine the horror if the only functioning kidney though ectopic is removed!

Quiz 5

What are the locations of the ectopic kidney?
1. One normal + one pelvic 1 in 3000
2. Crossed ectopia 1 in 7000
3. Ectopic thoracic kidney 1in 13000
4. Solitary pelvic kidney 1 in 22000.

Quiz 6

What are the features of the thoracic kidney?
1. Located in the thorax usually resting on the diaphragm
2. Adrenals are in their usual place
3. Not associated with stones and infections as with other sites if renal ectopy
4. Usually picked up during radiological workup—an ultrasound.

170. Left Atrial Enlargement

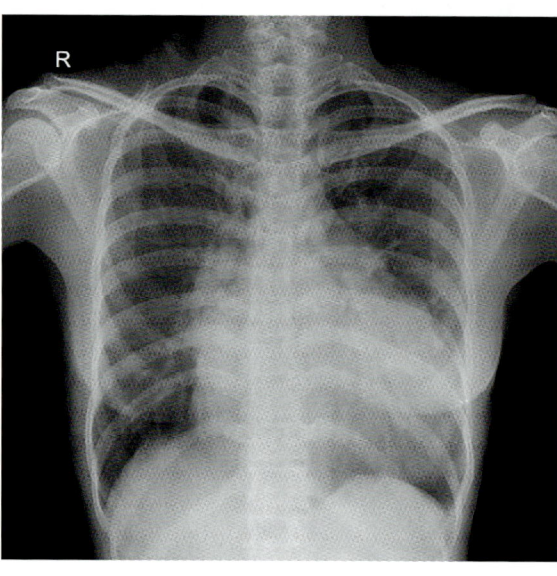

Quiz 1

What are the observations?
1. Double atrial shadow on the right side—inner shadow due to enlarged LA and the outer shadow due to enlarged RA.

2. Splaying of the carina—increase in the angle between the right and the left main bronchi due to enlarged LA occupying the places 1 and 2 indicate the enlargement of the body of the LA.

3. Straightening of the left heart border—constituted by aortic knuckle, pulmonary artery, enlarged LA (filling up the usual concavity between the PA and the ventricle) and the enlarged ventricle—indicates the enlargement of the LA appendage.

Other findings

4. Cardiomegaly.

5. Incresed upper lobe veins—indicating increased LA pressure.

6. Increased PA prominence—MPA and main branches indicating pulmonary hypertension.

171. Giant (Aneurysmally Dilated) Left Atrium

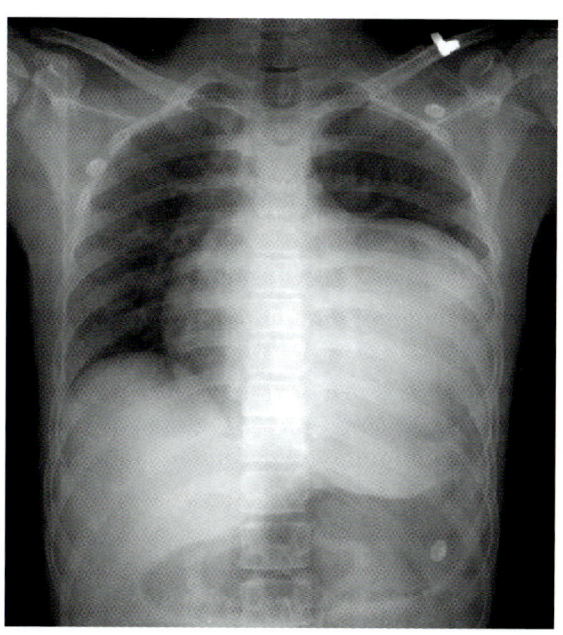

Quiz 1

What are the observations?

A very large bulge on the left heart border filling up the pulmonary bay and occupying the rest of the left heart border—indicating the origin from LA.

Quiz 2

It is seen in which condition?

Very rarely seen nowadays, it is due to severe mitral regurgitation.

Mitral regurgitation results in a volume and a pressure overload and is therefore capable of producing larger LA than what is seen in mitral stenosis where there is predominantly pressure overload.

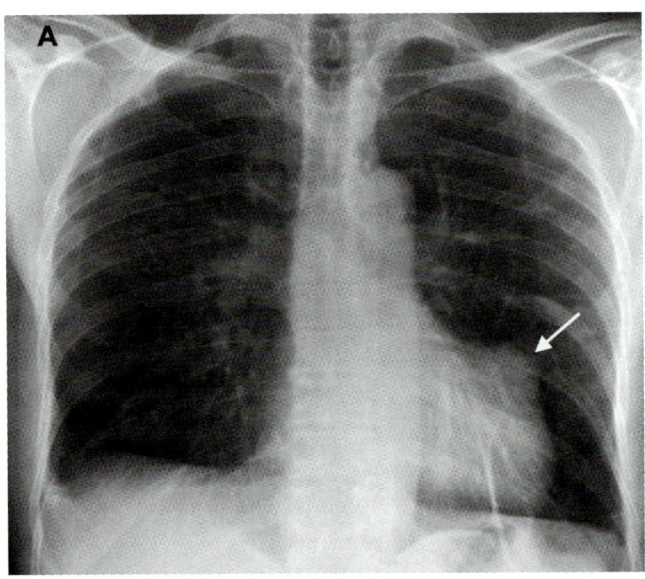

Quiz 3

What are the additional features of LA aneurysm in addition to those of LA enlargement?

a. Very much widened carina due to severe elevation of the left main bronchus
b. Severly displaced aorta to the left—Bedford sign
c. Highly enlarged LA almost touching the chest wall on the left side.

Quiz 4

What are the clinical features associated?

a. Symptoms
  • Dyspnoea
  • Dysphagia
  • Hoarseness
  • Cough.
b. Signs
  • Precordial pulsation—entire precordium pulsation
  • Presence of MR/MR + MS.

172. Third Mogul Sign—LV Aneurysm

A

Quiz 1

What are the observations?

• A bulge seen on the lower portion of the left heart border
• Location of the bulge indicates that it is arising from the left ventricle
• Outline of the bulge is smooth.

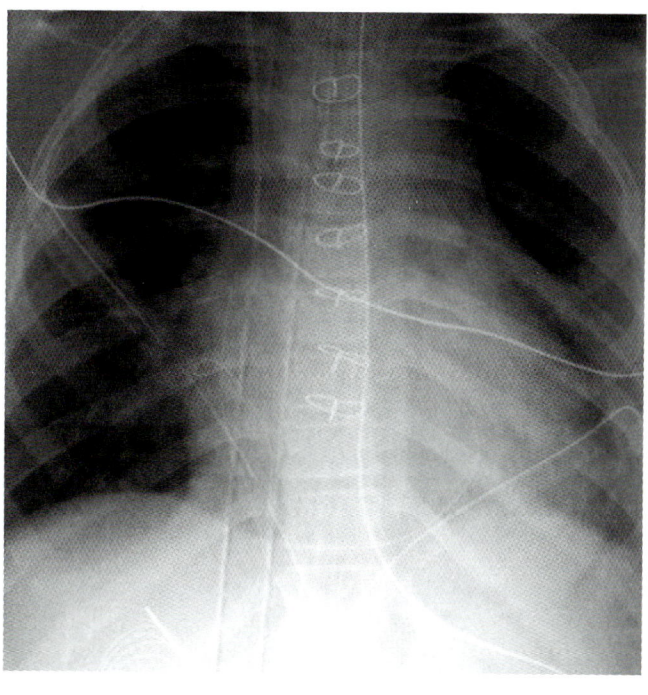

Quiz 2

What is the inference?

Overall findings suggest that it is an aneurysm arising from the wall of the left ventricle.

Quiz 3

What is the mechanism of production of LV aneurysm?

LV aneurysm is usually due to a bulge in the weakened portion of the myocardium following acute myocardial infarction.

Quiz 4

Which CXR clue helps pick it up?

This is a common cause of third mogul sign.

173. Free Air in the Pericardial Cavity—Pneumopericardium

OBSERVATION

1. Free air seen in the pericardial cavity—better seen outlining the left heart border.
2. Also seen (less distinctly) outlining the right heart border.
3. Pericardium is also seen nicely outlined—notice thick pericardium indicating the possibility of a chronic disease.
4. Observe evidence of open heart surgery.
5. Many tubes indicating ill patient—ICU setting.

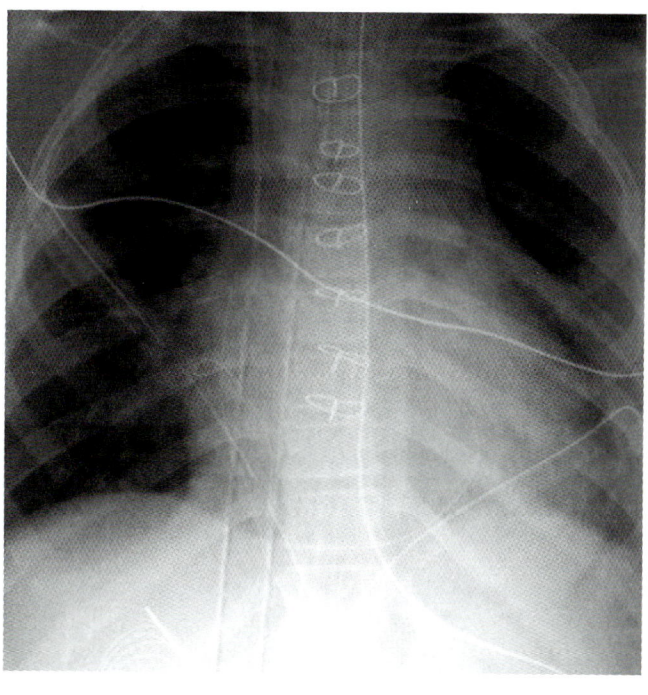

174. Westermark's Sign—Acute Pulmonary Embolism

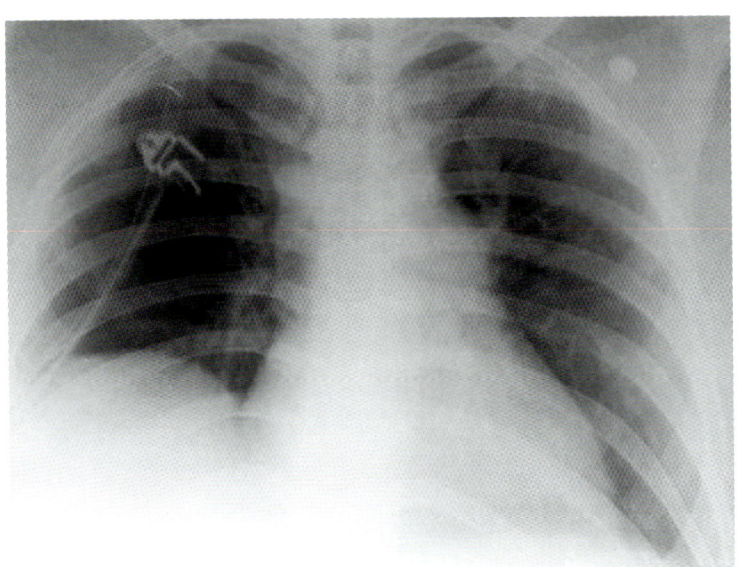

Quiz 1

What are the observations?

1. Relatively increased hyperlucency (Westermark's sign) on the right side due to blanching of the pulmonary vessels resulting in Wedge-shaped zone of pulmonary oligemia—suggestive of acute pulmonary embolism.
2. Elevated right hemidiaphragm.
3. A horizontal linear shadow seen above the mid portion of the diaphragm—Fleischner's line.

Quiz 2

What is the inference?

The overall appearances suggest acute pulmonary embolism.

Quiz 3

What are the various CXR features of PE?

1. Westermark's sign—wedge-shaped zone of local oligemia.
2. Pallas sign—dilated/prominent proximal pulmonary artery.
3. Knuckle sign—the dilated segment of the pulmonary artery just before the abrupt cut-off resembles a knuckle.
4. Hampton's hump—pleural based areas of increased opacity (representing intraparenchymal hemorrhage).
5. Melting snow sign—resolving infarct resolves from center to periphery like the melting.

Index